Tutorials in Palliative Medicine

Tutorials in Palliative Medicine

Edited by Peter Kaye,

MA, MB, FRCP, MRCGP

Consultant in Palliative Medicine

This book is available (by return of post) from:

EPL Publications
41 Park Avenue North
Northamptom NN3 2HT

Price £30.00, (Post and package free in the UK).
Books sent by return on receipt of cheque, payable
to EPL Publications.
© Peter Kaye 1997

ISBN 0-9519895-2-9

First published 1997

British Library Cataloguing-in-Publication Data
A Catalogue record for this book is available from the
British Library

Typeset by Land & Unwin (Data Sciences) Ltd.,
Bugbrooke, Northamptonshire.
Printed by MN Productions, Northampton.

This book
is
dedicated
with thanks
to
all the
(largely unsung)
medical secretaries
who work so hard
(mainly backstage)
to support
our health service

Preface

This book contains 17 tutorials, each one intended to provide an "update" in a particular aspect of symptom control. Each tutorial is designed to be long enough to provide an in-depth discussion of the subject, but short enough to be read at a sitting. Each author was chosen for their enthusiasm and special interest in the topic.

Each tutorial contains clinical case studies to bring the text to life.

The final chapter (Palliative Care – the next 10 years) looks to the future, but is also intended to put the other chapters into a broader perspective.

All the authors have their own particular style, but as the editor I have been vigorous in trying to make each tutorial as easy-to-read as possible. A big thank you to all the authors for their hard work, I think they have done a good job, and I hope you do too.

The topics covered in the tutorials are unashamedly concerned with physical problems. Symptom control remains the foundation of Palliative Medicine, and controlling any physical distress is always the first step towards achieving high quality palliative care for a patient and family. All the authors are very aware that effective symptom control can only be achieved in the context of good holistic care, but the emphasis here is on physical management. It would take another textbook to look at all the other aspects of palliative care ("Tutorials in the Psychosocial aspects of Palliative Care", perhaps).

Thank-you to Kirsten Hopkins, Jill Meredith and John Smith for their helpful comments, to Emily Kaye for her help with the index, to Hillary Austin from Land and Unwin for her skilful typesetting and especially to my secretary Ann Bates for her ongoing support.

I would welcome feedback from readers about the content of the book.

Peter Kaye
Northampton

Contents

Chapter 1

Palliative Surgery of the Thorax

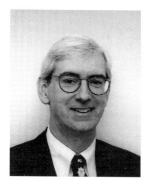

Mr Francis Wells
Francis Wells completed his training as Senior Research Fellow at the University of Alabama and was appointed Consultant Surgeon at Papworth Hospital 1985. He deals with all aspects of adult cardio-thoracic and oesophageal surgery. His special interests are conservative surgery of the mitral valve and the surgical management of lung cancer, gastro-intestinal dymotility and carcinoma of the oesophagus. He is the Programme Director of Lung Transplantation, Thoracic Services Director and the Training Director of the Higher Surgical Training of Registrars of the Anglia & Oxford Region. He has published many papers and books, and is the co-author of textbooks on Thoracic Surgical Techniques (Wells FC and Milstein BB, Longman Cartermill 1990) and Mitral Valve Disease (LM Shapiro and FC Wells, Heinemann-Butterworth, 1995).

INTRODUCTION

Palliative surgery for malignant disease of the thorax is commonly regarded as being too interventional for patients with incurable disease. Sadly this frequently leaves patients with distressing symptoms that could have been alleviated or abolished. Yet, it is within the thorax 'par excellence', that aggressive palliative intervention may yield the most gratifying results.

Best care is achieved through a multi-disciplinary approach. Ideally the team should consist of a Palliative Care Specialist, a Chest Physician, thoracic-surgeon, an oncologist/radiotherapist and a Nurse Specialist who can provide emotional and psychological support.

The most common malignant tumour within the thorax is that of the lung. As it is so frequent within the elderly population, and only 15-20% may be operable on presentation, a large number of patients continue to be seen outside a specialist centre.

Palliative interventions may benefit many, but cannot be applied if there is no access to specialist help. The centralisation of resources, as suggested by Calman,[1] made available in each region, may enable more patients to gain access to such specialist help. Patients with cancer of the oesophagus may also be referred to a variety of specialists or indeed, non-specialists (eg general gastro-enterologist, general physician or surgeon) as many areas do not have an identifiable team of experts.

Accurate histological diagnosis and staging of the disease ought to be available for all patients (other than those who are near to death). A specialist team, using protocol-driven care, can provide this service with the minimum of delay and cost.

Another benefit from this approach is the evolution of an evidence based practice. The concentration of patients with one expert team allows information to be derived from properly evaluated studies. The accumulation of significant data allows the planned introduction of new management strategies and the monitoring of their outcomes.

Further interventions may be needed as the disease progresses. Continued communication between the primary care physician and the specialist team is important.

Such an arrangement will enhance the ability to communicate in a more formalised way.

There are many tumours that arise primarily within the thorax or metastasise to intra-thoracic organs. The most important ones are as follows:

TUMOURS IN THE THORAX

Primary Tumours:

- **Lung Cancer**
- **Oesophageal cancer**
- **Mediastinal tumours** eg Thymomas

Extra-thoracic tumours causing intra-thoracic problems:

- **Breast cancer**
    - Pleuro-pericardial effusions
    - intra-bronchial stenosis
    - intra-pulmonary metastases
- **Uterine/Fallopian/Ovarian Cancer**
    - Pleuro-pericardial effusion
- **Osteogenic Sarcoma**
    - pulmonary metastases
- **Lymphoma**
    - residual disease within the thorax following chemotherapy

---

This list is not exhaustive but includes the most common malignant disorders that present in a regional thoracic centre. Any tumour causing symptoms within the chest may be managed using the techniques described below.

Investigation of the patient. All too often patients with advanced malignant disease are denied access to proper investigation on the grounds that it isn't worth it or that it is too much for the patient to suffer. There will of course, always be such cases, but all patients should at least be able to benefit from the opinion of a group of experts in the field. This may allow some patients to have well-targeted palliative care.

Specifically targeted investigations such as endoscopy, echo-cardiograms and CT scans are indicated in certain circumstances. Again, frequently these are denied to patients with advanced or disseminated disease on the grounds of inappropriateness.

These decisions ought to be made by appropriate specialists. Timely investigation may ultimately save money apart from also allowing better palliation of the patient.

LUNG CANCER

Airway Obstruction

Airway obstruction is a common occurrence in patients with advanced bronchial carcinoma. Symptoms may be caused by the loss of functioning lung, often accompanied by significant shunting of blood through un-aerated lung. Abscess formation, sometimes accompanied by empyema also occurs. Haemoptysis that can be life threatening is also commonly encountered.

Management of Airway Obstruction

There are several ways of clearing the obstructed airway. The first essential element is bronchoscopy to evaluate the extent of obstruction. CT scan will enhance this information by visualising the length of airway that is involved. With current 3-D reconstruction techniques, the quality of this information is extremely high (see photograph).

Provided there is a patent bronchus beyond the site of obstruction, a way through the narrowed areas can usually be found. If the whole length of the bronchus is occluded this may not be the case. Frequently though, definable obstructed segments can be opened up by a variety of techniques, include the following:

1. Dilatation (this usually applies to extrinsic compression)
2. Laser (to burn away endobronchial tumour)
3. Loop diathermy (to core out the tumour)
4. Removing the tumour with large biopsy forceps
5. Cryo-ablation
6. Local radiotherapy (brachytherapy) or locally implanted radioactive gold grains

Bleeding during these procedures can usually be controlled by the topical application of adrenaline. Most of these procedures need to be performed via a rigid bronchoscope. A team assessment of the most suitable technique is essential.

A 3-D RECONSTRUCTION FROM SPIRAL CT TO SHOW A LOCALISED BRONCHIAL STENOSIS. THIS CAN BE VIEWED FROM ANY ANGLE AND EVEN FROM INSIDE THE AIRWAY.

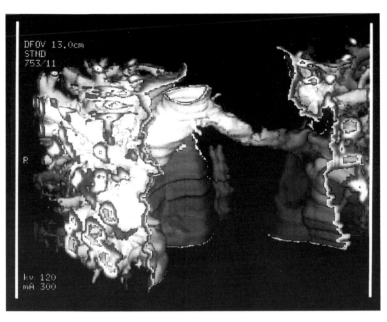

Stenting a bronchus

A 58 year old woman with tracheal squamous carcinoma presented with severe stridor and difficulty in self ventilation (even with helium added to her inspired gasses.)

CT scan demonstrated a local, near total, obstruction at the level of the third and fourth tracheal rings. The trachea was normal in diameter above and below this area. At rigid bronchoscopy it became impossible to ventilate her with the endoscope sited above the tumour. The residual lumen was too small to allow the adult bronchoscope to pass. Therefore, with a spiral movement of the bronchoscope, the instrument was thrust firmly through the tumour. A core was cut off by the endoscope which had acted as a cork-borer. The bronchoscope was rapidly removed, the obstructing tumour blown from the lumen and the endoscope re-introduced. The bronchoscope could then be passed easily into the distal trachea.

Vigorous suction and lavage cleared the main and distal bronchi. With slow removal of the bronchoscope the raw area (where the tumour had been removed) was treated with topically applied 1 in 10,000 strength Adrenaline and the bleeding stopped.

Later that day the bronchus was stented open using an expandable metal stent and later that week, treated with radiotherapy. The patient remains alive 18 months later.

Stents

As the case report illustrates, all of these techniques may be enhanced by the use of stents. There are now a variety of stents available. Tracheal compression or collapse may be held open with a Montgomery T tube – a silicone stent with a side arm that can be inserted through a tracheostomy incision, and the tracheostome, and is spigotted off to allow normal speech. It can be used for tracheal aspiration. This side arm also fixes the stent in place and prevents migration.

A variant of the Montgomery T tube has a bifurcated distal limb which will hold open the carina and both proximal major bronchi. This is also inserted by tracheostomy and has an upper side arm which protrudes through the tracheostome allowing tracheal toilet. This type is particularly useful when there is extensive sub-carinal lymph node enlargement.

Cooper and colleagues reported an extensive experience over 15 years.[2] Their paper demonstrates that excellent palliation can be achieved with airway stents. Further experience with Silicone prostheses for upper airway malignant obstruction is reported by Wassermann et al.[3] Although stent exchange was required in a number of patients, they clearly demonstrate the feasibility of such treatment.

Most recently, expandable metal stents have become available which can be placed in the correct position via a flexible bronchoscope and then dilated to give maximal air way opening.[2]

A 3-D RECONSTRUCTION FROM SPIRAL CT WITH MANIPULATION OF THE DATA TO SHOW THE STENT IN THE NOW DILATED BRONCHUS.

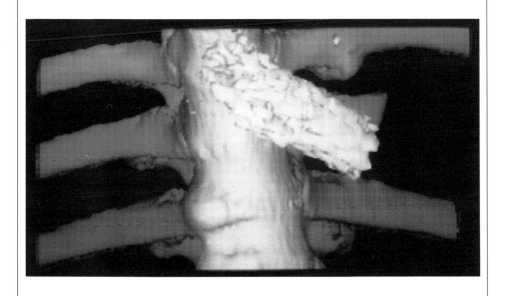

Local Radiotherapy

Local radiotherapy can open up obstructed airways and used in combination with the above methods, can relieve quite severe obstructions. Once the airway has been opened, the residual lung will re-expand. A study of patients at the Cleveland Clinic, of low dose endobronchial radiation alone or in combination with laser resection gave good to excellent symptom control.[4] However, laser therapy caused a significant mortality from exsanguination (an experience reported by others). In fact exanguination due to erosion of local blood vessels can occur with the use of stents alone.

Once the airway has been re-opened, constant monitoring of the patient will be necessary as it is likely with the passage of time that tumour will re-grow causing further obstruction It is possible to repeat these techniques on several occasions to keep the airway open for a considerable period of time.

Pulmonary Sepsis Lung abscesses should be treated with the appropriate antibiotics, but the mainstay of treatment, if possible, is to drain the abscess percutaneously. Fine bore catheters can be placed accurately using fluoroscopic control. The surrounding lung will then re-expand, collapsing the abscess. Once drainage ceases, the tube can be removed.

An empyema can also be drained percutaneously. Streptokinase instilled into the empyema cavity will break down adhesions and many empyemata can be resolved without resorting to more aggressive interventions. Open thoracotomy ought to be avoided if possible in these patients. The addition of simple saline irrigation is a useful adjunct, and will often speed up the resolution of fever.

Relief of Haemoptysis Haemoptysis is a common and disturbing accompaniment of airway involvement. It can often be well relieved with radiotherapy applied intraluminally (brachytherapy) or externally. Sadly in some cases it is a dreadful terminal event for which nothing can be done, other than make the patient as comfortable as possible.

Palliative Surgical Resection Surgical resection can be considered provided a good proximal clearance can be obtained. Even though this resection will not result in a cure it may bring about significant relief of symptoms. Selection of patients for this procedure however, is complex. Inappropriate use of surgery can worsen the situation. Break-down of the bronchial stump with post-pneumonectomy or post-lobectomy empyema is a thoroughly unpleasant situation, leading to chronic hospitalisation. Discussion amongst the specialist team in those circumstances is of vital importance.

Pleural Effusion Pleural effusion is a common complication of primary pulmonary malignancy and metastatic extrathoracic disease, e.g. breast or ovary. The effusion may be due to pleural involvement or due to obstruction of lymphatic drainage from the pleural space. In both cases – this represents advanced disease, is not manageable by surgical resection.

Palliative radical pneumonectomy

A 58 year old man (a chronic smoker) presented in a state of severe cachexia. Chest radiograph revealed a large abscess cavity in the left lower lobe with tumour placed centrally. The patient had a high, swinging fever and was anorexic. CT scan demonstrated large, mediastinal nodes. Although N_2 disease was present there appeared to be enough main bronchus clear of tumour to allow a satisfactory pneumonectomy. A palliative radical pneumonectomy with lymph node clearance was carried out.

Despite post-surgical staging suggesting advanced malignancy, the patient remains well with no sign of recurrent disease, two and a half years later. The patient has regained all his weight, looks well and is grateful to be alive.

Simple drainage is rarely enough and results in rapid re-accumulation of the fluid. It is therefore, almost always necessary to add something else to the procedure to prevent this happening. The choice of management will depend upon whether or not the underlying lung is capable of full expansion or not. If the lung is incapable of re-expansion, the space within the thorax will refill. Repeated pleural taps run the risk of introducing infection which will result in empyema.

Let us consider first, the situation where the lung will re-expand. In this situation, a pleurodesis either by mechanical scarification of the parietal pleura or insufflation of talc via a thoracoscope will, in the vase majority of cases, result in complete resolution of the problem with the lung adhering to the chest wall.[5]

If the lung will not expand because it is trapped by advanced tumour, then the decision on what to do next will depend upon the mobility of the mediastinum If the mediastinum is solidly fixed, then effusion will usually accumulate to a certain volume and then cease. Symptoms of shortness of breath in this circumstance is often due to the fixation of the intra-thoracic structures by tumour, and the removal of a pleural collection does not radically alter the way the patient will feel.

If the mediastinum and the diaphragm remain mobile, then the patient will become breathless as the fluid accumulates, due to increasing intra-thoracic pressure causing compression of the opposite lung. Under these circumstances, the use of a pleuro-peritoneal shunt would be appropriate.

These shunts are made of Silicone and consist of three parts. First, a central pumping chamber within which there is a simple flutter valve. When the chamber is compressed, fluid passes through the valve, which is similar to a finger of a surgical glove with the end cut off. The fluid cannot pass backwards. There is an inlet and outlet tube leading into and out of the chamber. Each of these tubes has multiple side holes to allow the fluid to enter or leave.

The inlet tube is placed in the thorax via a small purse-string suture in the intercostal muscle. The outlet tube is placed in a similar fashion through the peritoneum. The pumping chamber is then placed subcutaneously to one side of the incision over the costal margin.

The chamber will contain up to 5 mls of fluid, hence repeated pumping is required throughout the day. This can be accomplished through clothing however, once the patient has become accustomed to it. Pumping 40-50 times every 4-8 hours can keep the pleural space empty. Most patients are able deal with this without difficulty.[6]

The use of less aggressive agents such as Tetracyclines instilled into the pleural space via a small pleural tube are less effective. Some published information suggests they can be effective in up to 75% of patients whereas talc pleurodesis is effective in nearly 100% of patients.[7]

There is some evidence to suggest that the instillation of chemotherapeutic agents into the pleural space may have a good effect also, but some of these agents are absorbed and may make some infirm patients quite unwell.

Some situations are extremely difficult to handle optimally. The following case report demonstrates some of these difficulties.

An Effusion with a collapsed lung

A 63 year old man with extensive asbestos exposure, presented with a large, right sided pleural effusion. Pleural biopsies confirmed the diagnosis of mesothelioma. Shortly after this, the right lung completely collapsed leaving the patient very breathless. At thoracoscopy, it was clear that much of the lower lobe at the hilum was trapped by tumour, making full re-expansion of the lung impossible.

Satisfactory pleuradesis requires the lung to be fully re-expanded to fill the pleural space. In this case, full re-expansion was not likely to be achieved.

Simple aspiration of the pleural fluid would not be enough as rapid re-accumulation was bound to occur, and as the mediastinum was still mobile, mediastrial shift would compress of the left lung causing severe shortness of breath. Repeated aspirations were likely to result in an empyema.

In an attempt to produce the best compromise, the following management was adopted. First at thoracoscopy, all the pleural fluid was removed. Next the lung was reinflated as far as possible by positive pressure ventilation by the anaesthetist. Then sterilised talc was insufflated into the pleural space to encourage a pleurodesis between the opposing pleural surfaces. A drain was left on gentle suction to ensure that the re-inflated lung remained up to allow pleural adhesion. There was a moderate air leak, due to splitting of the visceral pleura, as the lung was forcibly re-expanded.

Although the presence of a chest drain is undesirable (as there is good evidence that mesothelioma may grow along the drain tract after removal) it was essential in this case to maintain inflation of the lung.

After a few days the intercostal tube drain was discontinued from suction and attached to a Heimlich valve to allow full mobility of the patient. After a further 5 days the drain was removed. Persistent re-inflation of the lung was achieved.

Later *a pleuro-peritoneal shunt* was placed in the basal pleural space to deal with the fluid accumulation around the lower lobe which could not be re-expanded because of tumour entrapment.

The cutaneous incisions made at thoracoscopy were treated with radiotherapy to minimise the possibility of tumour growth along the tube tracts.

Pericardial Disease

The pericardium may be directly involved from pulmonary tumours or from metastases from breast and other tumours. This commonly causes a pericardial effusion which may cause tamponade. Tamponade can be relieved by draining the fluid via the sub-xiphisternal approach (either needle aspiration or fine bore tube drainage).

Pericardial window

Recurrence of the effusion may necessitate a pericardial window. This can be carried out via a thoracoscope with video assistance (minimally invasive technique), or through a direct anterior mini-thoracotomy. By either route a 1-2 inch square of pericardium, usually anterior to the phrenic nerve, is resected leaving direct drainage into the pleural space. A drain is left in the pleural space in patients without significant pleural disease. On removal of the drain, fluid from the pericardium is absorbed by the pleura. If the patient has a pleural effusion, a pleural shunt can be placed at the same time.

Laham and colleagues have described their experiences with malignant pericardial effusions in 50 patients.[8] They describe a combination of methods and stress the importance of using the appropriate one in an individual patient.

OESOPHAGEAL CANCER

Oesophageal cancer is another formidable disease in that the majority of patients are incurable on presentation. The best palliation remains oesophageal resection provided there are no contra-indications (liver, brain or other distant metastases).

Local spread and lymph node involvement are not contra-indications to resection, because all other treatments are so inferior to a satisfactory oesophagectomy, which is the best palliative manoeuvre to restore normal swallowing.

The draw-back of oesophagectomy is that it is a substantial operation and carries with it a significant morbidity and mortality performed by an inexperienced team. With the correct selection of patients and skilled surgery some patients may be cured, even when pre-operative investigations suggest locally advanced disease.

If resection cannot be achieved or where distant metastases are present, oesophageal patency may be maintained in a variety of ways:

- Dilatation
- Intra-luminal stenting
- Laser therapy
- Radiotherapy
- Chemotherapy (+/- radiotherapy and stenting)
- Surgical bypass

Dilatation

The tumour may occupy only part of the circumference of the oesophageal wall. Simple dilatation may maintain adequate swallowing in many of these patients even when the disease is very systemically advanced.

Stenting
Endo luminal tubes

Prior to the availability of the more recent expandable stents, endo-luminal tubes were used. (Mousseau-Barbin tubes, Nottingham tubes, Celestin tubes, etc). None of them were entirely satisfactory, due to complications of dislodgement, regurgitation or distal displacement. The Mousseau-Barbin needed an open gastrotomy for placement (generally used when unexpected findings at laparotomy renders the oesophagus unresectable). The Celestin tube had a tendency to migrate onwards in the gastro-intestinal tract, and to break up causing intestinal perforation.

Expandable stents

Expandable metal stents, some covered by a plastic coating, have the advantage that they can be placed endoscopically over a guide wire and dilated to fit the oesophagus perfectly.[8] The covered stents are ideal for the management of tracheo-oesophageal malignant fistulae.[9] Although those stents are an improvement over their predecessors, they still can migrate. Also life-threatening haemorrhage can

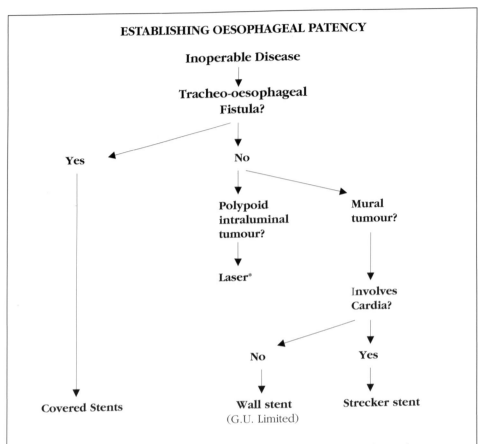

ESTABLISHING OESOPHAGEAL PATENCY

Inoperable Disease

Tracheo-oesophageal
Fistula?

Yes | No

Polypoid
intraluminal
tumour?

Mural
tumour?

Laser*

Involves
Cardia?

No | Yes

Covered Stents | Wall stent
(G.U. Limited) | Strecker stent

* A cheap and perhaps superior alternative to laser is piecemeal removal with biopsy forceps or cutting loop diathermy (similar to that used for T.U.R.P). After Mason, 1996[11]

occur from local pressure, due to erosion of a blood vessel.[10]

Tumour can grow over the ends of the stents (and in the uncovered variety, through the wall of the stent). This necessitates repeated endoscopy and resection of tumour by laser or biopsy forceps.

For difficult cases, it is possible to place a second stent within the first.

Laser therapy The use of laser to re-establish oesophageal patency is now quite widespread amongst gastro-enterologists and oesophageal surgeons. Although results can be very satisfactory, several treatments are usually required and it is not suitable for all tumours. If the oesophagus is completely occluded over a significant length, then laser therapy may be too time consuming and bear a significant risk of oesophageal perforation.

A recent paper by Mason comparing laser therapy with stenting, demonstrated a superiority of stenting, but not in all cases.[11] They suggest the treatment plan above (with chemotherapy added if the patient is fit enough).

Radiotherapy

Oesophageal tumours may be irradiated from within the lumen (brachytherapy) or with external beam irradiation. Brachytherapy allows more accurate targeting of the tumour and hence reduces collateral damage. The equipment however, is not widely available. External beam irradiation is used but involves more extensive exposure of normal tissues to the radiation beam. There is little prospective randomised information of either treatment modality.

There is a body of opinion which suggests that a combination of radiotherapy and combination chemotherapy protocols may provide the best hope for some patients, but their is a significant morbidity and mortality to this approach, especially in weakens patients.

Surgical bypass

Extra-anatomical bypass is much less frequently used today, but still has a place in some cases of tracheo-oesophageal fistula.

Stomach or colon are detached from their anatomical position and brought up to bypass the oesophagus which is left in its normal position. The oesophagus is stapled off above and below the tumour.

There is, in my view, an unacceptably high mortality from this procedure in debilitated patients and it should only be used in highly selected cases.

References

1. "A Policy Framework for Commissioning Cancer Services". A report by the expert advisory group on cancer to the Chief Medical Officers of England and Wales, April 1995 and accompanying EL (95) 51 A Policy Framework for Commissioning Cancer Services 21 April 1995
2. Cooper JD, Pearson FG, Patterson A, Todd TR, Ginsberge RJ, Goldberg M, Waters P. Use of Silicone stents in the management of air-way problems. Ann. Thor. Surg. 1989 Mar; 47 (3): 371-8

3. Wassermann K, Eckel H, Michel O, Muller R.P. Emergency stenting of malignant obstruction of the upper airways: Long-term follow-up with two types of silicone prosthesis. Journal of Thoracic And Cardiovascular Surgery 112 (4) October 1996: 859-66

4. Suh HH, Dass KK, Pagliaccio PA, Taylor ME, Saxton JP, Tan M, Mehta AC. Endobronchial radiation therapy with or without Neodymium Yttrium Aluminium Garnet Laser Resection for Managing Malignant Airway Obstruction. Cancer 73 (10) 1994 2583-2588

5. Yim APC, Chung SS, Lee TW, Lam CK, Ho JKS.Thoracoscopic Management of Malignant Pleural Effusions. Chest 109 (5) 1996 1234-1238

6. Petrou M, Kaplan D, Goldstraw P. Management of recurrent malignant pleural effusions. The complementary role of talc pleurodesis and pleuroperitoneal shunting. Cancer 75 (3) 1995: 801-805

7. Laham RJ, Cohen KJ, Kuntz RE, Bain DS, Lorell BH, and Simons M. Pericardial effusion in patients with cancer: outcome with contemporary management strategies. Heart 1996 75 : 67- 71

8. Winkelbauer FW, Schoft, R Niederle B, Wildling R, Thurnber S, Lammer J, Am. J. Roentgenol. Palliative treatment of obstructing oesophageal cancer with nitinol stents : value, safety and long term results. 1996 Jan. 166 (1) : 79-84.

9. Han YM, Song HY, Lee JM, Clio SI,Chung FH, Kim CS,Sohn MH,Choi KC. Esophago-respiratory fistulae due to esophageal carcinoma : palliation with a covered Gianturco stent. Radiology. 1996 April ; 199 (1) : 65-70

10. Acuras B, Rozanes I, Akpinar S, Tunaci A, Tunaci M, Acuras G. Palliation of malignant oesophageal strictures with self expanding nitinol stents : drawbacks and complications. Radiology. 1996 June; 199 (3) : 648-52

11. Mason R. Palliation of malignant dysphagia : an alternative to surgery. Ann. R. Coll. Surg. Eng. 1996; 78 ; 457-462.

Chapter 2

Palliative Radiotherapy

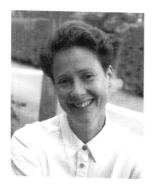

Dr Patricia Needham
Patricia Needham has been Consultant in Palliative Medicine at Dorothy House Foundation, Bath since 1995. During her training in Palliative Medicine she spent 12 months working in the Radiotherapy and Oncology Department at the Royal London Hospital looking at the palliative aspects of radiotherapy

INTRODUCTION

Radiation therapy has an important role to play in controlling and possibly preventing a wide range of symptoms.

Mechanism of action

There are 3 types of Radiotherapy: External beam, brachytherapy (the introduction of a radioactive source into, or close to the tumour) and radio-isotopes (eg Strontium-89).

All involve the targeted delivery of ionizing radiation (usually X-rays or gamma rays) to the malignant growth. This causes double-stranded breaks in cellular DNA, some of which are mis-repaired. The resultant chromosomal damage becomes evident at cell division, resulting in cell death.

3 TYPES OF RADIOTHERAPY
• External beam
• Brachytherapy
• Radio-Isotopes

Toxicity   Despite the targeting of RT, normal cells will also be exposed (to varying degrees) to the damaging effects of irradiation. Susceptibility to toxicity varies according to the tissues involved, and from patient to patient. Radiation damage is normally divided into early and late toxicity. Early damage occurs 1-3 weeks after irradiation has commenced, is reversible and usually only lasts a few weeks. Those normal cells which divide rapidly are most susceptible. See table below.

EARLY TOXICITY FROM RADIOTHERAPY

AREA TREATED	SYMPTOMS	MANAGEMENT	COMMENTS
Skin (Area Toxicity)	Redness, itching – ('dry desquamation')	No treatment may be needed, or 1% Hydrocortisone cream	Less with modern machines
	Ulceration – ('moist desquamation')	Controversial.	
Scalp	Alopecia	Early discussion about wigs	Will generally regrow (depending on the dose) after 3-6 months
Mouth	Mucositis	Difflam mouthwash Treatment of concurrent candidiasis	Dietary advice may be needed
Oesophagus	Oesophagitis and dysphagia	Mucaine, soft diet	Dietary advice may be needed
Small Bowel	Nausea and vomiting	Antiemetics, Steroids	Occurs immediately*
Large Bowel	Colitis/Proctitis with tenesmus, diarrhoea, bleeding and mucus	Antidiarrhoeals Local steroids Low fibre diet	
Bladder	Dysuria, frequency haematuria	Exclude UTI Encourage fluids	
Bone Marrow	Myelosupression	Supportive	

* Other symptoms generally occur 1-3 weeks after treatment started.

Late toxicity

Late toxicity (rarely seen with palliative regimens) occurs months to years after treatment and is generally a feature of slowly-dividing or non-dividing cells. Tissues such as the spinal cord (radiation myelitis), brain, lens of the eye, lungs and kidneys are therefore very sensitive to this type of damage, although any tissue can suffer severe late damage (eg rectum). It is caused by an obliterative endarteritis and fibrosis. It is generally irreversible, progressive and can be fatal.

Acute toxicity does not necessarily predict for late. Both are related to the total dose of radiation given and to the volume treated. Early damage is also related to the time period over which treatment is given. It is less likely if this is prolonged. Late toxicity is probably related to the size of the dose per fraction. Larger fractions are suspected to be more likely to cause problems.

Fractionation

To enable high total doses (with better destruction of tumour cells) to be tolerated, radiotherapy regimens are often fractionated.[1] This enables normal cells to recover from sub-lethal damage (*repair*) in between fractions. Normal cells which are capable of dividing are allowed to do so (*repopulation*). Malignant cells are less able to repair which provides a therapeutic advantage. Fractionation also allows the tumour to become better oxygenated (*re-oxygenation*) and oxygenated cells are more radio-sensitive than hypoxic ones. Finally, it increases the damage to malignant cells by allowing more of them to enter a susceptible phase of cell division (*reassortment*) – although unfortunately this also applies to actively dividing normal cells.

NEW AREAS OF DEVELOPMENT IN RADIOTHERAPY

Brachytherapy

In order to limit damage to normal tissues by more carefully targeting the tumour, brachytherapy is being increasingly studied in a variety of settings. It is starting to be looked at in the palliative setting, but its role is as yet limited.

Radiosensitisers

Radiotherapy regimens involving combinations with radiosensitisers such as razoxane and misonidazole, hyperbaric oxygen, hyperthermia and chemotherapy have all been looked at, but results have been disappointing and have therefore not found a role in palliative treatments.

Continuous hyperfractionated accelerated radiation therapy (CHART)

Each fraction of external beam irradiation is normally given on a daily basis in conventional regimens. CHART has been tried in various settings, generally curative, in an attempt to increase tumour cell kill without increasing late toxicity. This involves giving multiple daily fractions which are smaller than conventional fractions (to minimise late damage), over a shorter period of time than normal. This theoretically reduces the opportunity for malignant cell repopulation, which should increase the effectiveness of the radiation, without increasing late toxicity.

The interim findings from two large studies comparing CHART to conventional radical regimens have now been reported.[17] Improved survival at 2 years was found in patients with locally advanced NSCLC, but not in those with head and neck cancer, although the latter had an interesting trend towards improved local tumour control in more advanced disease. Toxicity was earlier, more severe, but quicker to settle, with no difference (at this stage) in late morbidity reported. CHART was completed in 12 days, compared to the 6–7 weeks of treatment with the conventional regimens.

Hypofractionation

An ideal palliative treatment is simple, non-time consuming, effective and non-toxic. *Radical regimens* – high total dose (40-60Gy), protracted course (4-6 weeks), with low dose per fraction (2Gy) – aim at eradication of all malignant cells with minimal late toxicity. When the aim is palliation less burdensome regimens are preferable, to achieve an effect at a lower total dose. *Hypofractionated regimes* are shorter with a higher dose per fraction (theoretically making late toxicity more likely, although this is unproven). However, the documented evidence is scanty and contradictory. The worries regarding hypofractionated regimens, can be summarized as:

- Less effective rates or quality of response. (Little evidence for this)
- Late toxicity (due to large fraction sizes) in patients surviving long enough to experience it (No supporting evidence).
- Shorter duration of response. (Some evidence, but RT can often be repeated).
- Problems re-treating (because of worries over late toxicity).

Optimum dose

Late toxicity is often not an issue (unless life expectancy is over 6 months, as it may be with metastatic cancer of the breast and prostate). Early toxicity can however have a major negative impact on patients quality of life and needs to be minimised. Palliative radiotherapy, given appropriately, rarely causes significant morbidity. The optimum regimen in many clinical situations remains unproven. Balancing the pros and cons of hypofractionation for each patient is often a matter for individual clinical judgement (taking into account departmental policy where applicable). There are many differences seen in clinical practice. Some patients may start a course of radical radiotherapy but are unable to complete it due to acute toxicity. We will now look at specific clinical situations in more detail.

SYMPTOM CONTROL

Bone Pain

Radiotherapy is most frequently used to relieve pain caused by bone secondaries[2] It can also be useful in pain related to infiltrative tumours eg pelvic and rectal tumours, neuropathic pain due to nerve compression or infiltration, and (rarely) liver capsule pain.

Localised external beam irradiation

Single fractions of local external RT have been shown in most studies to be as efficacious as fractionated regimens (suggesting that pain relief is not solely due to reduction in tumour bulk). Response rates in the region of 70-90% are generally reported. The optimum dose remains unproven. A dose of 8Gy is usually given, allowing subsequent treatments to be safely given. Studies to

---

USES OF PALLIATIVE RADIOTHERAPY

- **Pain control**
  - Primary tumours
  - Secondary tumours
  - Bone metastases

- **Haemorrhage**
  - Haemoptysis
  - Haematuria
  - Rectal bleeding,
  - Vaginal bleeding

- **Fungation**
  - Skin primaries
  - Skin secondaries
  - Head and Neck tumours
  - Breast carcinoma

- **Space occupying lesions**
  - Spinal Cord Compression
  - Cerebral secondaries

- **Obstruction of hollow viscera**
  - Superior vena cava
  - Obstruction
  - Dysphagia
  - Dyspnoea

- **Post-operative**
  - Following internal fixation of a long bone
  - Laminectomy
  - Craniotomy

---

date remain inconclusive regarding a potential higher relapse rate with single fractions and this is currently being looked at in a prospective randomised controlled trial.

Fractionated RT   Most radiotherapists continue to use a fractionated palliative regimen if the cervical spine is involved, due to fears of radiation myelitis (in long term survivors) and acute oedema with large single fractions, precipitating cord compression. Many would also use protracted regimens when there is a lytic lesion in a weight bearing bone, in order to promote recalcification, and in those with 'radio-resistant' tumours (eg melanoma and renal cell). This is not supported by the literature, in which recalcification has not been systematically looked at, and in which pain relief generally appears to be independent of histology.

Post-operative RT   There are no randomised studies of its use post-operatively in order to promote healing and prevent local relapse, and its use in this setting remains anecdotal although widely practised.

Large field irradiation

Hemi-body irradiation (HBI) is sometimes used to treat widespread bony metastases from prostate, myeloma, and occasionally breast cancer. It is usually given as a single fraction, limited to 6Gy to the upper body (due to the risk of pneumonitis), and 8Gy to the lower. If upper and lower HBI are given an interval is necessary in between to allow for recovery of the bone marrow. It can cause severe nausea and vomiting (despite pre-hydration) and steroids plus 5HT3 antagonists often prove useful. Other side effects include lethargy, myelo-supression, diarrhoea (if lower body) and alopecia (if skull involved in treatment field).

It usually requires a brief admission. 70-90% respond, most within 24-48 hours of a single fraction of HBI. Single local RT fractions can still be given safely at a later date. Fractionated HBI regimens have been found to give similar response rates, which last longer, but take longer to become apparent. They are more cumbersome. Single fraction HBI has been shown to delay the onset of new painful sites.

Radioisotopes

Strontium-89, is a radio-active calcium analogue administered IV. It concentrates at sites of osteoblastic activity and delivers a localised dose of radiation to the metastases, with relative sparing of normal tissues.[3] It is quick to administer, given in an out-patient setting, and can be repeated, (usually 3 monthly) if there is no bone marrow suppression. Its use is limited by its high cost. It has few side-effects. Myelosupression is the main one (especially thrombocytopenia, with a nadir at 5-7weeks), although it is generally not of clinical significance in most patients.

It is relatively contra-indicated in cases of renal failure or urinary incontinence, due to the risk of increased toxicity and radioactive contamination, as it is excreted renally. Response (10-29 days) is slower than with hemi-body irradiation but of an equivalent magnitude. When used in the adjuvant setting it has been shown to delay onset of symp-tomatic bone metastases.

It is used predominantly in multiple osteoblastic bone metastases from carcinoma of the prostate. It can also be used in osteoblastic lesions associated with carcinoma of the breast, lung and myeloma, where, although the X-ray lesion is predominantly lytic a bone scan demonstrates some osteoblastic activity.

The earlier radioisotope Phosphorus-32 is no longer used because of its lack of specificity in this situation and greater myelotoxicity. Iodine-131 although of use in metastatic differentiated thyroid carcinoma is probably less effective than external RT for symptomatic bone metastases due to this tumour.

Bisphosphonates Clodronate and pamidronate, used previously primarily for hypercalcaemia are now being used to treat multiple painful bone metastases. They inhibit osteoclast activity. They are also being used prophylactically to prevent skeletal morbidity.

A new compound 153-Samarium-EDMP is currently under investigation. This is a radioisotope which is incorporated into a bisphosphonate structure, which may prove to be a true 'magic bullet' targeting both symptomatic and asymptomatic bone metastases.

Pelvic Pain Pelvic pain can be caused by any tumour arising from the genito-urinary and GI tract and is often amenable to irradiation. *Fractionated regimens* are preferred. Several studies have reported significantly higher rates of late complications with high dose-per-fraction single and hypofractionated regimens. Single fractions are therefore reserved for those with a clearly limited survival. A study in pain associated with recurrent ovarian carcinoma showed both quality and duration of response to be better with more protracted higher total dose regimens.[4] Studies in bladder cancer have however been at variance. Results of the MRC study comparing 21Gy in 3 fractions with 35Gy in 10 fractions are awaited. Acute toxicity is greater with the fractionated higher total dose regimens, and include dysuria and frequency, diarrhoea and proctitis depending upon the treatment field.

Accelerated multiple daily fractions (44.4Gy in 12 fractions, 2 fractions per day, with two 2-4 week breaks during therapy – to minimise acute toxicity) produce good palliation, with less risk of late toxicity.[5]

Rectal Pain   Rectal pain caused by inoperable or recurrent rectal carcinoma is often helped by radiotherapy. Radical regimens are preferred where the patients condition allows as it gives a better chance of complete symptom control.[6]

PALLIATIVE RADIOTHERAPY OF RECTAL TUMOURS[6]

	Radical		Palliative	
	Complete Response	Partial Response	Complete Response	Partial Response
Pain	62%	30%	37%	49%
Rectal Bleeding	89%	46%	63%	22%
Mucoid Discharge	32%	55%	34%	52%
Diarrhoea	46%	38%	29%	52%

Acute toxicity (of which diarrhoea and tenesmus occur most frequently) is however considerable with these radical regimens, 81% experiencing problems in the above study. The palliative regimens, although less effective, are less toxic (39% experiencing toxicity) and better withstood by frail patients, and are often more appropriate.

Other symptoms associated with rectal tumours such as mucous discharge, tenesmus and obstruction also appear amenable to radiotherapy in a high proportion of patients. As more patients receive postoperative adjuvant irradiation, which reduces local failure rates after surgery, the need for palliative RT will be reduced.

Neuropathic Pain   When neuropathic pain is caused by compression or infiltration of nerve roots or peripheral nerves, (as with vertebral bone metastases, Pancoast's tumour of the lung, and axillary lymphadenopathy from carcinoma of the breast) palliative fractionated regimens are often used in conjunction with steroids, standard analgesics and co-analgesics.

Higher doses of palliative RT tend to be given but are based on anecdotal evidence rather than clinical studies.

Radiotherapy for Nerve Compression

Sue, 51, had widespread metastatic disease from adenocarcinoma of the lung. She was admitted to the local hospice for symptom control. One of her most distressing symptoms was weakness of the left arm of recent onset which limited her ability to self-care. X-ray of her cervical spine revealed a metastatic deposit a C5 which was felt to be responsible for her painless radiculopathy. She received 4 fractions of palliative DXT and her weakness recovered within a week. She died four weeks following the palliative RT.

Chest Pain   This generally arises from primaries or secondaries which involve the lung or oesophagus. Radiotherapy can often be helpful.[7,8]

PALLIATIVE RADIOTHERAPY FOR NON-SMALL CELL LUNG CANCER

	17Gy in 2 fractions (1 week apart)				30gy in 10 fractions/ 27Gy in 6 fractions[7]		10Gy single fraction[8]	
	1st study[7]		*2nd study*[8]					
	CR	PR	CR	PR	CR	PR	CR	PR
COUGH	37%	28%	19%	29%	37%	19%	24%	32%
HAEMOPTYSIS	79%	2%	64%	11%	84%	2%	54%	18%
CHEST PAIN	67%	8%	39%	20%	74%	6%	44%	28%

CR = Complete Response
PR = Partial Response

Hepatic Pain   Various fractionated palliative regimens have been tried for treating liver capsule pain. It is generally held in reserve for when pain is severe, and standard analgesics, NSAIDs and steroids have failed to work. It is associated with a significant incidence of nausea and vomiting (10-22% in reported surveys). Oesophagitis and pneumonitis are also reported, as is hepatitis and nephritis with certain regimens. Response rates of up to 95% for those completing treatment have been reported, the majority occurring within 2 weeks. Other symptoms associated with hepatic metastases such as night sweats, nausea and vomiting, jaundice, anorexia and ascites are less amenable.

Spinal Cord Compression   This is a radiotherapeutic emergency. The likelihood of improvement is related to the degree of disability preceding treatment. Those with significant motor impairment are much less likely to respond than those without.[9] Response rates to treatment vary considerably.

PALLIATIVE RT FOR SPINAL CORD COMPRESSION	Response Rates
PAIN RELIEF	38 – 92%
RECOVERY OF BLADDER FUNCTION	0 – 67%
RETAINING AMBULATION	66 – 100%
REGAINING AMBULATION	0 – 64%

(Overview of published studies)

Studies vary in how "response" is defined, and in the degree of pre-treatment neurological disability. The ideal regimen has yet to be established. Conventional regimens of 30Gy in 10 fractions or 20Gy in 4–5 fractions are generally used, but single fractions of 10-15Gy have been used with similar benefit. Concerns, as yet unsubstantiated, still exist over acute oedema and early relapse with these single large fractions.

Dexamethasone is generally recommended to counteract any acute oedema at doses ranging from 8-96mg. One study found that 96mg/day improved not only response rate but also its duration, when compared with patients not receiving steroids.[10] The optimum dose remains unclear.

Surgery for cord compression

Surgery is generally recommended if symptoms progress during (or relapses following) RT or when there is major structural compromise and the patients general condition is good. No randomised controlled trial has been possible to compare surgery and RT but retrospective studies suggest that results are equivalent. Structural instability following posterior laminectomy can be a problem. An anterior approach is however associated with greater surgical morbidity and mortality. There are no controlled studies to date looking at the role of post-operative RT. Retrospective studies would suggest it is beneficial.

Patients with cord compression who are fit enough for surgery should be seen urgently by both a radiotherapist and spinal surgeon, and have an urgent MRI Scan, before an individualised management plan is instituted.

Gliomas

Conventional radical regimens prolong survival in patients with high grade gliomas (increasing median survival from approximately 4 months to 8–10 months). Elderly patients and those with a poor performance status have a particularly poor prognosis and radical RT would seem inappropriate in this group. Hypofractionated regimens are effective in improving or stabilising function but have not been tested in a controlled trial.[11]

Solitary Brain Metastases

Management differs depending on whether brain metastases are single or multiple. Surgery is indicated if there is controllable local disease. Patients with good performance status, a long disease free interval from diagnosis, no other metastases, and radioresistant tumours should be treated aggressively with surgical excision, plus or minus post-operative whole brain radiation therapy (WBRT).

In a small proportion of patients survival can be prolonged (median survival 18 months). The majority however will deteriorate and die within the year. The advantage of post-operative radiation has been questioned, but it probably reduces local recurrence and possibly improves survival. For those not considered suitable for surgical excision, WBRT is indicated.

The optimum regimen remain unclear. Late damage of normal cerebral tissue limits total dose and fraction size. Clinical dementia has been reported in 10-19% of the few long term survivors who receive even 30Gy in 10 fractions. High total dose radiotherapy regimens which boost the site have not been shown to be beneficial.

Focal irradiation (by stereotactic external beam irradiation/radiosurgery or brachytherapy) for small(<3cm) solitary brain metastases enable high doses of radiation to be delivered to small target volumes within the brain, and can be fractionated. They are associated with less morbidity (no alopecia) and mortality, than surgery and WBRT. They may however need to be combined with WBRT to prevent relapse outside the limited treatment field. CHART has also been investigated.

Multiple Brain Metastases

RT is considered to restore function, control symptoms, or prevent progressive neurological dysfunction. Short courses (20Gy over 1 week) are as effective (in terms of response rate and duration, and survival) as conventional regimens (30-40Gy over 3-4 weeks).[18] One study[13] suggests that a single fraction of 10 Gy may well be adequate. The recent British Study comparing 12Gy in 2 fractions and 30Gy in 10 fractions found no difference in response rates, duration of response or complications. There was a suggestion that for those with a better prognosis, the longer regimen may have improved survival.[19]

Side-effects include dry desquamation of the scalp and some alopecia. Nausea, lethargy, headache and otitis media may occur. Alopecia, dermatitis and otitis media can persist. Dexamethasone is generally given to counteract the theoretical risk of increased intracranial pressure due to acute oedema with irradiation. A 'somnolence' syndrome has been reported, 6–12 week after irradiation.

Re-irradiation can be considered for initial responders who relapse, depending upon the initial regimen given.[20]

PALLIATION OF SYMPTOMS DUE TO CEREBRAL SECONDARIES[18]

	Standard Regimens (30-40Gy over 2-4 weeks)		Hypofractionated Regimens (20-40Gy over 1-3 weeks)	
	Complete Response	Partial Response	Complete Response	Partial Response
Headache	52%	30%	69%	13%
Motor Loss	32%	42%	37%	24%
Impaired Mentation	34%	37%	52%	17%
Cerebellar dysfunction	39%	36%	50%	14%
Cranial Nerve Dysfunction	40%	31%	44%	15%
Raised ICP	57%	26%		
Convulsions **– general**	66%	20%	87%	13%
– focal	58%	18%		
Sensory Loss	41%	36%		
Lethargy	39%	30%		

Treatment of Brain Metastases

Carol 47, had locally advanced breast carcinoma. She developed rib pain whilst receiving combination chemotherapy, and was given a single fraction of RT to her rib metastasis with good response. 18 months later she developed headaches, nausea and complex partial seizures. A CT scan confirmed the presence of multiple cerebral metastasis. She responded to steroids and a short course of cerebral RT with resolution of all her symptoms. The steroid dose was successfully reduced. Her symptoms recurred 3 months later but this time were unresponsive to steroids. She deteriorated rapidly and died (26 months after initial diagnosis).

SVC obstruction   Superior vena cava obstruction is no longer regarded as a radiotherapeutic emergency. Although causing distressing symptoms there is little evidence that unrelieved it is life threatening. Prognosis relates to the underlying pathology rather than duration of symptoms. Co-existing tracheal obstruction with stridor is however an emergency. There is generally time to make a tissue diagnosis before proceeding with treatment. This is important because chemotherapy is the treatment of choice for lymphomas and small cell lung carcinomas rather than radiotherapy.[15]

The optimal RT regimen is again unknown. Symptomatic improvement has been reported in 50-80% of patients, generally within two weeks, and often persists until death. Some have reported more rapid relief in those given initial high dose fractions. No correlation of tumour regression on X-ray with symptom relief has been found, and some improvement may well be due to the development of venous collaterals unrelated to therapy.

Dysphagia is the most troublesome acute side effect, reported in 26-57% of patients, depending upon the regimen used.

Thrombolysis or stent   Depending on the general condition of the patient, thrombolysis and stents have been employed in those where chemotherapy or radiotherapy was not possible, or who have relapsed despite these modalities. Steroids and diuretics may also be of help.

Dyspnoea   External RT and brachytherapy have much to offer for breathlessness from proximal occlusion (extrinsic or intrinsic) of an airway. This may be associated with distal collapse and/or post-obstructive pneumonia, due to primary lung cancer, secondaries or obstruction by lymphadenopathy. RT is *ineffective* for breathlessness due to:

- multiple lung metastases
- lymphangitis carcinomatosis
- pleural effusions.

Radical RT is often given to inoperable but early non-small-cell lung cancer in the hope of cure. 5 year survival is 20% (for stage 1) compared to about

5% for Stage IIIa. For those who are not regarded as potentially curable, treatment is reserved for symptomatic patients. Single fractions are as effective as the more protracted regimens with breathlessness improving in 41% of patients in the MRC study.[8] Further treatments can be useful for those who relapse.

Toxicity

The most troublesome acute toxicity is from oesophagitis. This appears to be less likely with a single fraction. Late radiation myelitis with paraplegia has been reported with hypofractionated regimens using large fractions although there is no firm evidence of a significant difference of incidence with 10Gy in one fraction as opposed to 30Gy in 10 fractions.

Intraluminal brachytherapy

Intraluminal brachytherapy has been increasingly studied. It is often combined with laser therapy. It requires bronchoscopy, and isolation whilst the radioactive source is in place. It has been reported to give good symptomatic relief, both as initial treatment and on relapse following external RT for haemoptysis (86-99% respond) and breathlessness (60-86%). It can be successfully repeated. Optimal dose and treatment times are yet to be established. It has been associated with better re-expansion of collapsed lung compared to external RT. It is often associated with a cough which settles within 2-3 weeks, but appears to cause less tiredness and oesophagitis. There are concerns over acute oedema causing stridor and the development of fistulae, haemorrhage and stenosis in the longer term. It is a more complex treatment requiring expensive machines and facilities. Some regimens have been given on an out-patient basis.

Steroids may give some temporary benefit by reducing peritumoural oedema. Laser therapy for intrabronchial tumours and stenting for intrinsic and extrinsic bronchial occlusion may also be considered.

Dysphagia

Radical RT for resectable oesophageal carcinomas (in patients unfit for surgery) results in equivalent 5 year survival rates to surgery (around 6%). Up to 20% of patients are unable to tolerate these regimens due to acute toxicity (mainly oeso-

Radiotherapy for Lung Cancer

Joan, age 64 had carcinoma of the lung, causing extrinsic compression to her (L) upper lobe and bronchus and (L) upper lobe collapse. She became bed bound with breathlessness, cough, chest pain, weight loss and weakness. Surgery was not technically feasible and she was not felt to be fit enough to withstand radical RT. She completed 30 Gy in 10# palliative RT, which in combination with Dexamethasone 8 mg, opiates and non-steroidal anti inflammatory drugs helped her cough, pain and breathlessness considerably. She experienced some dysphagia which was relieved by Mucaine. She was able to mobilise and get out of the house and experienced a markedly improved quality of life until her gradual deterioration 2 months later. She was considered for intraluminal brachytherapy but deteriorated rapidly and died 3 months following her palliative RT.

phagitis) and receive a palliative dose only. Those patients who require a large volume to be treated are also generally prescribed a palliative course because of toxicity with radical treatment. Studies have shown that the duration of palliation of symptoms is dose dependent. Response rates of around 70-90% are quoted with the palliative regimens.

Dysphagia due to extrinsic compression and invasion by lung carcinomas or hilar lymphadenopathy may also respond to external RT.[16]

Brachytherapy has been used both individually and in combination with external RT. It appears to give prompter relief of dysphagia. Dose and fractionation again remain unclear. It can cause severe oesophagitis. There is little data regarding late toxicity available yet.

Various endoscopic techniques are available, ranging from simple dilatation, alcohol , prosthetic intubation (for extrinsic compression as well as intraliminal obstruction) and laser therapy, both singly or in combination, and with or without radiotherapy.

Ureteric and Urethral Obstruction

Ureteric and urethral obstruction and secondary hydronephrosis can be relieved by external RT in certain cases, in combination with stents or nephrostomies, where appropriate.

Haemoptysis

Radiation therapy is extremely effective in treating haemoptysis from primary lung cancer. Single fractions may often be sufficient.[7,8]

Haematuria

Haematuria is a troublesome symptom often caused by cancer of the bladder or prostate. Single fractions have been shown to be effective, with less acute toxicity than more protracted regimens. Findings are equivocal as to whether larger protracted regimens increase response.

Vaginal Bleeding

Vaginal bleeding from advanced or recurrent carcinoma of the cervix, endometrium or ovary will often respond to a single fraction of external RT. Treatment of large volumes can cause severe late toxicity, and are generally only recommended when life expectancy is short. Intra-cavity isotope insertion is often used, especially if external RT has previously been given.

Rectal Bleeding

External RT has been shown to successfully treat rectal bleeding in the majority of patients.[6] Studies suggest that the more prolonged regimens produce a higher rate of complete responses in rectal carcinoma. They are however associated with greater acute toxicity.

Fungation

Fungating carcinomas of the breast, melanomas, skin secondaries and advanced head and neck tumours often respond to EBRT. Radical regimens are often used for these lesions in order to achieve long-term local control. Radical regimens are also often given to patients with extensive local disease of the head and neck who do not have disseminated disease in an attempt to cure (there are a few long term survivors) as well as to produce a durable improvement in function and body image through a greater reduction in tumour mass than is theoretically achievable with hypofractionated regimens.

Where a radical regimen is not likely to be tolerated (they are associated with considerable toxicity, especially oral mucositis) a fractionated palliative regimen may be preferred to a single fraction. Worries regarding high dose single fractions relate to the fact that the cervical spinal cord is usually encompassed in the treatment field with the risk of late radiation myelitis. Single fractions are generally reserved for those with a poor performance status and short prognosis.

Cough

A cough due to obstruction of an airway and distal infection may well respond to irradiation (EBRT or brachytherapy) whereas that due to multiple lung secondaries or lymphangitis carcinomatosis will not.[7,8] Response rates with brachytherapy range from 50-85%.

Retinal Deposits

Intraorbital metastases usually affect the choroid and are often bilateral. They may present as a visual disturbance, ranging from blurred vision to partial loss of sight, floaters, pain due to secondary glaucoma or proptosis. Early prompt recognition and treatment is important in order to retain or improve vision, as deterioration can occur rapidly. 30Gy in 10 fractions or 20Gy in 5 fractions are generally used. Worries over lower response rates and relapse with lower total doses have been highlighted in one retrospective study.

Kaposi's Sarcoma

As the incidence of AID'S has increased Kaposi's sarcoma has become more frequent. Skin lesions are generally treated for cosmetic reasons or when causing pain or oedema, usually with a single fraction when life expectancy is limited.

Small daily fractions are required for mucosal lesions because of an increased susceptibility to mucositis and necrosis with standard doses. Hyperpigmentation is also more of a problem than usual, taking many months to resolve.

Lymphoedema

When caused solely by pelvic obstruction to lymph flow (by primary or secondary tumour, or lymph node involvement) external RT may be helpful. It is however often disappointing, probably due to the extent of disease and lymphatic damage and existence of other contributing factors such as hypoalbuminaemia and dependence.

DISCUSSION

In the palliative setting the less intrusive and toxic an effective treatment is, the better. Single fraction and hypofractionated regimens are certainly more convenient for the patient than the more protracted regimens and put less demand on already overstretched radiotherapy departments, but have not always been shown to be equally effective or free from significant late toxicity.

Published response rates using differing regimens, or combinations of regimens, have to be interpreted with caution. They are often retrospective and uncontrolled, have low numbers of patients and fail to take into account concurrent therapies such as hormonal agents, chemotherapy and steroids, leading to considerable potential for bias in their findings. Criteria for response is often quite varied and may or may not take into account the patient's perspective. Toxicity is generally poorly addressed.

Randomised studies

Good controlled randomised studies in this area, although achieved in some instances (as described above) are extremely difficult to perform. Not only is recruitment difficult and attrition rates high, but standard, valid, reliable, user friendly instruments for measuring symptomatic improvement and toxicity, although increasingly available (often with specific modules relating to disease sites) can be cumbersome and difficult to analyze and interpret.

Much further work is needed in addressing the issues surrounding hypofractionation in each of the clinical scenarios described above.

Work is also needed to enable better selection of patients likely to respond to therapy, and in establishing the exact role of brachytherapy and CHART.

Until this is done confusion over optimum management and varied practice will remain.

SUGGESTED FURTHER READING

Walter J, Miller H, Bomford C.K. A short textbook of radiotherapy. Edinburgh, London and New York: Churchill Livingstone, 1979.

Hoskin P.J., Radiotherapy in symptom management. In: Doyle D, Hanks G, MacDonald N eds. Oxford Textbook of Palliative Medicine, first edition. Oxford, New York, Tokyo: Oxford University Press, 1993: 117-29.

References

1. Rodney Withers H. Biological basis of radiation therapy for cancer. Lancet 1992; 339: 156-59.
2. Needham P.R, Hoskin P.J. Radiotherapy for painful bone metastases. Pall Med 1994; 8: 95-104.
3. Hoskin P. Using radioisotopes for bone metastases. Eur J Pall Care 1994; 1(2): 78-82.
4. Corn B.W, Lanciano R.M, Boente M, et al. Recurrent Ovarian Cancer – Effective radiotherapeutic palliation after chemotherapy failure. Cancer 1994; 74: 2979 – 83.
5. Spanos W.J (Jr), Clery M, Perez C.A, et al. Late effect of multiple daily fraction palliation schedule for advanced pelvic malignancies (RTOG 8502). Int J Radiat Oncol Biol Phys 1994; 29(5): 961-7.
6. Taylor R.E, Kerr G.R, Arnott S.J. External beam radiotherapy for rectal adenocarcinoma. Br J Surg 1987; 74: 455 – 59.
7. Bleehen N.M, Girling D.J, Fayers P.M, et al. Inoperable non-small-cell lung cancer: a Medical Research Council randomised trial of palliative radiotherapy with two fractions or ten fractions. Br J Cancer 1991; 63: 265 – 270.
8. Bleehen N.M, Girling D.J, Hasleton P.S, et al. A Medical Research Council randomised trial of palliative radiotherapy with two fractions or a single fraction in patients with inoperable non-small-cell lung cancer and poor performance status. Br J Cancer 1992; 65: 934-41.
9. Bates T. A review of local radiotherapy in the treatment of bone metastases and cord compression. Int J Radiat Oncol Biol Phys 1992; 23: 217-221
10. Sorensen P.S, Helweg-Larsen S, Mouridsen H et al. Effect of high-dose dexamethasone in carcinomatous metastatic spinal cord compression treated with radiotherapy: a randomised trial. Eur J Cancer 1994; 30(1): 22-27.
11. Thomas R, James N, Guerrero D et al. Hypofractionated radiotherapy as palliative treatment in poor prognosis patients with high grade glioma. Radiotherapy Oncol 1994; 33: 113-6.
12. Coia L.R. The role of radiation therapy in the treatment of brain metastases. Int J Radiat Oncol Biol Phys 1992; 23: 229-38.
13. Borgelt B, Gelber R, Kramer S et al. The palliation of brain metastases: Final results of the first two studies by the radiation therapy oncology group. Int J Radiat Oncol Biol Phys 1980; 6: 1-9.
14. Harwood A.R, Simpson W.J. Radiation therapy of cerebral metastases a randomized prospective clinical trail. Int J Radiat Oncol Biol Phys 1977; 2: 1091-4.
15. Abner A. Approach to the patient who presents with superior vena cava obstruction. Chest 1993; 103:394S-97.

16. Bown S.G. Palliation of malignant dysphagia: surgery, radiotherapy, laser, intubation alone or in combination. Gut 1991; 32: 841-844.
17. Saunders MI, Dische S, Barrett A et al. Randomised multicentre trials of CHART vs conventional radiotherapy in head and neck and non-small-cell lung canger: an interim report. Br J Cancer 1996; 73: 1455–1462.
18. Borgelt B, Gelber R, Kramer S et al. The Palliation of Brain Metastases: Final results of the first two studies by the radiation therapy Oncology Group. Int J Rad. Oncol Biol Phys 1980; 6: 1–9.
19. Priestman TJ, Dunn J, Drada M et al. Final results of the Royal College of Radiologists' Trial Composing Two different Radiotherapy Schedules in the treatment of cerebral metastases. Clin Oncol 1996; 8: 308–315.
20. Wong WW, Schild S, Sawyer T et al. Analysis of outcome in patients reirradiated for brain metastases. Int J Rad. Oncol Biol Phys, 1996; 34: 585–590.

COMMENTS ABOUT THE REFERENCES:

1 provides an excellent, comprehensible explanation of how radiotherapy works.

2 and 3 give a comprehensive view of the role of radiotherapy and radioisotopes in the management of painful bone metastases, based on the current available evidence.

4 and 6 report on the palliation achieved by the external beam radiotherapy in patients with ovarian and rectal carcinoma, respectively.

7 and 8 report the 2 MRC trials comparing 2 versus 10 fractions, and 1 versus 2 fractions of RT in symptomatic patients with inoperable NSC lung cancer.

9 gives a helpful review if the role of radiotherapy in the management of bone metastases and spinal cord compression.

12, 13 and 14 look at the role of radiotherapy in the treatment of cerebral metastases. 12 provides the overview, 13 reports on the RTOG study with compared 5 different treatment schedules, and 14 reports on a study comparing 10 fractions with 1.

15 is a useful overview of the pathophysiology and management of superior vena cava obstruction.

16 discusses the role of the different therapeutic modalities available for managing malignant dysphagia.

Chapter 3

Palliative Chemotherapy

Dr Peter Kaye
Peter Kaye is Consultant in Palliative Medicine at Cynthia Spencer Hospice, Northampton. A Fellow of the Royal College of Physicians and a Member of the Royal College of General Practitioners. He has a special interest in the psychological aspects of illness.

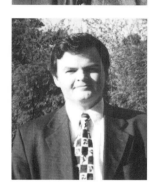

Dr David Levy
David Levy is Consultant Clinical Oncologist at Weston Park Hospital, Sheffield, previously a Consultant in Northamptonshire. His particular interests include palliative chemotherapy, brain tumours and education.

INTRODUCTION

"If the medical profession is to demonstrate its ethical and clinical competence, it must accept the challenge of developing clear guidelines for anti-cancer drug usage in patients with metastatic cancer".[1]

This chapter considers the appropriateness of palliative chemotherapy in advanced disease.

Palliative chemotherapy may be given to patients with locally advanced or metastatic disease in order to prolong life, to control symptoms or improve quality of life. Most chemotherapy is palliative from the outset.

Curative chemotherapy is only a possibility for leukaemia, testicular cancer, Hodgkin's and high-grade lymphomas and some childhood cancers. If relapse occurs further chemotherapy can prolong life but the chances of cure are then greatly reduced.

Most patients with disseminated cancer opt for chemotherapy treatment. Careful decision-making and monitoring are needed, because the main aim is to control symptoms using drugs that can actually *cause* symptoms.

CLASSIFICATION OF CYTOTOXICS

- Antimetabolites
  - 5FU
  - Methotrexate
- Alkylating agents
  - chlorambucil

- cyclophosphamide
- Intercalating agents
  - cisplatin, carboplatin
  - adriamycin

- Spindle poisons
  - vincristine, vinblastine,
  - vindesine
  - paclitaxel, docetaxel
- Others (? mode of action)

Chemotherapy and Tumour growth

Cytotoxic drugs inhibit cell division. However, by the time a tumour is detectable, at around the size of 1g (1cm on xrays or scans) it is already large in cellular terms. By the time a tumour is causing clinical symptoms, at around 0.5kg, it only needs a few doubling times before it causes death.

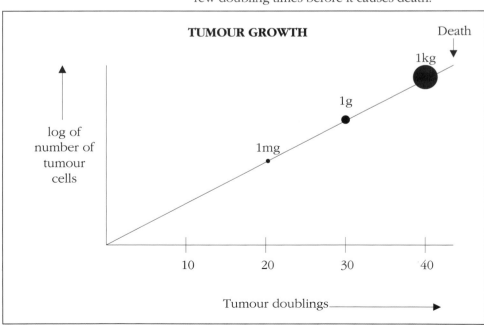

TUMOUR GROWTH

Death

1kg

1g

log of number of tumour cells

1mg

10   20   30   40

Tumour doublings

Tumours that are dividing rapidly, with short doubling times, tend to respond best to chemotherapy.

DOUBLING TIMES OF SOME COMMON TUMOURS	
	Days
Breast	60
Colon	80
Adenocarcinoma of lung	150
Hodgkins disease	5

Commonly treated cancers

Cancers most commonly treated with palliative chemotherapy include small cell and non-small cell carcinoma of the lung, breast, colo-rectal cancer, stomach, ovary, cervix, bladder, head and neck, soft tissue sarcoma, myeloma, melanoma and non-Hodgkin's lymphoma. The list of malignancies treated with palliative chemotherapy continues to grow. Newer drugs are being designed, some with lower toxicity. Newer techniques of giving chemotherapy (eg continuous infusions) may improve response rates and reduce toxicity.

Recent meta-analyses of results has shown:

● 10% survival benefit for patients with non small cell lung cancer.[7]
● Clinically significant response rates in patients with advanced colo-rectal cancer.[8,9]
● Benefit of platinum drugs in patients with ovarian cancer.[9]

ATTITUDES TO CHEMOTHERAPY

Even the experts disagree on the place of palliative chemotherapy for metastatic solid tumours. Here are the views of 2 medical oncologists[10]

DIFFERING VIEWS

"Most cancers are incurable once metastatic and often respond poorly to chemotherapy, which can result in side-effects, inconvenience, and a financial cost without improvements in symptoms or survival".

G M Mead

"Within specialist units, chemotherapy for advanced disease can be delivered safely and with appropriate selection of patients can improve quality and quantity of life"

D Cunningham

Attitudes of Patients   Cancer patients have different perspectives to healthy people. In one study[14] people were asked what chance of success would be needed for them to agree to *curative* chemotherapy which would also cause severe side-effects (severe nausea and vomiting, hair loss, frequent use of drips and needles, frequent tiredness, loss of libido and admission to hospital 3-4 days a month.) Cancer patients were willing to undergo such treatment even if there was only a 1% chance of cure:

Question: **What % chance of cure would encourage you to undergo intensive chemotherapy?**

	100 Healthy people	303 Cancer nurses	790 GPs	148 Cancer doctors	100 Cancer patients
Answer:	50%	50%	25%	10%	1%

(The % is the median of the answers given)

In the same study people were asked what chance of symptom relief would be necessary for them to consider a course of *palliative* chemotherapy, (causing slight nausea and vomiting, no hair loss, some tiredness, admission to hospital 1 day per month)? Again cancer patients were willing to consider treatment even if there was only a 1% chance of symptom relief:

Question: **What % chance of controlling symptoms would encourage you to undergo palliative chemotherapy?**

	100 Healthy people	303 Cancer nurses	790 GPs	148 Cancer doctors	100 Cancer patients
Answer:	50%	25%	25%	25%	1%

This study showed that patients accept side-effects more than doctors, nurses or healthy people (presumably because illness changes ones' philosophy of life). Slevin concluded:

> "A patient with cancer appeared to regard a minute chance of possible benefit as worthwhile, whatever the cost".

But another way of interpreting these results is that patients can be very vulnerable to accepting treatment that has little or no chance of giving benefit. Even when the evidence for benefit from chemotherapy is very meagre there is still a pressure on the patient to provide some sort of "hope" for themselves and their family, and on the doctor to "do something"

PATIENT SELECTION

A question of balance Chemotherapy is a two-edged sword. Given appropriately to a range of metastatic cancers it can be of great benefits in terms of prolonged life or symptom control. Given inappropriately, the side-effects can lead to poorer quality of life and may hasten death. The balance between advantages (improved survival, symptom control and quality of life) and disadvantages (toxicity and inconvenience) varies from disease to disease and from patient to patient.

Patient selection With such variability it is difficult to identify all patients who may benefit from chemotherapy. The careful selection of patients for palliative chemotherapy is of paramount importance. There are several factors which can help guide an Oncologist. The most important of these is the performance status of the patient. The most commonly used scale for performance status is that of the World Health Organisation (WHO). This is as follows:

W.H.O. PERFORMANCE STATUS

Grade 0   Normal activity

Grade 1   Ambulatory, can do light work.

Grade 2   Bed or chair up to 50% of waking hours, but self-caring

Grade 3   Bed or chair more than 50% of waking hours, limited self-care

Grade 4   Confined to bed or chair, no self-care, completely disabled.

Patients of poorer performance status are less likely to respond to palliative chemotherapy and more likely to die from it, whereas patients of good performance status (eg, grade 0 – 2) often have less bulky disease, are more likely to respond and so benefit from palliative chemotherapy.[12]

Bulk of disease   Bulk of disease is another useful factor in the selection of patients. This is certainly true for patients with carcinoma of the ovary who are more likely to respond and have a complete response if their disease has been optimally debulked prior to chemotherapy.

THE AIMS OF PALLIATIVE CHEMOTHERAPY

The main aim of palliative chemotherapy is improvement in quality of life. If a patient has no symptoms the use of palliative chemotherapy is questionable. Prolongation of life may be the hope, but may not be achieved. Until recently, apart from the moderately chemo-sensitive tumours, there was little evidence that palliative chemotherapy pro-longed life.

If metastases are life-threatening (eg diffuse pulmonary infiltration, fulminating liver disease) then chemotherapy can prolong life for a few weeks. Recent trials suggests chemotherapy can control symptoms and improve quality of life even when survival is not improved.[15]

Indications The main indication for palliative chemotherapy is symptom control. If a patient has no symptoms, its use is questionable, but it may occasionally be indicated to prevent symptoms, such as from rapidly progressive visceral lesions, or from imminent invasion of a nerve plexus.

Some indications for
Palliative Chemotherapy

- Metastases (if chemo-sensitive)
- Local spread (if chemo-sensitive)
- Tumour fungation
- Lymphoedema
- SVC compression
- Cord compression
- Lymphadenopathy
- Nerve invasion
- Re-opening compressed bronchus
- Improve bowel function (malignant obstruction)

Palliative Chemotherapy can improve symptoms

A 26 year old women presented with node-negative breast cancer and had a lumpectomy followed by adjuvant radiotherapy and chemotherapy (with malaise.) A year later she presented with jaundice and hepatomegaly. Staging investigations confirmed hepatic metastases only. As she was of good performance status (WHO=1) and had a very young family she was treated with epiadriamycin, given 3 weekly and with dexamethasone 4mg a day. After 3 courses her jaundice had resolved and the steroids were withdrawn. A CT scan showed some improvement. After 6 courses a further CT scan showed only a partial response but there had been a dramatic improvement in symptoms.

Lesson: Palliative chemotherapy can improve symptoms and performance status (without necessarily achieving an objective tumour response).

EXPLAINING CHEMOTHERAPY

Giving advice about chemotherapy is difficult. What is meaningful to the patient is an improvement in symptoms, survival, or quality of life. Unfortunately it remains difficult to predict the outcome for an individual patient, and few studies have compared the effectiveness of chemotherapy with supportive care alone.

Level of explanation

Explaining treatment options is a complex process, and explanation in terms of statistics and percentages is often very difficult to understand. Doctors have to give accurate information (for informed consent) but also want to avoid removing hope and demoralising the patient. This involves judgement about what information will be helpful for a particular patient. The careful explanation of the disease and the aims and possible side-effects of treatment can be very supportive when done sensitively, but the level of detail explanation depends on the patient's:

- ability to understand
- main concerns
- desire for information
- expectations of treatment
- emotional state
- family support

Ideally care is shared between a Palliative Care Physician and an Oncologist. In advanced disease, it may be better to offer the option of skilled symptom control and emotional support rather than palliative chemotherapy, which may arouse false hope and subsequently a sense of failure because the tumour "failed" to respond to treatment. Discussion needs to focus on the advantages and disadvantages of the treatment being offered:

PALLIATIVE CHEMOTHERAPY

Advantages	Disadvantages
Symptom Relief	Toxic side-effects
?Prolonged survival	Time lost to treatment
Objective response	Psychological morbidity
Improved activity	Social disruption

GIVING CHEMOTHERAPY

Oncologists give palliative chemotherapy under careful supervision, so benefits and side effects can be carefully assessed.

When to Start? It can be helpful to think in terms of a "therapeutic window of opportunity" for palliative chemotherapy. Treatment at the right stage in the disease can be helpful, whereas treatment earlier or later may be unhelpful. If one leaves the patient too long then, the bulk of the disease will increase and performance status will deteriorate and, the chance of response is less likely. There is a body of opinion that patients who present with metastatic disease should be treated sooner rather than later.

The relationship between tumour progression and symptoms remains poorly understood. It is possible that earlier palliative chemotherapy may reduce the frequency of symptoms even though survival is not prolonged.[13]

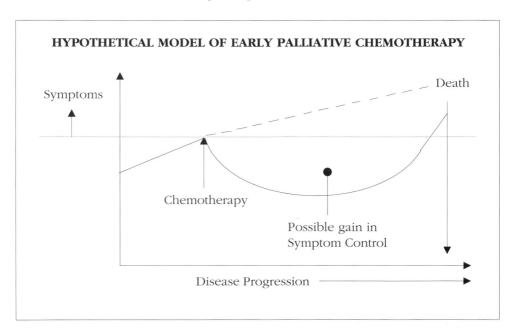

HYPOTHETICAL MODEL OF EARLY PALLIATIVE CHEMOTHERAPY

Symptoms

Death

Chemotherapy

Possible gain in Symptom Control

Disease Progression

Nevertheless, there are a large number of patients with metastatic disease who are often best treated with symptom control and an observational policy.

The options should be discussed with the patient. Some patients particularly in the older age group, may not wish to undergo potentially toxic chemotherapy treatments.

NB Patients having palliative chemotherapy deserve optimism from their professional carers that it will be effective.

Quality of life Very few studies have looked at quality of life in patients receiving palliative chemotherapy (though many are currently ongoing) but one study of breast cancer patients suggested there is no diminution in quality of life with palliative chemotherapy. In some patients who responded there was an improvement in quality of life scores.[15]

Sometimes a compromise is the best approach, for example to agree with the patient to try 1 or 2 treatments of chemotherapy and if no benefit ensues (in terms of physical or psychological well being) to change the focus of management to symptom control and emotional support. The concept of "appropriate hope" can be helpful at this point: hoping for something that is realistic and achievable raises morale.

Investigations Investigations may be needed before, during or after treatment to assess the extent of disease, to monitor the blood count and hepatic and renal function, so that the drugs can be given safely, and afterwards to monitor the response to treatment or diagnose any intercurrent problems (the most important being neutropenic sepsis). Special tests may be needed for research if the treatment is part of a trial.

Drug trials *Drug trials* are necessary to test new drugs which have shown promise in the laboratory in phase I and II studies. Ethically they have to be tested in patients who have no prospect of benefiting from other treatments. Patients enter into trials for new experimental drugs because of the (very small) chance of benefit and so they can contribute to furthering medical knowledge. They may also benefit from the increased level of medical interest in them.

Larger phase III studies are looking at drug combinations for common malignancies such as non small cell lung cancer, breast cancer and colorectal cancer to assess which drugs are best for these patients. These studies should have quality of life analysis built in, as well as health economic evaluation.

TRIALS OF NEW DRUGS (in volunteer patients)

Phase 1: Toxicity studies

Phase 2: Treatment of individuals (where other agents have failed)

Phase 3: Randomized trials (multi-centre)

Phase 4: Routine anti-cancer treatment

ASSESSING THE RESPONSE

Until very recently the outcome of chemotherapy was traditionally measured in terms of tumour response. A complete response is rare, so this usually means assessing a partial response.

DEFINITIONS

- **Complete Response**: Disappearance of all detectable disease for at least a month.

- **Partial Response**: Reduction in tumour diameter of 50% for at least a month (eg skin nodule, scan or Xray shadow)

- **Progressive disease**: The development of new lesions or increase in tumour diameter of 25%.

Response rates for the common tumours are:

Advanced Tumour	Approximate Response Rates
– Small cell Lung	40-80%
– Breast	40-50%
– Ovary	30-60%
– Stomach	Up to 80%
– Colo-rectal	20%
– Head and Neck	30%
– Bladder	20-50%
– Sarcoma	30%
– Melanoma	25%
– Cervix	40%

A 50% response rate means 50% of tumours will show a response, but this does not mean 50% of patients will automatically benefit from treatment. Shrinkage of the tumour often has little effect on survival.

On the other hand many patients report their symptoms have improved when scans are unable to detect any measurable tumour shrinkage, and some patients with no objective response may feel better during and after treatment.

Drugs are now being marketed with other factors than tumour response being measured, including quality of life, reduction in analgesic consumption and improvement in performance status. These more subjective measures may be more important, not just to the patient but to the doctors, giving a truer reflection of the value of the treatment that is on offer.

For several tumour sites (eg, colorectal cancer, ovarian pancreatic cancer), there is an increasing use of tumour markers which can be used to help determine response.

PSA	–	prostate
CEA	–	colorectal
CA125	–	ovary
CA19-9	–	pancreas

How long to continue?

Treatment is usually given 1-2 times a month, for 3-6 months, but the optimum length of treatment is rarely known. If there is evidence of progression of the disease after 6 weeks, treatment is usually stopped. However, if the disease is responding (eg tumour markers are falling) symptoms have been controlled and the patient is tolerating the chemotherapy well, treatment may be continued up to 6 months.

When to stop?   There is a common fear that deciding to stop chemotherapy may upset the patient, by removing hope. If the disease is obviously progressing despite chemotherapy it should be stopped, but often the effect is not clear, and everyone continues to hope for a response. The key question then becomes: "Does the chemotherapy make the patient feel better?"

If the patient feels better, either physically or psychologically, then chemotherapy should usually be continued. If it is making the patient feel worse, it is time to rest from the chemotherapy and to focus on symptom control and the quality of remaining life. There comes a point when it can be a great relief for a patient and family to discuss this and to stop unhelpful treatment.

NB. It is much easier to stop chemotherapy if the goals of treatment have been clearly explained from the start.

Palliative Chemotherapy can prolong life.

A lady of 67 years presented with a cough, weight loss of a few stone and malaise. She was shown to have Small Cell Lung Cancer with cervical lymphadenopathy. Her performance status was limited (WHO=3). After a frank discussion she agreed to have chemotherapy. In view of her performance status she received etoposide and vincristine with Septrin prophylaxis. Within 2 courses she was well enough to be discharged home and there was an improvement in her performance status (WHO=1). She received a total of 4 courses of chemotherapy. 3 months after the completion of treatment her disease began to progress again

Lesson: Appropriate palliative chemotherapy may offer important improvement in survival and quality of life.

SIDE-EFFECTS OF CYTOTOXIC DRUGS

- Nausea and vomiting   (1-2 days)
- Marrow suppression   (7-10 days)
- Malaise   (7-14 days)
- Mucositis   (7-14 days)
- Hair loss   (7-21days)
- Neuropathy   (weeks)
- Lung fibrosis   (weeks)
- Reduced libido   (weeks to months)
- Headache   intrathecal drugs

SPECIFIC SIDE-EFFECTS OF SOME DRUGS:

Vinca alkaloids
- peripheral neuropathy
- jaw pain
- constipation
- colic

Platinum compounds
- high tone hearing loss
- neuropathy
- nephropathy

Alkalating agents
(eg, cyclophosphamide, nitrosureas)
- infertility
- neuropathy
- lung fibrosis

Anthracyclines
- arrhythmias
- heart failure
- mucositis

Bleomycin
- lung fibrosis
- Raynaud's phenomenon

Methotrexate
- stomatitis
- cystitis
- diarrhoea
- pneumonitis
- neuropathy

5FU
- oral mucositis
- diarrhoea

Taxol
- neutropenia
- alopecia
- neuropathy

Nausea and vomiting can be severe with cisplatin, dacarbazine, cyclophosphamide, lomustine, carboplatin and doxorubicin. This is now fortunately, much better controlled with the use of the new 5 HT3 antagonists (eg, Ondansetron). The delayed nausea and vomiting, sometimes seen with Cis-platinum and anthracyclines is helped by steroids (Dexamethasone 2-4 mg tds) for a few days.

QUALITY OF LIFE ISSUES

Quality of Life   The impact of chemotherapy can be complex, with social, psychological, emotional, marital, family and spiritual dimensions, as well as physical effects. On the other hand, chemotherapy may have little impact in terms of the patient's routine and adverse effects, and some patients maintain a positive attitude throughout. Assessment of new palliative chemotherapy regimes, using multi-centre trials and meta-analysis, must focus on quality of life as well as response rates.

EFFECT OF CHEMOTHERAPY ON QUALITY OF LIFE

Negative aspects
- Side-effects
- Fear of treatment (social "myths" re chemo)
- Reminder of disease
- Time lost (clinics etc)
- Loss of independence
- Altered body image (eg hair loss)
- Loss of libido
- Continued uncertainty
- Decreased self-esteem
- Role change ("under treatment")
- Guilt/failure (failure to respond)
- Number of relationships (professional team)
- Separation anxiety at end of treatment
- Seeing effects on other patients (good and bad)
- Disruption of family life.

Positive aspects:
- Hope of improvement
- Physical well being
- Mental well being
- Treatment routine may help structure time

PALLIATIVE CHEMOTHERAPY FOR SPECIFIC TUMOURS

Small cell lung

Very early disease may be curable with chemotherapy and radiotherapy. 70% present with extensive disease (ie spread beyond one hemithorax), when chemotherapy can prolong median survival from 2 to 9 months (and 5% can survive 2 years). Assessment is important. Patients with poorer performance status are at risk of death if inappropriate chemotherapy is given.

Standard treatment is now oral etoposide and IV vincristine for patients with poor performance status and extensive disease.[18]

Non-small cell lung

30 years of research has failed to show a role for chemotherapy in non-small cell lung cancer, but a recent overview of 52 randomized trials[10] suggested that regimes including cisplatin may confer some benefit.[6] Further research is being performed nationally and internationally using Cisplatinum regimes and newer drugs including Gemcitabine and Taxol. Gemcitabine, has shown an improvement in performance status for patients with non small cell lung cancer.[16] A currently favoured regime includes Mitomycin, Ifosphamide and Cisplatinum (MIC) which is being used in a large Phase III trial.[19]

Breast

Palliative chemotherapy is usually reserved for patients who fail to respond to hormone therapy, but is used earlier in younger patients where there is less likely to be a response to hormones and also those with aggressive visceral metastases, such as diffuse pulmonary metastases causing dyspnoea or liver metastases.

A commonly used regime is CMF (Cyclophosphamide, Methotrexate and Fluorouracil). Other drugs that are sometimes used include single agent Doxorubicin (or Epiadriamycin), Mitomycin or Mitozantrone.

Taxotere is also now licensed for use in younger patients with metastatic disease.

Palliative chemotherapy has a response rate of up to 50% with a median duration of 6–8 months. Treatments usually continue for 4-6 months, with no evidence that longer treatment have any benefit. Secondary regimes (such as IV mitozantrone) give lower response rates of about 20% with a median duration for 2-3 months.[20] Even with advance disease in elderly patients, quality of life can occasionally be improved by chemotherapy.

Ovarian

Early disease (stage I, confined to the ovary) may be cured with surgery and adjuvant chemotherapy. Combinations of cytotoxic[11] drugs show no advantages, as yet, over single platinum agents. The most active drugs are cisplatin, carboplatin and Taxol. For patients with a poorer performance status, particularly elderly patients, Carboplatin is the drug of choice as this can be given on an out-patient basis with less toxicity and appears well tolerated. Ultrasound scanning or CT is needed to monitor response, though, the serial measurements of plasma antigen CA 125 can give valuable information.

Treatments usually continued for up to 6 cycles in patients who respond. If there is no response after 3 cycles treatment is stopped. 40% of patients show a response to palliative chemotherapy, which can reduce ascites, reduce tumour bulk and occasionally can prolong life. A new trial is shortly to commence looking at the role of second line chemotherapy in those patients who relapse more than 6 months after first line chemotherapy.[21]

Stomach

20–40% of patients respond to 5 FU with folinic acid. Ascites and pain may be reduced, but survival is not significantly improved. More aggressive regimes (in better performance status patients) have been used including a newer infusional regime using Epiadriamycin, Cisplatinum and 5 fluorouracil.

Response rates of up to 80% have been documented, though there appears to be no improvement in median survival as yet.[22] Care must be taken giving chemotherapy to these patients particularly as they are often in a catabolic state.

Colo-rectal

Intravenous 5FU with folinic acid remains the mainstay of treatment. 5FU and folinic acid relieves symptoms even though only about 23% have an objective tumour response.[8] Continuing IV infusion via indwelling central venous line (eg Hickman) and using a portable electronic pump is more expensive but may be less toxic and may improve response rates slightly. Raltitrexed (Tomudex) is a new drug which is marketed for advanced colo-rectal cancer. It has similar response rates to 5 FU and folinic acid.

All three regimes outlined above are now the subject of an MRC trial to establish what is the best regime for patients with advanced colorectal cancer and also how long they should continue.[17]

No advantage has been shown as yet for using hepatic artery infusion which remains a research technique.

A meta-analysis of patients with advanced colorectal cancer suggests those with metastatic disease limited to the liver have significantly improved survival compared to those with more extensive disease.[8]

Cervix Combination therapy (eg bleomycin, cisplatin, methotrexate and ifosphamide) achieves response rates of around 40% but at the risk of significant side-effects. Medium duration of response is 5-6 months.

Chemotherapy is indicated for relief of symptoms such as pain or leg oedema. It is monitored with serial CT scans or ultra-sound scans, but symptom relief can occur even when there is no objective tumour response. There is no routine place for second line cytotoxic therapy.

Bladder Chemotherapy is reserved for patients with symptoms such as pain or oedema (but it does not control haematuria as well as radiotherapy). Combination therapy (eg methotrexate, vinblastine, doxorubicin and cisplatin can produce a 60% response rate but side effects can be severe. Recent evidence suggests that Cisplatinum is a very important part of any combination.[23]

Head and Neck Chemotherapy is usually reserved for symptomatic local recurrence after radical surgery or radiotherapy (though it has been given in adjuvant settings). Combinations of cisplatin and 5FU or methotrexate give response rates of about 20 to 30% for about 3 months, but side-effects can be severe.

Non-Hodgkins lymphomas

Disseminated low grade non-Hodgkins lymphomas are relatively resistant to eradication by chemotherapy. Gentle chemotherapy (usually chlorambucil with or without prednisolone) may control symptoms for many years as may radiotherapy.

Myeloma

Melphalan and Prednisolone remains the most useful combination and can provide useful control of symptoms.

Soft tissue sarcomas

Chemotherapy is used where local symptoms such as pain or ulceration are beyond the scope of radiotherapy, or for lung metastases causing dyspnoea which are not suitable for resection. Regimes using doxorubicin and ifosfamide give response rates of about 30% but side-effects can be troublesome.

PRINCIPLES OF GIVING PALLIATIVE CHEMOTHERAPY

- Avoid chemo-resistant disease
- Limit investigations
- Use least toxic agents
- Avoid toxic doses
- Short courses

- Consider home treatment?
- Symptom control also needed
- Consider hormonal therapy
- Frequent review
- Consider impact on quality of life

HORMONE THERAPY

Introduction

The observation that inoperable breast cancer responds to oophorectomy is 100 years old. 50 years later it was discovered that prostate cancer responds to bilateral orchidectomy or oestrogen treatment. Most hormone therapies involve the antagonism or supplementation of natural hormones. This "endocrine manipulation" can result in control of the disease.

Hormone therapy is now used in cancers of breast, prostate, endometrium and thyroid, (and stomach, melanoma and kidney, with less proven benefit). *Duration of response* may last years, whereas response to chemotherapy is often measured in months. Side effects of hormone therapy tend to be much less severe than with chemotherapy. Hormone therapy tends to be used before chemotherapy, except in younger patients.

Breast Cancer   Oestrogens are produced by the ovaries and also in small amounts by the adrenal glands. In post menopausal patients, the ovaries and adrenal glands produce androgens which are then metabolised (by the peripheral enzyme "aromatase") to oestrogens. The aim is to reduce circulating levels of oestrogen (since oestrogens stimulate breast cancer cells to grow).

1. Anti-oestrogens (tamoxifen, toremifene)
2. Progestogens (medroxyprogesterone, megestrol)
3. Aromatase inhibitors (anastrozole, aminoglutethimide)
4. LHRH agonists (goserilin)

Tamoxifen 20 mg daily. Is the drug of first choice it has a minimum of side effects, but can commonly cause menopausal symptoms (flushing, vaginal dryness, vaginal bleeding) and weight gain. Second line treatment is considered after relapse, particularly in patients who responded for more than 6 months to tamoxifen.

NEW ENDOCRINE THERAPIES FOR BREAST CANCER[27]

Anti-oestrogens (block the oestrogen receptor)

- Tamoxifen   — Agonist/antagonist
- Droloxifene   — *Non-steroidal.* Less agonist

- Faslodex   — *Steroidal* (derivative of oestrogen) with no agonist properties.

Aromatase inhibitors (block peripheral synthesis of oestrogen)

- Anastrazole ⎫
- Letrozole   ⎬ *Non-steroidal.* Oral, minimal toxicity and no steroid replacements needed (unlike
- Vorozole   ⎭ the old aromatase inhibitor aminoglutethimide)

- Exemestane   *Steroidal.* Oral (whereas Formestane required IM injection)

Anastrazole (Arimadex) 1mg daily, is an aromatase inhibitor increasingly being used as second line therapy. It is given orally and does not cause adrenal suppression (unlike aminoglutethimide which must be given with hydrocortisone).

Side-effects include hot flushes, vaginal dryness and nausea. Weight gain is not seen.

Progestogens, such as megestrol acetate 160mg daily, are mainly used as third-line therapy. They tend to cause fluid retention and weight gain.

LHRH agonists are only used for pre-menopausal patients to suppress ovarian function (the response rate post-menopausally is less than 10%).[2]

Hormone Therapy in Breast Cancer

A 48 year old lady, known to have had breast cancer resected 2 years previously, presented with increasing shortness of breath. She was found to have a pleural effusion and staging investigations revealed bony metastases. She was changed from Tamoxifen to a progestogen and had a pleural aspiration performed. She remained asymptomatic for 3 years then developed further bony pains and was changed to aminoglutethimide plus hydro-cortisone with good effect. She continues on follow up.

Elderly women with locally advanced disease who are unfit for surgery can be treated with hormone therapy. The response rate is only 30-40% but it avoids the potential hazards of surgery. In patients who are otherwise well surgery is the best option rather than have a 60-70% risk of progression of disease.

Prostate Cancer Prostate cancer is the second most common cause of cancer death in men. Approximately 9000 men die each year from prostate cancer in the UK. 50% present with metastatic disease when hormone therapy is of proven benefit. The tumour usually has androgen receptors and hormone therapy is to reduces the activity of endogenous androgens. 80% of patients respond to hormone therapy with a median duration of 18 months. Choice of treatment is guided by side effects and patient preferences. Methods correctly used include:

1. Anti-androgens (cyproterone acetate, flutamide)
2. Bilateral orchidectomy
3. LHRH agonists (Goserelin, Leuprorelin)

Anti-androgens can cause impotence (flutamide less so) and hot flushes and carry the risk of diarrhoea and abdominal upset. Cyproterone acetate has been associated with disturbance of liver function tests, which should be monitored, if the drug is used for more than a few months. Flutamide can, less commonly cause hepatic damage.

Bilateral orchidectomy (which is a relatively simple procedure) is used less commonly. It results in a permanent reduction in endogenous androgen and thus causes impotence and occasionally hot flushes.

LHRH agonists are given by monthly (or 3 monthly) depot injection and should be given with an oral anti-androgen for the first 2 weeks, to prevent a tumour flare. They are a popular choice with patients.

Total androgen blockage (LHRH agonists plus anti-androgens) should theoretically improve survival[3] but this has not been confirmed by meta-analysis, and cannot be currently recommended.[4]

After failure of first line hormone therapy (ie disease progression) the median survival is 6-12 months. Only 20% will respond to second line treatment (unlike Breast Cancer), usually Prednisolone or Dexamethasone. Otherwise the best possible treatment for the patient is symptomatic control with analgesia, radiotherapy and other appropriate measures.

Endometrial Cancer

Most patients present early and undergo hysterectomy (and may receive adjuvant radiotherapy). A few patients present who are medically unfit for operation or have metastatic disease at presentation. They may benefit from Provera, though the response rate is only in the order of 30-40%.

Thyroid Cancer

The management of thyroid cancer usually involves surgery, possibly radio-active iodine and radiotherapy. Thyroxine plays an important role in the management of such patients. Papillary of follicular carcinomas are often treated with high dose Thyroxine to suppress TSH production, which can stimulate these tumours to grow. Typical doses of Thyroxine vary between 200-300 mcg per day and must be carefully monitored.

Carcinoid Tumours

Octreotide, a Somatostatin analogue, may relieve symptoms and result in regression of disease. A dose of 50mcg BD subcutaneously is used initially. Disease may progress in the majority after 6 months but symptoms may be controlled for longer. Side-effects include nausea, abdominal pain and gallstone formation with longterm use.[5]

Renal Cancer

Progestogens give a response rate of approximately 10% or less in patients with metastatic disease.

Stomach Cancer

It was suggested at one time that Tamoxifen may improve survival though this is now not thought to be so.

Melanoma

Tamoxifen improves the response rate to DTIC in patients with metastatic disease. There is no evidence that long term tamoxifen is of any benefit.

CONCLUSION

Palliative Chemotherapy is not just tumour-orientated. It is one part of a therapeutic partnership between patient and professionals. In patients with far-advanced disease the aim is to obtain symptom relief with minimum side-effects and inconvenience.

Less toxic regimes are selected whenever possible, although the more potent anti-emetics now allow a wider range of cytotoxics to be used for palliative purposes. Whenever possible chemotherapy should be given as part of a clinical trial.

Palliative chemotherapy is beneficial to many patients with cancer, but decision-making about palliative chemotherapy is complex, and the potential advantages and disadvantages of treatment have to be discussed individually with each patient, in terms of their ideas and beliefs, present concerns, expectations and priorities. The process can be summarized as:

- Patient selection
- Explanation
- Administration
- Monitoring response
- Decision to stop
- Overlap with palliative care team

Careful assessment of new palliative chemotherapy regimes will continue, using multi-centre trials and meta-analysis, focusing on quality of life issues rather than simply on response rates.

The use of very intensive chemotherapy with stem cell transplants, for patients with less bulky chemo-sensitive disease, (eg, breast cancer), may improve survival in well-motivated patients with good performance status.[13]

New cancer treatments will need to be assessed for cost-effectiveness (in terms of quality of life outcomes, not just survival) as more and more expensive treatments become available. The use of growth factor analogues such as GCSF (granulocyte colony-stimulating factor) and possibly in future growth factors for red cells and platelets, may prevent marrow toxicity and allow higher dose chemotherapy to be used for palliation.

The Calman Report on the Commissioning of Cancer Services should bring improvements in the organisation of cancer services. The use of protocols will ensure optimal use of palliative treatments and evidence-based medicine for all patients.

REFERENCES

1 Stein RC et al. Total Oestrogen Blockade. British Journal of Cancer 1990; 62:679-683
2 Crawfurd ED, Isenberger MA. A controlled trial of Luprolide with and without Flutamide in prostatic cancer. New England Journal of Medicine 1989; 321:419-24
3 Maximum Androgen Blockade in advanced prostate cancer: an overview of 22 randomised trials with 3283 deaths in 5710 patients. Lancet 1995 July 29; 346 (8970): 265-9
4 Arnold R, Frank M, Cajdan U. Management of gastroenteropancreatic endocrine tumours, the place of Somatostatin analogues. Journal Digestion 1994; 55, supplement 3: 107-113
5 Editorial: Is there a better way? Bioethical reflections on palliative cytotoxic drug use. Palliative Medicine 1995; 9: 269-271
6 Moertal CG, Fleming TR, MacDonald JS et al. Levamisole and Flurouracil as adjuvant therapy of resected colon cancer. New England Journal of Medicine 1990; 3: 352-358
7 Stewart LA. Chemotherapy in non-small cell lung cancer: a meta-analysis using updated data on individual patients from 52 randomised clinical trials. BMJ 1995; 311: 899-909
8 Advanced colo-rectal cancer. Meta-analysis project. Modulation of Fluorouracil by Leucovorin in patients with advanced colo-rectal cancer. Evidence in terms of response rate: Journal of Clinical Oncology 1992; 10: 896-903
9 Meta-analysis of randomised trials of biochemical modulation of 5 FU by Methorexate in metastatic colo-rectal cancer. Journal of Clinical Oncology 1994; 12: 960-969
10 Controversies in Management: Chemotherapy for Solid Tumours BMJ 1995; 310: 246-8
11 Stewart LA. Chemotherapy in advanced ovarian cancer, an overview of randomised clinical trials. BMJ 1991; 303: 884-893
12 Stephens RJ, Girling DJ, Machin D. Treatment-related deaths in small cell lung cancer trials: can patients at risk be identified? Medical Research Council Lung Cancer Working Party. Lung Cancer 1994; 11 (3-4): 259-74
13 Improving Efficiency in Healthcare. New approaches in non-small cell lung cancer. Published by St Mary's Hospital Medical School.
14 Slevin ML, Stubbs L, Plant HJ et al. Attitudes to chemotherapy: comparing views of patients with cancer with those of doctors, nurses and general public. Br Med J 1990; 300: 1458-60
15 Fraser SCA, Dobbs HJ, Ebbs SR, Fallowfield LJ, Bates T, Baum M. Combination or mild single agent chemotherapy in advanced breast cancer? CMF versus Epirubicin measuring quality of life. British Journal of Cancer, 1993; 67: 402-406
16 Thatcher N, Anderson H, Betticher DC, Ranson M. Symptomatic benefit from Gemcitabine and other chemotherapy in advanced non-small-cell lung cancer: Changes in performance status and tumour related symptoms. Anti-cancer drugs, 1995; 6, supplement 6: 39-48
17 MRC CRO6 Study. Chemotherapy choices in advanced colo-rectal cancer. (A randomised trial comparing two chemotherapy regimes in the palliative treatment of advanced colo-rectal cancer.)
18 Comparison of oral etoposide and intravenous multi-drug chemotherapy for small cell lung cancer: A stopped multi-centre randomised trial. MRC Lung Cancer Working Party. Lancet 1996; 348: 563-566
19 The Big Lung Trial. Does short term chemotherapy improve the survival of patients with non-small cell lung cancer? A major randomised trial to determine the value of cisplatinum based chemotherapy for all patients with non small cell lung cancer supported by the British Thoracic Society 1996
20 Gregory WM et al."Chemotherapy of advanced breast cancer: outcome and prognostic factors" British Cancer Journal 1993; 68: 988-995
21 A randomised trial of Taxol with platinum versus platinum-based chemotherapy for relapsed ovarian cancer. MRC Gynaecological Cancer Working Party. ICON 4, 1996

22 Findlay M, et al. A phase II study in advanced gastro-oesophageal cancer using epirubicin and cisplatin in combination with continuous infusion 5-fluorouracil. Annals of Oncology 1994; 5(7): 609-16

23 Meed GM, et al. Medical Research Council, randomised trial comparing MV (Methotrexate and Vinblastine) with CMV (Cisplatinum plus MV) for metastatic transitional cell carcinoma of the bladder. American Society of Clinical Oncology, 1996; Abstract 600

24 Bezwoda WR, Seymour L, Dansey RD. High dose chemotherapy with haemopoetic rescue as primary treatment for metastatic breast cancer. Journal of Clinical Oncology 1995; 10: 2483-2489

25 Rubens RD, Towlson KE, Ramirez AJ et al. Appropriate chemotherapy for pallating advanced cancer. Br Med J 1992; 304: 35-40

26 Payne S. Coping with palliative chemotherapy. Journal of Advanced Nursing 1990; 15: 652-658.

27 Howell A, Dowsett M. Recent advances in endocrine therapy of breast cancer. Br Med J 1997; 315: 863–6.

Chapter 4

Update on AIDS

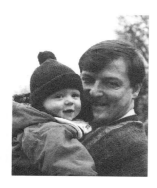

Dr Liam O'Siorain

Liam O'Siorain is Medical Director of Our Ladys Hospice, Caritas Unit, in Dublin. He is a consultant in palliative medicine to St. James's Hospital and lecturer in palliative medicine to Trinity College, Dublin. As medical director of the home care services for AIDS patients in Dublin, he has a special interest in the palliative care of patients with AIDS.

INTRODUCTION

The greatest challenge to palliative care as we approach the new millenium is the extension of specialist palliative care services to patients with non-malignant diseases. Of all the illnesses categorised as non-malignant, Acquired Immune Deficiency Syndrome, (AIDS), presents the greatest challenge to palliative care.[1]

Similarities   There are many similarities between the care of patients with AIDS and those with advanced cancer. Common issues include pain, anorexia, nausea, weight loss, psychosocial problems, isolation, loneliness and depression.[2] The lessons learnt from cancer patients can be directly transferred to patients with AIDS, but with some important differences.[3]

AIDS v CANCER – SOME DIFFERENCES

- Younger age group
- Misery of coexisting diagnoses
- Polypharmacy
- Unpredictable course – difficulty in predicting terminal phase
- Lengthy dying process
- Need for active palliation or maintenance treatment
- Rapidly changing patterns of disease and treatment
- Differing symptom profile
- Wider variety of medical presentations and problems
- Psychosocial issues
  - isolation, stigma
  - lack of family support
  - housing problems/poverty
  - drug abuse
- More complicated networks of families/carers
- Lower degree of GP involvement
- Spend more time in care
- Occupational health issues for staff

The diagnosis of AIDS

A 20 year old man with AIDS was admitted to the Palliative Care Unit from home. He was beginning to die from progressive cerebral lymphoma which had been diagnosed by brain biopsy 4 months earlier. He had 3 brothers and 4 sisters and both parents were alive. He did not want his diagnosis discussed with either his brothers or his parents. His sisters were aware that he had AIDS and that he was homosexual. His parents and brothers were only aware that he had a brain tumour.

He died peacefully in the Hospice without ever discussing his illness with his parents or brothers. After his death his sisters had great difficulty in bereavement and felt that the collusion had caused a division in the family that had previously shared very open communication.

This case illustrates issues concerning patient autonomy and confidentiality and the importance of bereavement support to families.

Symptom control   Symptom control is the cornerstone of good palliative care. In patients with AIDS, symptoms are often a presenting feature of opportunistic infections and their early diagnosis and specific treatment can greatly improve both quality and length of life.[4] The interrelationship between acute medical treatment and palliative treatment is complex in HIV and AIDS and boundaries may be indistinct. The changing nature of the HIV epidemic may lead to a different pattern of morbidity with less hospitalisation and more demand for specialist home care teams to provide maintenance therapy at home and to monitor symptoms. Closer liaison with the hospital based acute medical teams will also need to be developed.

Continued advances in anti-retroviral therapies and in the prophylaxis and treatment of opportunistic infection will radically alter the clinical manifestations of symptomatic disease.[5] In patients with AIDS, the symptom pattern differs from patients with cancer.

THE DIFFERENT SYMPTOM PROFILE IN AIDS

- Blindness
- Paralysis
- Neuropathy
- Dementia

- Myopathy
- Skin Disorders
- Severe Diarrhoea
- Recurrent Chest Infections

CMV retinitis

Over the course of the AIDS epidemic, some symptoms have become more prevalent, eg blindness due to the increase in CMV retinitis. This changing pattern challenges palliative care in new ways. Treatment of CMV retinitis may continue until the final hours or days of a patient's life in an attempt to prevent much feared blindness. This may require high dose IV treatment with blood tests, central lines etc. This requires a more interventionalist approach that is usual in palliative care.

Anti-retroviral drugs

Prognosis is harder to determine in AIDS and patients may be referred for palliative care at an earlier stage than cancer patients. Some patients, referred in anticipation of a short prognosis, now respond so dramatically to new anti-retroviral treatment, that the palliative care teams role is primarily that of support and surveillance. Many patients with HIV and AIDS suffer from a 'roller-coaster of health" with serious opportunistic infections, good responses to treatment, then another dip due to the next infection.[2] The course of cancer is more predictable and the boundaries between active therapy and palliative care are more easily distinguished.

Challenges   As AIDS in the Western world becomes a chronic illness due to the success of new therapies, palliative care will need to be sensitive to patients and carers new expectations.

Most patients will now be treated with several anti-retroviral drugs and knowledge of their interactions and side-effects is becoming more important.

The epidemiology of AIDS is changing with increasing prevalence in women and in the heterosexual population. Psychosocial issues can predominate and in patients who are active drug users, new challenges are faced by the palliative care team.[6]

HIV IN IV DRUG USERS

The symptoms of continued drug abuse (anorexia, weight loss, cough, dyspnoea, ataxia and changes in mental state) may mimic those of HIV disease. Substance abuse in HIV positive patients and pain control in patients on methadone maintenance (or abusing other opiates) present challenges and difficulties.

Some families of active drug users will have suffered multiple deaths from AIDS and in some cases grandparents or siblings are left to care for children. Appropriate bereavement follow up and support can have a critical role.

Palliative care professionals need to be very clear on what they can offer and need to be current in their knowledge of:

1. opportunistic infections
2. symptom control management
3. new drug treatments

HIV IN IV DRUG ABUSERS

- Chaotic life style, unpredictable interaction with staff and/or other patients
- Lack of support structures/homelessness
- Non-compliance with medication
- The need to get a fix – theft/prostitution
- Manipulative behaviour
- Financial pressures
- Methadone maintenance

- Symptom control in patients on other opiates
- Specific complications of IV drug use
  - overdose
  - skin infection site abscesses
  - endocarditis
  - hepatitis C
  - recurrent bacterial chest infections
  - increased psychiatric mobidity

AIDS in drug abusers

A 24 year old IV drug user with AIDS was dying at home under the home care team. He was on a methadone maintenance programme and as he deteriorated, the decision to switch him to subcutaneous diamorphine was made. After two days it was noted by the home care team that his syringe driver had been tampered with. He had also become more agitated and it was felt that two of his siblings who were active drug users may have used his syringe driver.

He was switched from subcutaneous diamorphine to a Fentanyl patch and this was closely supervised. He settled within 12 hours and died peacefully 4 days later.

Families who have multiple members who are actively abusing drugs can present difficult challenges to the palliative care team.

OPPORTUNISTIC INFECTIONS

Opportunistic infections are the major cause of morbidity and mortality in patients with AIDS.[7] Because of immunosuppression, opportunistic infections may present in unusual ways and as disseminated infection. Over the course of the AIDS epidemic, survival from opportunistic infections has improved with the increased availability of anti-retrovirals and prophylactic agents.

This section will cover some of the common opportunistic infections with an emphasis on clinical presentation and new developments:

COMMON INFECTIONS IN AIDS

- **Protozoal**
  - Toxoplasmosis
  - Cryptosporidium
- **Mycobacterial**
- **Viral**
  - CMV
  - Herpes simplex
  - PML
  - Kaposi's sarcoma
- **Fungal**
  - Pneumocystis
  - Candida
  - Cryptococcus

Toxoplasmosis

Toxoplasma gondii infection in AIDS patients involves CNS, lungs and eyes. CNS involvement is the most common presentation. There is often multifocal involvement of the CNS, with many presentations –

- Altered mental status
- Seizures
- Motor weakness
- Cerbellar signs
- Meningeal involvement
- Movement disorders
- Neuropsychiatric manifestations

The most common presentation is subacute onset of focal neurological signs such as hemiparesis or speech abnormalities. Persistent headache is a common symptom and occasionally patients may present with seizures.

Differential Diagnosis:
- Primary CNS lymphoma
- PML
- Other CNS infections
  - CMV
  - Herpes simplex
  - HIV
  - Bacterial infections
  - Fungal infections – aspergillus

Diagnosis Diagnosis is based on the clinical presentation and neuroradiological appearance of CT scan/MRI scan. CT findings of multiple bilateral ring enhancing lesions are present in 80%. Characteristic lesions on CT/MRI scanning is not pathognomic. Cerebral lymphoma can be particularly difficult to distinguish. Other infectious agents may need to be excluded by brain biopsy particularly in cases of a solitary lesion.

Treatment: Most centres will give a trial of treatment without proceeding to brain biopsy.

TREATMENT OF TOXOPLASMOSIS

pyrimethamine	for 3–6 weeks with CT scan at 3 weeks to monitor response
sulphadiazine	
folic acid	

Alternative treatment is clindamycin and pyrimethamine/atovaquone.

Prophylaxis Relapse of toxoplasmosis will occur in up to 80% of patients within months of stopping therapy. Even with maintenance therapy relapse rates of 20% are reported. Non-compliance is an important consideration in relapsed cases.

Maintenance Therapy is with pyrimethamine and folinic Acid plus one of the following:

- sulphadiazine
- clindamycin
- azithromycin
- clarithromycin

- atovaquone
- dapsone

Cryptosporidium

Cryptosporidium muris is an intracellular protozoan parasite that can infect epithelial cells lining the digestive or respiratory tract. The classical presentation is diarrhoea with or without crampy abdominal pain. It may be intermittent and scant or voluminous and watery. In some patients diarrhoea can amount to 12 – 16 litres a day leading quickly to dehydration. Fever is an associated symptom and nausea and vomiting also occur.

Other clinical manifestations include cholecystitis, hepatitis, pancreatitis, reactive arthritis and respiratory problems.

Differential Diagnosis

Shigella, Salmonella, Campylobacteria, Clostridium Difficile, Giardia Lamblia, Entamoeba Histolytica and Isospora Belli, Cytomegalovirus, Mycobacterium Avium and Microsporidia.

Diagnosis

Stool cultures, duodenal aspirate culture, sigmoidoscopy and biopsy if CMV is suspected and cultures are negative.

Treatment

No reproducibly effective therapy. The disease is usually self limited but dehydration requires careful management (see Diarrhoea).

Tuberculosis

Mycobacterium tuberculosis

Mycobacterium tuberculosis has become much more prevalent since the AIDS epidemic. Its course, in patients with AIDS, is more rapid with an increase in the number and severity of symptoms and a short prognosis without treatment.

Presentation

Presentation depends on site of disease. Extrapulmonary disease occurs frequently and presents as lymphadenitis or disseminated disease. Symptoms include:

- fever
- weight loss
- sweats
- cough
- chest pain
- abdominal pain

Diagnosis

Diagnosis may prove difficult. Sputum culture, broncho-alveolar lavage or transbronchial biopsy may be needed. TB should be considered in the differential diagnosis of –

- unexplained fever
- cough
- pulmonary infiltrates
- lymphadenopathy
- meningitis
- brain abscess
- pleural effusion
- intra-abdominal abscess
- skin abscess

Treatment

Isoniazid, pyrazinamide, rifampicin and ethambutol are all used for treatment. Rifabutin is recommended in preference to rifampicin in patients who are on protease inhibitors. Of the protease inhibitors, indinavir appears to have the least drug interactions with anti-tuberculous treatment.

Atypical mycobacteria

Organisms belonging to the Mycobacterium Avium complex (MAC) are the most commonly recovered atypical mycobacterium in AIDS patients. Disseminated M.avium disease is usually a late opportunistic infection in patients with a CD4 count less than 100. Symptoms include:

- Severe fatigue
- Weight loss
- Chronic malaise
- Fevers/Rigors
- Mild to severe diarrhoea

Diagnosis involves blood cultures, bone marrow culture and nodal cultures.

Treatment

Treatment should be reserved for the patient with symptomatic clinical disease. Standard therapy should include either azithromycin or clarithromycin with at least one other agent, i.e. ethambutol. Addition of rifabutin has also proved of benefit and in patients with diarrhoea ciprofloxacin is beneficial.

Prophylaxis

Prophylaxis is now accepted and current practice recommends use of clarithromycin and azithromycin either alone or in combination with rifabutin.

Treating infections in AIDS

A 35 year old woman with AIDS presented with nausea and vomiting. Her AIDS defining illness was PCP and she had acquired HIV hetero-sexually. She had recently commenced triple therapy with Epivir (3TC), stavudine and indinavir. While her CD4 count and viral load showed response, her general condition deteriorated.

On admission to the Palliative Care Unit she complained of nausea, anorexia, abdominal pain and diarrhoea. During her admission she became febrile. All cultures were negative. Her condition worsened and she was transferred back to the referring acute hospital.

A presumptive diagnosis of atypical mycobacterial infection was made. She commenced treatment and within 5 days her symptoms had resolved. She remains well at home today, 9 months later.

This case illustrates the importance of good communication between the acute hospital and the Palliative Care Unit. It also illustrates the necessity to treat empirically on occasions without a definitive diagnosis.

VIRAL INFECTIONS IN AIDS

- Cytomegalovirus
- Herpes Simplex
- Progressive Multifocal Leukoencephalopathy
- Kaposi's Sarcoma associated Herpes Virus

Cytomegalovirus

Up to 45% of patients with AIDS will have evidence of CMV disease. Serious CMV infection is an increasing problem as patients live longer. Retinitis, colitis, oesophagitis and pneumonitis are the most common presentations. Hepatitis and neurological involvement are also reported.

CMV retinitis

Patients with lesions near the macula or optic nerve commonly present with decreased visual acuity or visual field defects. Lesions further away from the fovea or optic nerve often present as floaters or loss of peripheral vision. Patients do not complain of pain or photophobia. Retinal detachment is a common complication in CMV retinitis. Symptoms include:

- sudden onset of floaters
- flashing lights
- loss of visual field
- decreased visual acuity

Diagnosis   Diagnosis is made on the characteristic perivascular fluffy, yellow-white retinal infiltrates often associated with retinal haemorrhage. CMV retinitis usually presents unilaterally but untreated will progress to involve both eyes. The presence of serum antibodies to CMV is usual and their absence makes a diagnosis of CMV retinitis doubtful. Differential Diagnosis includes:

- Acute retinal necrosis 2^0 to herpes zoster or simplex
- Intraocular lymphoma
- Toxoplasmic chorioretinitis
- Pneumocystis carinii chorioretinitis
- Rare causes – syphilis, mycobacterium TB, cryptococcus, candidiasis.

Treatment   Standard therapy consists of induction therapy with high dose ganciclovir or foscarnet IV for two weeks followed by life-long maintenance therapy. Oral ganciclovir has been used as maintenance therapy but may result in a shorter time to progression of retinitis. It does however have the distinct advantage of avoidance of indwelling central lines and the associated risks of infection.

IV cidofovir has also been used to treat relapsing retinitis and seems to delay onset of progression compared to ganciclovir or foscarnet. It has a prolonged intra-cellular half life and can be given conveniently once a week for induction treatment and once every 2 weeks as maintenance treatment. Intraocular implants containing ganciclovir have also been used, however, there is a risk of retinal detachment at operation of up to 18%.

Herpes simplex   The frequency of HSV-1 infection in patients with AIDS does not differ greatly from the general population. Rates of infection of HIV-2 are however particularly high in homosexual and bisexual men with AIDS. Vesico-ulcerative lesions may occur at any mucocutaneous site. HSV-1 commonly affects the mouth or lips, HSV-2 affects the genital or perianal area. However primary genital lesions can be caused by HSV-1 and vice versa. Symptoms of ano-genital ulceration can include:

- pain
- itching
- painful defecation
- tenesmus
- discharge
- constipation
- fever
- sacral root pain

Diagnosis is by virological studies. Treatment reduces the symptoms and duration of infection. Acyclovir has been the mainstay of therapy but valaciclovir is increasingly of value as it can be taken as a once daily preparation. Prophylaxis is recommended.

Progressive Multifocal Leukoencephalopathy

Progressive multifocal leukoencephalopathy (PML) is a demyelinating disease of the CNS due to infection of oligodendrocytes by JC virus. The classical features of PML are focal neurological signs without a mass effect on neuro-radiological imaging. White matter disease is however present on imaging.

Presentation

Weakness (usually hemiparesis), limb and truncal ataxia, visual defects – homonymous hemianopsia, qauadrantanopsia, cortical blindness, cognitive impairment (usually much more rapidly progressive than in HIV encephalopathy).

Diagnosis is strongly supported by radiographic imaging but require brain biopsy for definitive diagnosis. Differential diagnosis includes HIV encephalopathy and CMV encephalopathy. There is no treatment. There are some reports of improvement in PML after newer anti-retroviral therapy, but this is a controversial area.

Kaposi's sarcoma

Kaposi's sarcoma, (KS), is the most common cancer occurring in patients with AIDS and is now thought to be caused by a new herpes virus – Kaposi's sarcoma associated herpesvirus. KS may affect skin, mucous membranes, lymph nodes, the gastro-intestinal tract and in some cases the liver, lungs and spleen.

Skin lesions tend to present on the upper trunk, head and neck. Involvement of the mucous membranes and GI tract is common. In general, patients with KS may be quite asymptomatic. However lesions can progress leading to ulceration and fungation often on the lower limbs. Pulmonary involvement may also lead to dyspnoea or haemoptysis. Lymphatic involvement by KS can lead to oedema. The course of the disease varies from slow and indolent to rapid and fatal.

Treatment Treatment will depend on the degree of sympto-matic discomfort. Modalaties available include laser therapy, radiotherapy, chemotherapy and immuno-therapy. Chemotherapy used includes vincristine/vinblastine/bleomycin and doxorubicin. New approaches include the use of liposomal chemo-therapy, i.e. doxorubicin, to reduce toxicity.

FUNGAL INFECTIONS IN AIDS
● Pneumocystis
● Candidiasis
● Cryptococcosis

Fungal infections are extremely common in AIDS patients. They may vary in severity from mild discomfort associated with oral candidiasis to life threatening fungal meningitis.

Pneumocystis pneumonia Pneumocystis carinii is a eukaryotic microbe related to the Astromycetes yeast family. Its morphological features and response to antiprotozoal drugs suggested for years that it was protozoal. The onset of pneumocystis pneumonia in AIDS patients is usually gradual with symptoms present for 3 – 4 weeks. The cardinal manifestation is a chronic, non-productive cough. Retrosternal chest tightness intensified by coughing or inspiration is also very common. Fever occurs in 80 – 90%. Dyspnoea is a late feature. Patients may present actively with severe respiratory distress but this is now unusual.

Diagnosis   Bronchoalveolar lavage is the cornerstone of diagnosis. The addition of transbronchial biopsy yields a diagnostic rate approaching 100%. Chest Xray may show diffuse alveolar and interstitial infiltrates. Early diagnosis and treatment improves survival significantly.

STANDARD THERAPIES FOR PCP

Mild – Moderate

Low dose oral:

- Trimethoprim/Sulphamethoxazole
- Trimethoprim and Dapsone
- Atovaquone
- Primaquine and Clindamycin

Moderate – Severe

- IV Trimethoprim – Sulphamethoxazole
- IV Pentamidine
- Adjunctive steroids

Patients who have previously presented with pneumocystis will have an approximate relapse rate of 5% per month. Patients with CD4 counts <200 are also at increased risk. Prophylaxis is recommended with either oral TMP-SMX or nebulised pentamidine.

Candidiasis   Candidia albicans is the most common strain found in patients with AIDS. Most HIV positive patients become colonized with Candidia, especially in the oral cavity, at rates that increase as CD4 count decreases and viral load increases. Symptoms of oropharyngeal candidiasis include:

- burning pain
- altered taste sensation
- dysphagia

Oral candidiasis   The oral manifestations of candidiasis are classified into four categories:

1 pseudomembranous (thrush)
2 acute atrophic (erythematous)
3 chronic atrophic (angular cheilitis)
4 chronic hyperplastic (leukoplakia)

Differential diagnosis of oral candiadiasis includes:

- Aphthous ulceration
- Herpes virus infection
- Epstein-Barr virus – Hairy leukoplakia
- Histoplasmosis

Treatment

Local and systemic therapies are available. Fluconazole is now the systemic treatment of choice. Higher doses are used for treating oesophageal diease. Clinical response usually occurs within 7 days in 90-100% of patients. The relapse rate is high but prophylactic fluconazole is not recommended because of the emergence of resistant strains. In resistant cases or if oral intake is compromised, IV Fluconazole or IV Amphotericin may be necessary.

Vaginal candidiasis

Vaginal candidiasis usually presents with a creamy-white abnormal vaginal discharge. Symptoms include:

- vaginal or vulvar pruritus
- burning pain
- dyspareunia

Fluconazole is an effective systemic treatment in most cases.

Cryptococcosis

Cryptococcus neoformans is an encapsulated yeast-like fungus that is an important cause of infection and mortality in patients with AIDS. Presentation is with subacute meningitis or meningoencephalitis. Patients often have an insidious, progressive course of 2 – 4 weeks before presenting wth:

Symptoms of meningitis

- Fever
- Malaise
- Headache
- Nausea and vomiting

These overt meningeal symptoms are present in only 25%. Patients may present with symptoms of encephalopathy including:

Symptoms of encephalitis

- Lethargy
- Altered thinking
- Personality changes
- Memory loss

Focal signs and seizures occur in less than 10%.

Diagnosis requires culture of CSF or blood.

Treatment is with specific antifungal therapy, i.e. fluconazole, itraconazole or amphotericin B. Prophylaxis with fluconazole is recommended at high dose of 400 mgs. daily.

SYMPTOM CONTROL MANAGEMENT

This section covers some common symptoms in AIDS. It is not possible to cover all the many symptoms that patients with AIDS may have, hence making a diagnosis whenever possible is critical to improving symptom control.

COMMON SYMPTOMS IN AIDS

- Pain syndromes
  - Abdominal pain
  - Neuropathic pain
  - Arthralgia/Myalgia
  - Headache
  - Oral pain
  - Anal pain
- Anorexia/Cachexia
- Dysphagia/Odynophagia
- Diarrhoea
- Dementia
- Dyspnoea
- Visual loss

Pain   Pain is a common symptom in patients with AIDS and is both under-reported by patients and under-treated by professionals.[8] Accurate diagnosis of the cause of pain can be a challenge but is important because of the frequency of opportunistic infections amenable to specific therapy. Non-opioids such as paracetamol are drugs of first choice in the managment of pain. Where arthralgia and myalgia predominates, a trial of an NSAID is appropriate. If this does not provide adequate relief, then a weak opioid such as codeine or dextropropoxyphene should be added. Failure to control pain with weak opioids will necessitate the introduction of a strong opioid such as morphine. These principles are the same as the WHO recommended guidelines for managing cancer pain.

Delays in optimum analgesic therapy are not acceptable while awaiting results of investigation. Treating the pain does not compromise an accurate diagnosis. Patients with AIDS may have total pain and careful attention must also be paid to the social, psychological, emotional and spiritual factors underlying total pain.[9]

Concern is often expressed about the use of opiates in patients with a current or past history of IV drug use. Where patients are on methadone maintenance, introduction of another opioid such as morphine or fentanyl is preferable in treating pain rather than increasing the methadone. It is important to separate the treatment of the addiction from the treatment of the pain.

Where patients on methadone are entering the terminal phase, withdrawal symptoms occur unless the methadone is replaced by an equivalent dose of a strong opiate. A single dose of 5 mgs. methadone is equivalent to morphine 7.5 mgs. Regular methadone is 3–4 times more potent than oral morphine and has a duration of action of 8–12 hours.[10] Benzodiazepines also need replacing in patients who have a dependency and midazolam is an effective choice.

Abdominal pain

Abdominal pain in AIDS has a large differential diagnosis.[11]

Management

Management depends on isolating a specific cause. An approach to the patient with gastrointestinal disease involves[12]:

- Having a wide differential diagnosis of possible infective agents (see table)
- Consider new pathogens in common sites
- Consider common pathogens in new sites
- A multiplicity of causes is often the rule
- Be thorough and persistent
- If no gastrointestinal pathology is found, look elsewhere
- When infection is found remember
    - it may not respond to standard therapy
    - it may relapse frequently
    - it may require permanent prophylaxis
- Not all problems are HIV related

CAUSES OF ABDOMINAL PAIN IN AIDS

- **Enteritis**
  - Cryptosporidium
  - Shigella/Salmonella
  - Campylobacteria
  - CMV
  - MAC

- **Cholecystitis**
  - Biliary tract obstruction
  - KS
  - Stones
  - Lymphoma

- **Infections**
  - CMV
  - Cryptosporidium
  - Cryptococcus

- **Peritonitis**
  - Infections
  - Gram negative pathogens
  - MAC
  - TB
  - Pneumocystis

- **Bowel obstruction**
  - MAC
  - Kaposi's Sarcoma
  - Lymphoma
  - Severe constipation

- **Drug-induced pancreatitis**
  - Didanosine
  - Zalcitabine
  - Pentamidine
  - Trimethoprim – sulphamethoxazole

- **Malignancy**
  - KS
  - Lymphoma

- **Hepatitis**
  - Infections
  - Hepatitis A,B,C
  - MAC
  - CMV

- **Retroperitoneal Lymphadenopathy**
  - Infections – MAC, TB
  - Malignancy – KS, Lymphoma

Neuropathic pain

Presentation   The most common neuropathy in patients with AIDS is a symmetrical, predominantly sensory, painful, peripheral neuropathy.[13] Patients may present with tingling, pins and needles, hyperaesthesia and shooting pains. The pain may be very severe and patients will often describe an unpleasant burning sensation in the soles of the feet which prevents them from walking.

Clinical signs of absent or reduced ankle jerks, reduced perception of vibration and painful stimulation are usual.

Differential Diagnosis   CMV infection can also present with progressive neuropathy usually affecting several nerve roots and confined to the lumbar and sacral nerve roots. Sensory and motor functions are involved and sphincter involvement is an early feature of an unrelenting progression.

Treatment   Treatment with amitriptyline 25–100 mg daily can be very effective. Oral mexiletine or IV lignocaine given under cardiac monitoring repeated as needed up to every 4 – 6 weeks can also be an effective measure.

Arthralgia and arthritis   The most frequent reported arthritis is a reactive arthritis which may prove to be severe, persistent and unresponsive NSAIDS. Diarrhoea is a common precipitant for the reactive arthritis present in HIV positive patients. The most common clinical picture is a severe persistent oligoarthritis primarily affecting the large joints of the lower extremities. Patients may also have sacroilitis or other features of Reiter's Syndrome (urethritis, conjunctivitis, circinate balanitis, keratoderma blenorrhagica and painless oral ulceration).

Arthralgias are common and may occasionally be the persisting feature of acute HIV infection. Septic arthritis is rare although occasionally opportunistic infections have been isolated from joints. The main causes of arthralgia are:

- Infective arthropathies
- Joint stiffness due to immobility
- Other arthropathies

Treatment   The approach is broadly similar to the management of any musculoskeletal pain, namely general measures including physiotherapy and more specific measures such as NSAID therapy. Frequently pain does not respond as well to NSAIDs and requires low dose opiates.

Headache   Headache in patients with AIDS is a frequent symptom and may indicate a serious underlying cause or may be unrelated to the diagnosis. Therefore it can prove to be a significant diagnostic challenge.

Differential Diagnosis
of Headache

- Encephalitis
  - HIV
  - Cryptococcal
  - Herpetic
- Meningitis
- Toxoplasmosis
- Cerebral Lymphoma

Other causes

- Migraine
- Tension
- Medications
- Muscle spasm
- Sinusitis

Toxoplasmosis and cryptococcal meningitis are the 2 most common opportunistic infections of the CNS seen in patients with HIV disease.

Mouth problems

Oral symptoms are common and include:

Presentation

- Altered taste
- Halitosis
- Mucositis
- Gum recession
- Tooth decay
- Oral ulceration
- Xerostomia

Causes of mouth problems

- Infections
  - Candidiasis
  - Cheilitis
  - Dental abscess
  - Gingivitis
  - Herpes simplex
  - Herpes zoster

- Medications
  - Chemotherapy
  - Radiotherapy

- Malignant
  - KS
  - Squamous cell carcinoma

The oral problems of HIV are well described.[14] They can cause distressing symptoms and can contribute to poor food intake and to general debility. Oral candidiasis is common and responds well to antifungal measures and oral hygiene. Bacterial infections and dental abscesses are not uncommon. Oral ulceration is also a common finding and may be caused by HSV, EBV, CMV, and atypical or typical myobacterial infection. Kaposi's sarcoma is also a common feature presenting with disease on the palate which is usually asymptomatic.

Treatment of mouth problems

Herpes simplex stomatitis can be treated with Acyclovir or Valaciclovir

Apthous ulceration can be treated with:

- Hydrocortisone lozenges
- Adcortyl in Orabase

} applied directly to ulcer base

- Benzydamine mouthwash (Difflam)
- Thalidomide 50 – 100 mgs. daily

Peri-anal pain

Patients may present with severe tenesmus on attempts to micturate or to open the bowel.

Causes

Infections
  - Perirectal abscess
  - Candidasis
  - Herpes simplex or zoster
  - CMV proctitis
  - Warts
  - STDs

Malignant
  - KS
  - Squamous cell anal carcinoma
  - Lymphoma

Others
  - Fissure
  - Fistulae
  - Haemorrhoids

Management

Appropriate diagnosis and treatment of specific infection.

Symptomatic measures include stepwise analgesia, lignocaine 2% jelly TDS and before/after bowel movements.

Attention to hygiene with frequent bathing.

Appropriate laxatives if constipated.

Topical steroids must be avoided in the presence of herpetic lesions. (see opportunistic infection).

Anorexia/cachexia   The main causes of anorexia/cachexia are:

- HIV wasting syndrome
- Opportunistic infections
- Lymphoma
- Kaposi's Sarcoma
- Malabsorbtion
- Medications
- Poor dietary intake
- Psychosocial issues – poverty, deprivation

Treatment   Treat reversible causes (eg. oral candidiasis).

Review and reduce medication where appropriate.

Involve the dietician

To stimulate appetite consider:

- – alcohol before meals
- – progestational hormones – megestrol 80–160 mg BD
- – periactin 4 mg TDS
- – dexamethasone 4 mg daily

Dysphagia   Over one third of patients will develop oesophageal symptoms of dysphagia or odynophagia. Presence of these symptoms often contribute to poor oral intake and consequent debility.

Treatment   General treatment includes:

- – Minimise oral medications
- – Consult dietician
- – Consider swallowing assessment – speech therapist
- – Manage gastro-oesophageal reflux

Specific measures include:

- – analgesics
- – anaesthetics – oxethazaine, aluminium and magnesium hydroxide mouthwash (Mucaine), 15 – 30 mls t.d.s. before eating.

CAUSES OF DYSPHAGIA IN AIDS	
● **Infections**	● **Malignancy**
– Candidiasis	– Kaposi's sarcoma
– CMV	– Non Hodgkins Lymphoma
– Herpes simplex	● **Other causes**
– Herpes zoster	– Oesophageal ulceration due to HIV
– Atypical TB	
– Cryptosporidium	– Excess alcohol
– Pneumocystis carinii	– Hiatus hernia
● **Neurological**	– Post radiation therapy
– HIV encphalopathy	– Drugs – zidovudine
– PML	

- decrease acidity – ranitidine 150 mg BD, famotidine 30 mg daily, omeprazole 20 – 40 mg daily
- alginic acid (gaviscon)

The most common cause of symptomatic oesophageal disease is candidiasis. The absence of oral candidiasis does not exclude oesophageal candidiasis. The presence of persistent oesophageal symptoms after treatment for presumptive candidiasis or gastro-oesphageal reflux will require further investigation. Diagnosis of a specific cause is important as symptoms will respond well to treatment. Other causes of oesophageal ulceration include CMV or HIV associated oesophageal ulceration.

Kaposi's sacroma is the most common oesophageal malignancy but rarely causes significant symptomatology.

Diarrhoea

Treatment Specific therapy will depend on isolation of an infective cause (see opportunistic infections). Treatment involves careful attention to fluid balance and specific treatment of the infective cause.

CAUSES OF DIARRHOEA IN AIDS	
● **Infections**	● **Malabsorbtion**
– Cryptosporidium	– HIV enteropathy
– Microsporidia	– Lactose intolerance
– MAC	– High osmotic feeds
– Salmonella	
– Clostridium difficile	● **Other**
– Campylobacter	– Medications
– Entamoeba histolytia	– Constipation with overflow
– Giardia Lamblia	– Rectal incontinence
– Shigella	
– Isospora belli	
– CMV	

In patients who are terminally ill, symptomatic management with loperamide 4–8 mg QDS and SC octreotide 600 mcg/24 hours is often effective. Abdominal cramps may respond to the addition of hyoscine butylbromide.

Dementia

AIDS dementia complex is one of the more frightening aspects of the illness for patients and carers.[15] In the early stages, the patient may have considerable insight into short-term memory loss, poor concentration and occasional episodes of confusion. Presentation is as a continuum from short-term memory loss to mutism.

Causes of dementia

● HIV encephalopathy
● Opportunistic infections i.e. toxoplasmosis
● Progressive multifocal leucoenophalopathy (PML)
● Cerebral lymphoma

Differential diagnosis is important as it will determine therapy. Usually MRI/CT scan are diagnostic but brain biopsy is occasionally needed. The presence of neuropathic pain has been suggested as a useful clinical marker in differentiating HIV encephalopathy from other causes of cognitive impairment.[12]

FEATURES OF DEMENTIA

- **Early features**
  - Short term memory loss
  - Blunted effect
  - Mental slowing
  - Decreased concentration

- **Late features**
  - Psychomotor retardation
  - Confusion
  - Ataxia

  - Sundown syndrome
  - Withdrawal
  - Hypomania
  - Loss of co-ordination

- **End stage**
  - Dysarthria
  - Confusion
  - Mutism
  - Incontinence

Treatment   Newer anti-retroviral therapy can benefit patients with HIV encephalopathy, and some patients have had a significant improvement in cognitive function.

Methylphenidate 5–20 mg orally 4 hourly has been used to improve alertness in patients who are severely withdrawn. When agitation is a factor, oral halo-peridol is the neuoleptic of choice starting at 0.5 mgs 8 hourly. Patients with AIDS have a significantly higher risk of developing *malignant neuroleptic syndrome* and this needs to be kept in mind.

Respite   The inpatient palliative care unit can have an important role in providing respite admission and day care to patients with AIDS dementia complex giving carers a much needed break.

Dyspnoea   In the patient with AIDS, dyspnoea can be caused by multiple factors. Specific AIDS related causes include opportunistic infections (especially pneumo-cystis pneumonia and TB) Kaposi's sarcoma, Non Hodgkins lymphoma and anaemia secondary to marrow suppression. The symptomatic manage-ment of dyspnoea is similar to that of patients with cancer. Accurate diagnosis is critical and early instigation of treatment is necessary.

Visual loss   Visual loss may develop gradually with blurring of central vision and loss of peripheral vision. Causes include:

- CMV retinitis
- Herpes simplex or Zoster
- PML
- Pneumocystis
- Toxoplasmosis
- Malignant cerebral lymphoma

Changes in a patients vision should always provoke a quick response as permanent blindness may develop quickly in cases of CMV retinitis. Patients with AIDS in a palliative care unit should have fundi examined routinely every 2–3 weeks. If in doubt referral to a specialist ophthalmologist is recommended.

DRUG THERAPY

Recent advances in the drug treatment of HIV have lead to more new agents becoming available in the past twelve months than in the past ten years.[16] These new agents are classified into:

- Reverse Transcriptase (RT) inhibitors
- Protease inhibitors
- Non-nucleoside RT inhibitors

Reverse Transcriptase inhibitors

Lamivudine (3TC) is the latest addition to a group including zidovudine (AZT) didanosine, zalcitabine (DDC) and stavudine. Lamivudine reverses viral resistance to zidovudine and the combination provides sustained falls in plasma HIV RNA. Toxicity of the combination is no greater than that of zidovudine alone.

Protease inhibitors

3 new drugs were released in 1996 – Saquinavir, ritonavir and indinavir.

Saquinavir is the best tolerated protease inhibitor at current dosage guidelines but has the least antiretroviral activity. High dose therapy is more effective but gastro- intestinal side effects and raised aminotransferase may be limiting.

Ritonavir has greater effect on both HIV RNA and CD4 count than saquinavir but often causes gastrointestinal symptoms and transient paresthesias. It also induces the cytochrome P45O system leading to significant drug interactions.

Indinavir has similar potency to ritonavir with fewer gastrointestinal or neurological side effects but can cause renal stones and indirect hyperbilirubinemia.

Combinations

The combination of saquinavir, zidovudine and zalcitabine has been shown to reduce plasma HIV RNA to a greater extent than any combination of two of these drugs.[17]

The combination of indinavir, zidovudine and lamivudine has shown the greatest sustained fall in plasma HIV RNA, and is less likely to allow emergence of resistant strains.

Non-nucleoside reverse transcriptase inhibitors

Nevirapine is the first of a new class of drugs to be licensed. It has been shown to be very effective in reducing plasma HIV RNA in combination with zidovudine and didanosine. Rash is the most common side effect and may be serious in up to 9% of patients.

OCCUPATIONAL EXPOSURE TO HIV

The risk of infection after the average percutaneous needlestick injury is 0.3%. The centre for disease control now recommends prophylaxis for high and medium risk exposure. A 3 drug combination (zidovudine – lamivudine – indinavir) is recommended for high risk and a 2 drug combination (zidovudine – lamivudine) for medium risk. No drug prophylaxis is recommended for low risk exposure.

Prophylaxis should commence as soon as possible and a 4 week period of treatment is recommended. Procedures should be in place in all units allowing access for exposed health care worker to treatment 24 hours a day.

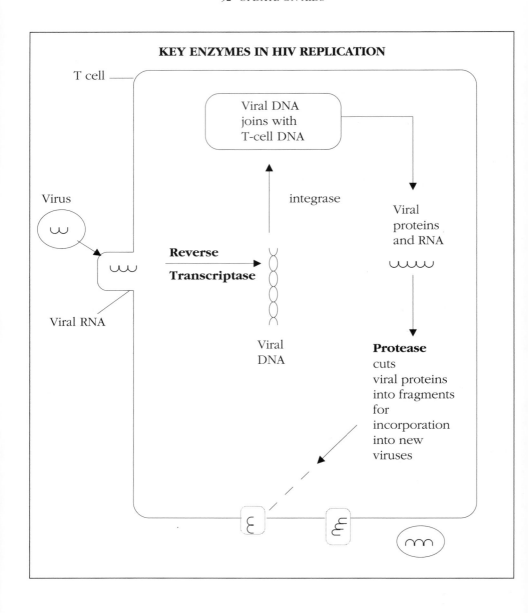

KEY ENZYMES IN HIV REPLICATION

CONCLUSION

AIDS patients are often well informed and articulate. Access to the internet means availability of up-to-date information from support groups and the results of new drug trials. Expectations are often very high and giving palliative care in this situation is in itself a challenge. Palliative care professionals have much to offer patients with AIDS in terms of their holistic approach and skills in symptom control. However, the model for care of patients with AIDS is changing as new treatments and improved survival become realistic.

REFERENCES

1   Foley F J, Flannery J, Graydon D, Flintoft G, Cook D. 'Aids – Palliative Care' – Challenging The Palliative Paradigm Journal of Palliative Care 1995; 11.2: 19–22
2   Grothe T M and Brady R V 'Palliative Care for HIV disease' Journal of Palliative Care 1995; 11.2: 48–9
3   Walsh T D 'An overview of Palliative Care in Cancer and AIDS'. Oncology. September 1991 161 5.9 p. 7–11.
4   Moss V, 'Palliative Care in advanced HIV disease: presentation, problems and palliation', AIDS 4 1990 S235–S242
5   Beiser C. Recent advances in HIV infection – 2 Br. Med J; 314: 579–583
6   O'Connor P G, Selwyn P A, Shotlenfeld R S. 'Medical care for injection drug users with human immunodeficiency virus infection' N. Engl J Med. 1994; 331 p.450–459
7   Broder S, Merigan T, Bolognesi D. Textbook of Aids Medicine, 1994. William and Wilkins, Baltimore Maryland (an extremely useful reference book)
8   Breitbart W, Patt R E. Pain management in the patient with AIDS. Haem/Onc Annals 2; 1994 p. 391–99
9   O'Neill W and Sherrard J S. 'Pain in human immunodeficiency virus disease: a review'. Pain 54 (1993) p. 3–14
10 Sims R and Moss V. 'Palliative Care for people with AIDS'. 2nd edition, 1995 (an indispensible starting point to learning the multifaceted approach to patients care).
11 Ferris F D, et al. 'Palliative Care: A comprehensive guide for the care of persons with HIV disease'. 1995 Mount Simai Hospital/Casey house hospice ISBN 0 – 662 – 22924 – x (a superbly comprehensive palliative care approach to the care of patients with AIDS)
12 Dietrich D T, et al. 'Gastrointestinal manifestations of HIV disease'. Textbook of Aids Medicine (see reference 7)
13 Evaluation of recalcitrant pain in HIV infected hospitalised patients' Anand A, Carmosino L, Glatt A. Journal of Acquired Immune Deficiency Syndrome 7: 1994 p.52–56
14 Cook G C, 'The mouth in Human Immunodeficiency Virus (HIV) Infection' Cl. J. Med., 76 (1990) p. 655–657
15 McKeogh M. 'Dementia in HIV disease'. A challenge for Palliative Care. 1995 11: 2, p. 30–33
16 Cohn J A, 'Recent advances in HIV infection – 1'. Br. Med. J. Vol. 314, p. 487 – 491
17 Collier A L, et al. 'Treatment of human immunodeficiency virus infection with saquinavir, ritonavir and zalcitabine'. N. Engl J. Med. 1996; 334. p. 1011 – 1017

Chapter 5

Update on Analgesics

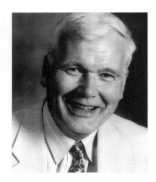

Dr Robert G Twycross
Robert Twycross is Macmillan Clinical Reader in Palliative Medicine, Oxford University (1988).
He graduated from Oxford University Medical School in 1965, was appointed Research Fellow in Therapeutics at St Christopher's Hospice, London in 1971 and returned to Oxford in 1976 as Medical Director of Sir Michael Sobell House, Chirchill Hospital, Oxford. He has written over 200 articles, chapters and editorials, and is author of several books on palliative medicine. He is: Director, WHO Collaborating Centre for Palliative Cancer Care (1988); Chairman, International School for Cancer Care (1988); Trustee, Global Cancer Concern (1995).

SOME DEFINITIONS	
Analgesic:	A drug which reduces the perception of pain without loss of consciousness.
Primary analgesic:	A drug which is marketed primarily for relief of pain, e.g. aspirin, paracetamol, codeine, morphine.
Secondary analgesic:	A drug which relieves pain but which is marketed primarily for some other purposes, e.g. tricyclic anti-depressants and anti-convulsants (synonyms: adjuvant analgesic, co-analgesic).
Opioid:	A generic term for all substances which bind specifically to endogenous opioid receptors and produce some agonist actions. Such drugs may or may not have a pharmacological profile similar to that of morphine.
Allodynia:	Pain caused by a stimulus which does not normally provoke pain.
Hyperalgesia:	An increased response to a stimulus which is normally painful.

INTRODUCTION

The WHO Method for Relief of Cancer Pain using a 3–step analgesic ladder and regular by-the-clock administration has helped countless doctors to become scientific and systematic in their use of analgesics.[1, 2] Recent criticism of the WHO Method[3] rightly met with strong countercriticism.[4-6] When used imaginatively, the WHO method results in excellent or satisfactory pain relief in about 90% of patients.[7]

Broad Spectrum Analgesia

One of the key concepts in the WHO Method is that of 'broad-spectrum' analgesia, exploiting the analgesic potential of various classes of drugs by using them in combination in a scientific and imaginative way.

Dorsal horn sensitization

Opioids are less effective when the dorsal horn of the spinal cord becomes sensitized.[8] This occurs to a variable degree with:

- chronic nociception
- inflammation
- damaged nerves.

With inflammation, the nociceptors are sensitized by the chemicals in the inflammatory soup. There is then a knock-on effect and peripheral sensitization leads inexorably to central (dorsal horn) sensitization.

Damaged nerves are also hypersensitive and discharge spontaneously, again resulting in central sensitization.[9] In these situations opioids generally need help from other drugs to achieve satisfactory relief.

With inflammatory pain, a nonsteroidal anti-inflammatory drug (NSAID) is the drug of choice because it corrects peripheral sensitization, the precursor to central sensitization. Thus, for many patients, broad-spectrum analgesia means combining a NSAID and an opioid.[10] In nerve damage pain, a logical broad-spectrum approach would be to use an anticonvulsant to dampen down the spontaneous activity associated with nerve injury and to enhance inhibitory GABA-nergic neurones in the dorsal horn and/or a tricyclic anti-depressant to facilitate descending inhibitory pathways.

NMDA receptors

The N-methyl D-aspartate (NMDA) receptor-channel complex plays a key role in the induction of dorsal horn sensitization. This explains why ketamine, a dissociative anaesthetic and an NMDA antagonist, is of benefit in patients whose pain fails to respond to other measures.[11]

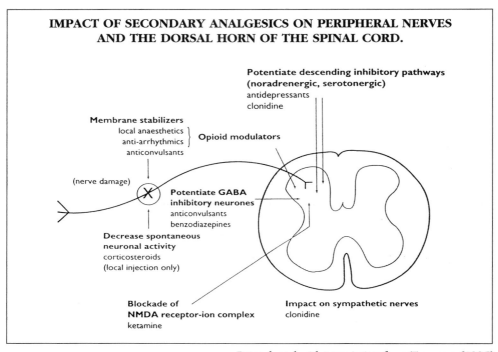

IMPACT OF SECONDARY ANALGESICS ON PERIPHERAL NERVES AND THE DORSAL HORN OF THE SPINAL CORD.

Reproduced with permission from Twycross (1995)

Pain as an experience

But it is essential to remember that pain is a somatopsychic experience, and is always modified by the subject's cognitive and emotional reaction to the noxious stimulus. Pain management is always more than the prescription of an analgesic – indeed sometimes may not even require one. At other times, a drug without specific analgesic effects may provide relief in situations where morphine or other analgesic has proved ineffective, as illustrated by the following case history.

Some pains are not morphine responsive

A 17 year-old with a bone tumour required repeated debridement. Patient-controlled analgesia (PCA) with morphine failed to relieve the pain. IV diazepam was then tried. After this he became relaxed enough to discuss his anxiety and the details of his care. He subsequently refused opioids and had only minimal pain during further debridement.[13]

MORPHINE

There is a strong international consensus that morphine is the strong opioid analgesic of choice for cancer pain management.[14] When correctly used, morphine is not only remarkably effective but also remarkably safe.[15]

Psychomotor effects

A controlled study of the psychomotor impact of morphine on cancer patients demonstrated no significant negative impact on function such as might impair driving.[16] In two tests of high-level concentration, however, a significant dose-dependent relationship was observed between plasma concentrations of morphine and its glucuronide metabolites and poor performance. Even so, overall results in the cancer patients (with and without morphine) showed no differences from those in physically healthy adults of comparable age.

Other studies have reported comparable results.[17,18] A few patients, however, are adversely affected. Work still needs to be done to elucidate the possible role of psychostimulants (such as dexamphetamine or methylphenidate) in these patients.[19] In patients most susceptible to morphine-induced cognitive failure (delirium), it may be necessary to switch to another opioid.

Global use of morphine

Despite its general safety, morphine is often underused. There appears to be an unholy trinity of reasons for this, namely:

- Doctors' lack of knowledge about the correct use of morphine for cancer pain
- Cultural and professional fears about addiction and diversion of medicinal morphine into illicit hands
- A failure by drug regulatory authorities to recognize their obligation under the 1961 UN Single Convention on Narcotic Drugs to ensure that adequate supplies of morphine and related drugs are available for medicinal use.

Even so, the use of morphine globally has increased over the last decade. Further increases can be expected as a result of two publications, one a consensus statement by an Expert Working Group of the European Association for Palliative Care (EAPC) and the other the second edition of the WHO Method for Relief of Cancer Pain.[20, 2]

Oral to parenteral ratio

There is disagreement between the EAPC and the WHO on several points. The WHO document states that the dose of morphine is the same SC, IM and IV and that the oral conversion ratio is 2–3 (i.e. double or treble the parenteral dose).

The EAPC consensus, however, distinguishes between IV and SC (and discourages IM use) and recommends an oral convertion × 2 from SC and × 3 from IV. It is pointed out, however, that the 'precise' conversion ratio from SC to PO probably lies somewhere between 1:2 and 1:3.

Two recent studies suggest that the oral to parenteral ratio is the same for both SC and IV routes. A single dose comparison of SC and IV morphine in volunteers failed to detect a significant difference between the two routes (Hanna M, personal communication). In a non-blind one-way crossover study of continuous infusions of morphine, 32/40 patients did not require any adjustment in dose when changed from IV to SC.[21] In the other 8 patients the SC dose was approximately one third greater than the IV dose. These 8 patients required higher does of morphine (on average 2.5 × greater than the other 32 patients), suggesting that, at higher doses, there may be significant non-equivalence between the two routes. Alternatively, given the higher starting doses, these patients probably had pain which was more difficult to control, and the increase could reflect worsening pain – which cannot be compensated for in a one-way crossover study. The EAPC advice would still seem reasonable given the inevitable approximate nature of a whole-number conversion ratio.

Individual variation

There is no single 'precise' oral to parenteral dose ratio for the whole population; there is variation around the mean. In some patients, it will be necessary to adjust the dose after converting from one route to another. Those with very good oral bio-availability will need a dose reduction (because free of pain and feeling drowsy), those with very poor oral bio-availability will need a dose increase (because of a resurgence of pain).

Modified-release morphine

The EAPC consensus favours initial titration with 4 hourly morphine tablets or solutions, and then conversion to modified-release (m/r) morphine. This is unnecessarily restrictive. Many doctors prescribe a 'best guess' initial dose of m/r morphine when converting from a weak opioid to morphine. This is backed up with rescue doses of the weak opioid, or ordinary morphine tablets or solution.

For example, a patient converting from co-proxamol 2 tablets QDS or dihydrocodeine 60mg QDS would be transferred to m/r morphine 20mg BD – using an approximate conversion ratio of 10 :1 for dextropropoxyphene, dihydrocodeine and codeine and increasing the dose by about 50% to obtain greater analgesia. If the patient had been taking these drugs every 4 hours and using rescue doses as well, then m/r morphine 30mg BD would be appropriate.

Rectal use

The WHO document hardly mentions m/r morphine tablets but recognizes their possible value if given *rectally* in vomiting or moribund patients. In contrasts, the EAPC consensus actively discourages this manoeuvre even though it could make all the difference between comfort and distress in the home situation. Indeed, the study which is used to support a statement that rectally there is reduced bioavailability and haphazard absorption is open to alternative interpretation (see figure below).

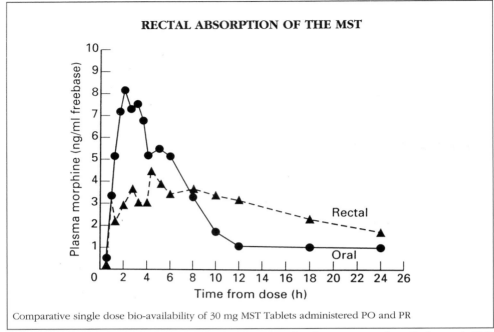

RECTAL ABSORPTION OF THE MST

Comparative single dose bio-availability of 30 mg MST Tablets administered PO and PR

Reproduced with permission from Kaiko et al. 1989

Rectally the peak plasma concentration is lower and delayed (a potential advantage) and, after 24h, an average of 90% has been absorbed (i.e. much the same). Rectal absorption varies, from about 70% to 120% of the oral absorption, and knowledge of this variability is important but it does not in itself mean that rectal use should be vetoed.

Starting modified release morphine

When changing from ordinary morphine tablets (or solution) to m/r morphine, it is still sometimes taught that the last dose of the 'immediate release' preparation should be given at the same time as the first of the m/r tablets. This view, however, is not borne out by the results of a randomized controlled trial.[22] In practice it would seem best to advise a patient to change to m/r morphine at bedtime with no overlap.

Formulations

Several different formulations of m/r morphine are now available. MXL capsules are a once-a-day morphine preparation which produces similar plasma levels to 4 hourly or 12 hourly preparations (see figure below). Morcap/Kapanol (an alternative m/r preparation manufactured in Australia,[24]) is now also available in the UK licensed for once or twice a day usage.

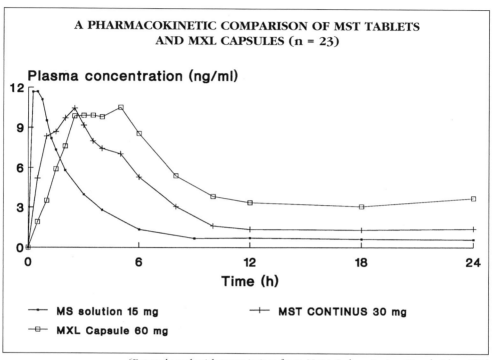

A PHARMACOKINETIC COMPARISON OF MST TABLETS AND MXL CAPSULES (n = 23)

(Reproduced with permission from Napp Laboratories, Cambridge, UK.)

Variation in morphine requirements

The dose of morphine to relieve cancer pain varies considerably from very small doses (e.g. 30 mg in 24h) to very high doses, either by mouth or by injection. In addition to this well-recognized inter-patient variation, there appears to be wide inter-centre variation.[25] Some of this variation is undoubtedly an artefact relating to the use of *mean* or *median* maximum doses (the mean is often much higher). Small or atypical samples may also play a part. Thus, at Sobell House, a morphine census in 1994 (the first 100 patients to receive morphine) yielded a mean daily dose of *oral morphine equivalents* of 86 mg one week before death; in 1995 the figure was 316 mg.

SOBELL HOUSE DATA	
	Mean morphine dose/day
1994	86 mg
1995	316 mg

The only difference between the two years, was several patients in 1995 received high dose epidural diamorphine. These had a disproportionate effect on the mean. Further data from 1994 and 1995 are shown in in the box and table below.

Another factor in inter-centre variation in the doses of morphine may be variation in the concurrent use of NSAIDs, secondary analgesics and non-drug measures.[26, 27] Recognition of the influence of non-physical factors on pain and investment in psychological support may explain the lower doses at some centres. Such comments, of course, are speculative. An agreed protocol for reporting morphine requirements is clearly necessary to provide a definitive answer to the puzzle of inter-centre variation.[28]

THE USE OF MORPHINE IN 200 PATIENTS

- First 100 patients receiving morphine in 1994 and 1995
- The median time from referral to death was 1 month (range 1 day to 34 months)
- *At referral* 47.5% were taking morphine (83/95 on oral morphine, 10 parenteral and 2 epidural)
- 97.5% received morphine in the 24h before death
- All doses were converted to oral morphine equivalents (IV or SC diamorphine × 3 and epidural diamorphine × 10 to give oral equivalents)
- *The median 24h dose* of oral morphine equivalents was:
    - 60mg at referral
    - 85 mg 2 weeks later
    - 80 mg 1 week before death
    - 90 mg 24 hours before death
- *In the final 24h*, 9 patients received oral morphine or SC diamorphine only 'as needed'; 11 took regular oral morphine; 172 received parenteral diamorphine and 8 epidural diamorphine

Combined data from two annual censuses at Sir Michael Sobell House

MORPHINE EQUIVALENT DOSES IN THE FINAL 24H

Route	Number of patients[1]	Dose (mg/h)		
		Median	Mean	Range
Oral	11	60	53	15–80
Subcutaneous[2]	172	90	135	15–900
Epidural[2]	8	1000	2388	100–6000

1 First 100 patients in each of 1994 and 1995 referred to Sir Michael Sobell House, Oxford, who received morphine at any time between referral and death; 9 patients received morphine only 'as needed' in the final 24h and are not included.

2 To obtain oral morphine equivalents, subcutaneous *diamorphine* doses have been multiplied by 3 and epidural diamorphine/morphine doses by 10.

METHADONE

Methadone differs from morphine in several ways. Its long half-life is the most important difference. The relationship between plasma concentration and analgesia is not straightforward. With single doses, analgesia is maximal after 1–2h, whereas peak plasma levels occur after 4–6h. By 6h pain relief has fallen to 25% or less, even though the plasma concentration is still near maximal.[29] Clearly, plasma concentrations

METHADONE: DIFFERENCES FROM MORPHINE

- Mu-delta agonist with NMDA receptor antagonism
- No active metabolite
- Long variable plasma half-life (approximately 8–80h)
- Cumulation when given regularly
- Non-linear relationship between plasma concentration and analgesia
- Longer duration of action (maintenance doses generally need to be given only twice daily)
- Renal failure does not alter pharmacodynamics
- Faeces are a major route of excretion
- SC injection more likely to cause local reaction

do not reflect the effective concentration at the receptors.[30] With chronic dosing, close supervision is needed until a patient's response to methadone has been fully evaluated. The plasma concentration may not reach a steady state for 2 to 3 weeks and accumulation and drowsiness may gradually develop. Particular care should be taken when psychotropic drugs are being administered concurrently.

Routes of adminstration

Methadone is well absorbed rectally; doses of up to 600 mg per suppository have been used. The cost of methadone suppositories is about one tenth that of parenteral morphine or hydromorphone.[31] Methadone can also be given by the buccal or sublingual routes. One third of the content of 1 ml of a methadone solution was absorbed in 10 minutes.[32] If the pH of the mouth was raised to 8.5, the absorption increased to three quarters. Methadone can be given epidurally.[33]

Drug interactions

Methadone is displaced from its protein binding by high concentrations of propranolol, phenothiazines and tricyclic antidepressants.[34] This interaction is probably not relevant with normal doses of these drugs. Several clinically important interactions between methadone and other drugs, however, have been reported. Rifampicin speeds up methadone metabolism and has occasionally precipitated withdrawal symptoms[35]. Cimetidine inhibits the metabolism of methadone; this may lead to drowsiness or even coma[36].

Spectrum of activity

Given the fact that methadone is more broad-spectrum than morphine, it might seem to be a better analgesic:

	mu	*delta*	*kappa*	*NMDA*
Morphine	++	+	+	−
Methadone	++	++	−	+

Its variable and prolonged half-life, however, is a significant drawback. Dose titration is more complicated than morphine – with the possibility of overdosage occurring after several days of excellent pain relief. The price of success with methadone is even greater vigilance than with morphine. Most of my patients transferred to methadone have been on high doses of oral morphine (1000mg or more per 24h) when mu receptor tolerance has been suspected.[37]

Dosage

Because of its broad-spectrum properties, the dose of methadone is generally much less than anticipated from single-dose postoperative studies, sometimes only 1/10 of the former dose of morphine. In practice, therefore, I generally start with 30–40mg twice a day and every 3h as needed. After 3–4 days, the dose of methadone is increased if additional doses are still needed. This does not always prevent problems (drowsiness, delirium) at a later stage. Patients who subsequently report drowsiness should be advised to reduce the dose of methadone by 50%. Much smaller doses, eg 5–10 mg BD and as needed, can be used in patients with severe renal failure in whom morphine is causing troublesome toxicity.

The use of methadone

A 52 year-old man with squamous cell cancer of the pharynx developed progressive head, neck and chest pain from an enlarging tumour mass. Oral morphine 270 mg/day eased the pain but the patient experienced hallucinations and was sedated. With oral methadone 80mg/ day (20 mg q6h), however, the patient had almost complete relief of pain and no adverse effects [38].

FENTANYL

Drug profile:
- mu agonist
- Plasma half-life 22 hours (transdermal)

- High lipid solubility
- High potency
- Trandsdermal route has slow onset and offset of action
- Less constipating than morphine[107]

Metabolism

Fentanyl is a synthetic mu opioid agonist chemically related to pethidine. IV, it is about 100 times more potent than morphine and has a plasma half-life of 3–4 hours.[39] It is widely used as a perioperative analgesic. Because of its high lipid solubility, fentanyl is widely distributed throughout the body. This accounts for the brief duration of action after a single IV dose (0.5–2 hours) and the potential for toxic cumulation with repeated or continuous administration. Elimination is predominantly by hepatic metabolism to inactive norfentanyl, with subsequent urinary excretion.

Patch use

Fentanyl patches are available for dermal application.[40] It is an ideal drug for transdermal absorption because it is both lipid and water soluble and, because of its high potency, only small amounts are needed. Transdermally the minimum effective blood concentration is reached after 3–23h and steady state after 36–48h.[41] After removal of a transdermal patch, the elimination halflife of fentanyl is 22h.[42]

Fentanyl patches deliver 25, 50, 75 or 100 mcg/h over three days.[42, 43] The manufacturer provides a conversion table based on potency ratio with oral morphine of 150 (although one study recommends a ratio of 100 – Donner et al, 1996). Patients who have not previously taken morphine or other strong opioid should always be started on the lowest dose, i.e. 25 mcg/h. The patches do not permit rapid dose titration because of the slow onset of activity. The first patch should overlap with the last regular does of morphine. Rescue medication with oral morphine may still be necessary particularly during the first 24 h. A reduction of laxative medication is necessary when switching from morphine.

The benefit of transdermal fentanyl

A 40 year old woman with metastatic lung cancer had severe pain caused by collapse of a thoracic vertebra. She was prescribed m/r morphine 90mg b.d., m/r diclofenac 75mg b.d., cyclizine 50mg TDS, ranitidine 300mg daily and senna tablets nocte. After 2–3 months cyclizine was supplemented by ondansetron 4mg BD, ranitidine changed to omeprazole 40mg daily, and senna supplemented by co-danthramer and magnesium hydroxide. She also took etidronate and calcium supplements, and various other opioids at different times. She was severely constipated.

She was then changed to transdermal fentanyl 75mcg/h, later increased to 100mcg/h. For the next four months she remained mostly painfree. All her other medication was stopped when fentanyl was started except cyclizine. She was no longer constipated and required no laxatives. The use of transdermal fentanyl meant that she had about 18 fewer doses of medication to take each day.

This case history is a good example of the potential benefits of transdermal fentanyl.

Cost

Fentanyl patches offer an alternative to a syringe driver in patients whose opioid dose is constant and who cannot take oral medication regularly. However, rigorous pharmaco-economic studies are not available. Transdermal fentanyl clearly reduces drug administration and book-keeping times, and there is less need for laxatives and other bowel measures. It is not clear, however, whether these savings compensate for the greater cost of the fentanyl patches.

A few patients obtain relief for less than the intended 72 hours. The manufacturer recommend increasing the patch strength in this situation. High fever and exposure to external heat sources (e.g. heat pads, electric blankets) can increase the rate of delivery of fentanyl.

Withdrawal symptoms

Some patients experience withdrawal symptoms (colic, diarrhoea and nausea together with sweating and restlessness[45,46]) when changed from oral morphine to transdermal fentanyl despite satisfactory pain relief.

Morphine and fentanyl are both predominantly mu-opioid agonists so the development of opioid withdrawal phenomena seems bizarre. However, fentanyl is far more water and lipid soluble than morphine and crosses the blood-brain barrier with relative ease. Thus, only small amounts of peripheral fentanyl are needed to achieve a central analgesic impact. In contrast large amounts of morphine are needed in the vascular system to achieve comparable central penetration. When

A DIAGRAM TO EXPLAIN PERIPHERAL MORPHINE WITHDRAWAL PHENOMENA AFTER SWITCHING TO TRANSDERMAL FENTANYL
(fentanyl penetrates the blood-brain barrier more easily)

Blood-brain barrier

Vascular system

Central nervous system

(Based on animal data)

fentanyl is substituted for morphine, there will be a massive reduction in the amount of opioid available at *peripheral* opioid receptors, which may well result in peripherally mediated withdrawal phenomena – as occurred in the case reports.[45, 46]

When transferring from morphine to transdermal fentanyl, it is important to reduce the dose of laxative (eg by half or even stop it temporarily) then re-titrate according to bowel activity.

Fentanyl can also be used subcutaneously. 11 patients with adverse effects with morphine (e.g. nausea and vomiting, delirium, excessive drowsiness), all had a reduction in adverse effects when switched to fentanyl.[39]

Alfentanil, has also been used successfully in patients with renal failure who became agitated on SC diamorphine.[47] The starting dose for alfentanil was 1/10 that of the diamorphine Its plasma halflife is about 90–100 minutes and it is converted by the liver to inactive metabolites.

TRAMADOL

Drug profile:
- Synthetic analgesic
- Centrally active
- Opioid + non-opioid
- Inhibits noradrenative re-uptake
- Well absorbed orally
- Less constipating than morphine

Tramadol has only recently been introduced into the UK, although it has been used extensively in many countries for several decades. It is a synthetic centrally-acting analgesic with both opioid (mainly mu receptor) and nonopioid properties,[48] (inhibiting presynaptic re-uptake of noradrenaline and serotonin). Naloxone only partially reverses the analgesic effect of tramadol. Its binding at opioid receptors is about one tenth that of codeine, yet it is twice as potent as codeine clinically. This can be explained by postulating a synergistic effect between its opoid receptor affinity and its inhibition of mono-amine re-uptake. A synergistic interaction is necessary to explain its analgesic effect.

INHIBITION OF OPIOID BINDING AND MONO-AMINE UPTAKE[49]

	K_i values (µM)				
	mu	delta	kappa	Noradenaline	5-HT
Tramadol	2.1	57.6	42.7	0.79	0.99
Codeine	0.2	5.1	6.0	inactive	inactive
Morphine	0.00034	0.092	0.57	inactive	inactive
Dextropropoxyphene	0.034	0.38	1.22	inactive	inactive
Imipramine	3.7	12.7	1.8	0.0066	0.021

Note: The smaller the k_i value the more potent the drug

Tramadol is readily absorbed from the Gl tract and has an oral bio-availability of about 70%. It can also be given rectally. Parenterally, it is 1/10 as potent as morphine;[50] orally it is 1/5.[51] By mouth, therefore, it can be regarded as double-strength codeine. An open study of tramadol in cancer pain has been published.[52] Tramadol is an alternative to codeine (or other step 2 analgesics); it can also substitute for morphine, up to 120mg/24h.

Desmethyl-tramadol, an active metabolite produced in the liver, is 2–4 times more potent than tramadol. It is produced only in small quantities and probably does not contribute much to the analgesic effect of tramadol. Bio-transformation is mainly inactive metabolites which are excreted by the kidneys. Tramadol has a plasma half-life of 6h. Duration of analgesic effect is 4–6h depending on the dose and the intensity of pain. Typical *oral doses* are 50–100mg q4h-q6h; higher doses can be given.[53] Tramadol is as effective as codeine as an anti-tussive.[54] It causes less constipation and respiratory depression than equi-analgesic doses of other opioids,[50,55] Its dependence liability is considerably less;[56] it is not a Controlled Drug.

Tramadol has been used for patient-controlled analgesia postoperatively. A randomized controlled trial with over 500 patients emphasized the importance of initial 'loading'.[57] Of a mean of some 350mg administered IV in the first 24h post-operatively, more than half was required in the first 90 minutes.

NALOXONE

Naloxone is a specific opioid antagonist. It should *not* be used to correct opioid-induced sedation in patients on regular opiords for pain control. In these circumstances, the next dose of the opioid should be delayed and/or reduced, and the drowsiness allowed to wear off spontaneously.

The BNF contains two entries for naloxone.[59] The first relates to overdosage by addicts and recommends *0.8–2mg* IV every 2–3 minutes up to a total of 10mg if necessary (with the possibility of an ongoing IV infusion).

Reversal of respiratory depression

The second relates to reversal of respiratory depression caused by the medicinal use of opioids (an extremely rare situation in palliative care). *100–200mcg* IV should be given, with increments of *100mcg* every 2 minutes until respiratory function is satisfactory. Further doses should be given after 1–2h by IM injection if there is concern that late absorption of the opioid will result in delayed respiratory depression. The American Pain Society recommends even lower doses.

Epidural morphine

With epidural morphine naloxone reverses respiratory depression without reversing analgesia and it is safe to give 0.4mg.[60] Given *by mouth*, it may have a small part to play in the management of severe opioid-induced constipation.[58]

NALOXONE FOR OPIOID OVERDOSE

- If respiratory rate ≥ 8/minute and patient not cyanosed, 'wait and see'
- If life-threatening respiratory depression, dilute a standard ampoule of naloxone 400 mcg/1ml to 10 ml with saline
- Give 0.5 ml (20 mcg) IV every 2 minutes until the patient's respiratory status is satisfactory
- Further boluses may be necessary every 30–60 minutes because naloxone is shorter acting than morphine (and other opioids).

  N.B.   Measure response by respiration rate (not level of consciousness) because giving enough to wake the patient up will cause a return of pain and may cause severe physical withdrawal symptoms, and marked agitation.

  (*Based on American Pain Society recommendations*)[61]

KETAMINE

Drug profile:
- IV anaesthetic agent
- Non-opioid
- Analgesic via NMDA antagonism
- Effective SC or PO
- Metabolized to norketamine
- Plasma half-life 3 hr

Ketamine is mainly used as an IV anaesthetic induction agent. It depresses the cerebral cortex but is unusual in that it also activates the limbic system. Its analgesic effect is mediated mainly at spinal level where it acts as a N-methyl D-aspartate (NMDA) receptor antagonist. (There may also be an effect on the medial thalamic nuclei.) Sub-anaesthetic doses have been used as an analgesic in injured, post-operative and cancer patients by SC, IM, IV, epidural and IT routes.[62, 63] It has also been given PO. Oral bio-availability is <20%. Ketamine has a plasma half-life of about 3h. Norketamine is the main metabolite and is about one third as potent as ketamine. The maximum blood concentration of norketamine is greater after oral administration than after parenteral.

Case report of ketamine

The use of ketamine in cancer pain management has been reviewed.[64] Several case reports have also been published.[65, 66] These detailed accounts are useful for guiding the would-be prescriber. For example, in one patient with neuropathic pain unresponsive to either opioid escalation or spinal morphine and bupivacaine, ketamine 150mg/day by SC infusion provided good pain relief and allowed a dramatic reduction in oral morphine from 5G to 200mg daily.[66] After 13 months the patient continued to have good pain relief despite evidence of progressive disease; by then he needed ketamine 400mg/day and morphine 200mg/day, both by SC infusion.

Dosage

Most centres start with low dose ketamine 100–200mg/day and increase by 100mg/day up to 500–600mg. Some centres start high, e.g. 500–600mg/day then reduce rapidly by 50% over the next few days. If this approach is used, the dose of morphine should be halved when the ketamine is commenced. Further reductions can be made according to progress. Because ketamine is irritant, a more dilute solution of ketamine may be preferable (i.e. 10mg/ml rather than 50mg/ml). If necessary, this can be diluted further with an equal volume of physiological saline.

In one case report of a patient with cancer of the maxillary sinus, the starting dose of ketamine was *100mg/h IV*. Two weeks later when the patient died, he was taking double this together with morphine 1000mg/h and midazolam 12mg/h.[65] I have not heard of comparable doses being used in the UK. At the other end of the scale, it is claimed that some patients have benefited from *oral* doses as small as 10–50mg every 4 hours , equivalent to 2–10mg by injection.[64]

Bedbound patients have been given boluses of IV ketamine to prevent movement-induced pain during nursing procedures.[64] They also received IV diazepam 2–10mg or IV haloperidol 1–3mg two to three minutes before ketamine in order to prevent the hallucinosis or bad dreams commonly seen as 'emergent' phenomena after ketamine anaesthesia. One patient continued to experience bad dreams despite IV midazolam 7.5mg or IV haloperidol 2.5mg. She refused further IV ketamine but subsequently tolerated SC ketamine 120 mg/24h for 30 days.

Ketamine, however, is not just of value for movement induced and neuropathic pain. In the following case history, ketamine was used to treat intractable pain associated with *en cuirass* metastatic breast cancer.

The value of ketamine

A 49 year-old woman was admitted with constant severe burning pain, affecting the upper half of her torso and her left arm to the elbow. Its site corresponded to cutaneous recurrence of breast cancer. On admission she was in severe pain despite 10,000 mg of oral morphine daily, together with a tricyclic antidepressant and a corticosteroid. Within 24 h of starting a SC infusion of ketamine at a rate of 0.5 mg/kg/h she said she was comfortable. *The morphine was reduced to 100 mg daily.* She remained on ketamine infusion for 48 days, had improved mobility and slept well. The infusion was maintained between 0.25–0.5 mg/kg/h with boosts of SC ketamine before the dressing was changed. She died peacefully seven weeks after starting ketamine[67]

Assuming that the woman weighed around 55 kg, the daily dose of ketamine (excluding boluses) varied from 300–720 mg. It is possible she might also have benefited from an NSAID rather than the corticosteroid and tricyclic antidepressant prescribed.

OPIOID TOXICITY SYNDROMES

Common side-effects of opioids

Like most drugs, opioids often cause adverse effects. Emesis and drowsiness are the most common immediate ones: constipation is the most common longterm one. Initial drowsiness generally diminishes after 3–5 days on a steady dose. Nausea and vomiting may settle spontaneously but often require longterm anti-emetic therapy. On the other hand, constipation almost always persists and requires longterm laxatives. With such measures, however, most cancer patients who require strong opioids take them without other major inconvenience.

Two idiosyncratic adverse effects

Occasionally, however, a patient has an idiosyncratic adverse effect which necessitates a reduction in dose or a change to an alternative opioid (see Table below). Opioid-induced *cognitive failure* and *hyperexcitability* (myclonus, hyperalgesia and allodynia) are particularly important to recognize, because they can have such dire consequences. Most reported cases have occurred with morphine or hydromorphone but other opioids are occasionally implicated, including fentanyl.[72, 73] Both syndromes respond to reducing the dose of opioid or switching to an alternative ('opioid rotation').[74]

1. Opioid-induced cognitive failure

Delirium can occur with high doses of morphine,[75] as with other psycho-active drugs. In one case, however, a patient manifested psychomotor disturbance and cognitive impairment with a low oral dose.[76] In another report of 13 patients who developed delirium on typical doses of morphine, 9 experienced a resolution when switched to oxycodone. All but one (a 'poor metabolizer' of oxycodone to the active metabolite, oxymorphone) reported less pain and nausea and vomiting.[77]

At one centre, it is standard practice to administer the Mini-Mental State Questionnaire (MMSQ) about twice a week, and to switch opioids and hydrate by SC fluids if the MMSQ score deteriorates. As a result, 'opioid rotation' increased from 21% in 1988–89 to 41% in 1991–92 and agitated delirium decreased from 26% to 10%.[78]

MORPHINE INTOLERANCE

Type	Effects	Initial Treatment	Comment
Gastric stasis	Epigastric fullness flatulence, anorexia, persistent nausea	Metoclopramide 10–20 mg q4h cisapride 10–20 mg b.d.	If the intolerance persists, change to an alternative opioid
Sedation	Intolerable sedation +/- delirium	Reduce dose of morphine; consider methylphenidate 10mg once to twice a day	Sedation may be caused by other factors; stimulant rarely indicated
Cognitive failure	Agitated delirium with hallucinations	Reduce dose of morphine and/or prescribe haloperidol 3–5mg at once and at bedtime; if necessary switch to an alternative opioid	Some patients develop intractable delirium with one opioid but not with an alternative opioid
Myoclonus	Multifocal twitching +/- jerking of limbs	Reduce dose of morphine but revert to former dose if pain recurs; consider clonazepam 0.5–2mg at once and at bedtime	Unusual with typical oral doses; more common with high dose IV and spinal morphine
Hyperexcitability	Abdominal muscle spasms and symmetrical jerking of legs; whole-body allodynia and hyperalgesia manifesting as excruciating pain	Change to an alternative opioid	A rare syndrome in patients receiving intrathecal or high dose IV morphine; occasionally seen with typical oral and SC doses
Vestibular stimulation	Incapacitating movement-induced nausea and vomiting	Cyclizine or dimenhydrinate or promethazine 25–50 mg q8h-q6h	Rare. Try an alternative opioid or levomepromazine (methotrimeprazine)
Histamine release • **cutaneous**	Pruritus	Oral antihistamine	If it does not settle in a few days, prescribe an alternative opioid
• **bronchial**	Bronchoconstriction → dyspnoea	IV/IM antihistamine (e.g. chlorphenamine 5–10mg) and a bronchodilator	Rare. Change to a chemically distinct opioid immediately e.g. methadone or phenazocineeaooxmrnuvm.

Hallucinations Visual hallucinations have also been reported in four patients receiving hydromorphone without impaired cognition as determined by the Mini-Mental State Questionnaire.[79] The hallucinations occurred after a minimum of 10 days, and in 2 cases after more than 3 weeks. All responded to haloperidol; in 3 cases this was stopped after 5–7 days. In three the opioid was changed to morphine or diamorphine. In the fourth patient, however, a short course of haloperidol alone was sufficient to stop the hallucinations until they recurred 5 weeks later. The nature of the hallucinations suggests that psychological factors (fear of death etc.) may have played a role in their development. The authors, however, considered hydromorphone to be the major determinant and wondered whether the hallucinations were the first manifestation of an evolving (otherwise undetectable) delirium.

Morphine-induced hallucinations

A 61 year-old woman with breast cancer developed visual hallucinations, insomnia and impaired attention after morphine m/r was increased from 20mg to 30mg b.d. to relieve pain from spinal metastases. Decreasing the dose and administering haloperidol 2mg/day did not improve her condition. The visual hallucinations continued intermittently for about 3 weeks until the morphine was discontinued after a course of radiotherapy [76].

2. Opioid-induced Hyperexcitability The earliest reports of opioid hyperexcitability related to pethidine. A combination of anticholinergic properties and a toxic metabolite (norpethidine) are considered to be the cause. For many years, hyperexcitability was thought to be unique to pethidine.

PETHIDINE AND CNS EXCITATION

- Pethidine was synthesized in 1939. It has structural similarities to atropine and comparable anticholinergic effects, e.g. mydriasis, dry mouth, tachycardia, flushing and delirium.[80.]

- Its main metabolite is norpethidine.

- Excitatory effects have been observed after pethidine 75–150mg IM regularly for several days:
    - tremors or twitching (i.e. mild myoclonus)
    - marked myoclonus and agitated delirium,
- occasionally seizures
    - petit mal
    - grand mal[81; 82]

- Pethidine and norpethidine have plasma halflives of about 3.5h and 15–30h respectively.

- The half-life of norpethidine is longer in renal failure.

- Norpethidine appears to be the causal factor of the excitatory phenomena; plasma concentrations are considerably higher in patients manifesting marked myoclonus or seizures than in those with shaky feelings or tremors. The phenomena clear 2–5 days after stopping pethidine without any other intervention.

- Naloxone does not correct the excitatory effects. Indeed, by reversing the central depressant effect of pethidine, naloxone may precipitate seizures. [83, 84]

- As with atropine, pethidine-induced delirium is reversible with physostigmine 1mg IM, given as needed once or more times.[85]

- In order to prevent pethidine-induced hyperexcitability, the use of pethidine should be restricted to a maximum of 48h and to doses of 600 mg/24h.[61]

More recent reports, however, indicate that a similar syndrome occurs with other opioids, notably morphine and hydromorphone. Initial reports linked opioid hyperexcitability to intrathecal or high dose IV morphine, e.g. 1–2g/h.[86] Subsequent reports, however, have implicated considerably lower doses including one 55 year-old woman receiving only m/r morphine 60mg/day.[87]

OPIOID HYPEREXCITABILITY SYNDROME[86–88]

- **Myoclonus**
  - twitching
  - jerking lower limbs
  - abdominal muscle spasms (painful)

- **Hyperalgesia**
  - exacerbation of pain

- **Whole-body allodynia**
  - pain on touch
  - pain at all points of body contact

- **Delirium**
  - agitation
  - screaming in agony

- **Grand mal seizures** (with megadoses)[88]

DEFINITION

Myoclonus: Sudden, brief, shock-like involuntary movements caused by primary muscle contractions or CNS stimulation. Myoclonus may be focal (a single muscle or group of muscles), regional or generalized; unilateral or bilateral (either asymmetrical or symmetrical); mild (twitching) or severe (jerking). Myoclonus may be physiological, primary ('essential') or secondary to neurological and metabolic disorders, or drug or other toxicity. Secondary diffuse myoclonus is pre-epileptiform.

Animal studies   Animal studies have demonstrated that behavioural features suggestive of allodynia and hyperalgesia occur when morphine, morphine-3–glucuronide or morphine-6–glucuronide is injected into the cerebral ventricles.[89] However, M–3–G is several hundred times more potent than morphine in eliciting hyperactivity even though it is inactive at opioid receptors. Generally the more potent an opioid is as an analgesic, the less likely it is to cause hyperexcitability.[90] Further, naloxone exaggerates the abnormal behaviour, strongly suggesting that a

Morphine induced allodynia

A 61 year-old woman with a chordoma in the sacrum had deep aching local pain, dysaesthesia in the perineum and spontaneous stabbing pain in the left thigh. The pains were controlled with a combination of m/r morphine 30mg TDS, a NSAID, two tricyclic antidepressants and an anticonvulsant. After 3 years the dose of m/r morphine had risen to 500 mg TDS. Various neurolytic procedures were tried and failed, including epidural morphine and bupivacaine. An implanted dorsal column electrode relieved the pain for a few weeks but then, because of excruciating pain and anxiety, all oral medication was discontinued and IV morphine and methotrimeprazine commenced. Doses rose to 4.2g and 200mg respectively over the first 12h. Although mostly asleep, the patient's skin became painful when touched (allodynia). The next day IV morphine was increased to 15g/day and levomepromazine to 1.2g. The skin sensitivity persisted and the patient was more uneasy, awake and hallucinating. Frequent distressing symmetrical spastic contractions of her lower abdominal muscles, arms and legs developed, with exacerbation of her pains. Several doses of IV diazepam 20mg stopped the spasms. The next day, however, the patient complained of constant excruciating pain and continuing whole body allodynia. She became more agitated and began to scream. The IV morphine was doubled and she received 'substantial' doses of benzodiazepines and methotrimeprazine until she died a few hours later[86].

non-opioid receptor system is primarily responsible for opioid hyperexcitability.[90] In humans, normorphine has also been implicated[91] and, in relation to hydromorphone, hydromorphone-3–glucuronide.[92]

Animal studies show that high doses of methadone, fentanyl, alfentanil and sufentanil do not produce hyperactivity.[88, 93] This has led some to conclude that these drugs are free from comparable effects in humans. Unfortunately, although probably less neurotoxic than other opioids, this may well not be

Morphine hyperexcitability

A 49 year-old man with lung cancer developed severe right-sided chest pain. Morphine was administered by continuous intrathecal infusion. Intrathecal morphine was increased progressively to 80mg/day. He then developed multifocal **myoclonus** particularly in the legs with pain and **allodynia** in the lower half of the body. After reducing the dose of intrathecal morphine to 50mg/day and prescribing diazepam, the allodynia and myoclonus remitted. The patient died of a pulmonary haemorrhage one week later. (Reproduced with permission from De Conno[94])

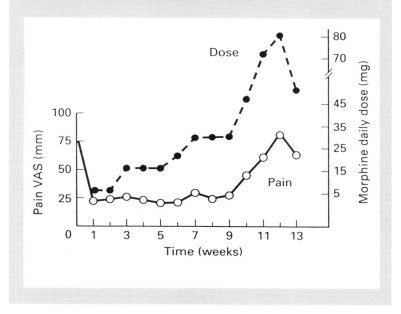

the case. For example, bilateral synchronous myoclonic jerks involving the extremities and trunk have been reported in an 87 year-old woman treated with transdermal fentanyl 75 mcg/h.[73]

Glycine Antagonist Strychnine, a glycine antagonist, can produce similar behaviour.[88] Glycine mediates postsynaptic inhibition on dorsal horn neurones. It is possible, therefore, that opioids and/or their metabolites act via a spinal anti-glycinergic effect.

Sodium bisulfite Sodium bisulfite, a preservative in ampoules of morphine sulphate, may be responsible for some cases of hyperexcitability.[96] 2 patients who received respectively 9g and 12g/24h of morphine sulphate by continuous IV infusion for 2 days both developed grand mal seizures. In one patient, the prodrome was typical of pethidine hyperexcitability (shakiness, tremors and hallucinations) whereas, in the second patient, the prodrome was typical of morphine hyperexcitability (jerking of the abdominal muscles and lower limbs). Apart from these two cases seizures have not been a feature of morphine or hydromorphone hyperexcitability, suggesting sodium bisulfite was at least partly responsible in these two cases.

Sulfites are used as anti-oxidants in foods and pharmaceutical preparations and also have antimicrobial activity, making them suitable for as a preservative. They have been reported to cause seizures in animals and humans at very high doses[97, 98] and in humans with congenital sulfite oxidase deficiencies at normal doses.[99] Generalized seizures have also been reported in patients receiving 10–21 1/day of peritoneal dialysis solution which contained 0.5mg/ml of sulfites.[98]

Management

Management options for opioid hyperexcitability include:

- Reduce dose of opioid
- Clonazepam (see case history below)
- Switch opioid ('opioid rotation')

Myoclonic Jerks

An 87 year-old woman developed distressing myoclonic jerks (without allodynia or hyperalgesia) 2 weeks after starting m/r morphine 20mg b.d.[100] In this case, clonazepam 1mg nocte stopped the myoclonus. It did not recur even when the dose of morphine was subsequently increased to 180mg/day.

Opioid rotation

Numerous articles have appeared in recent years encouraging 'opioid rotation', ie switching from one strong opioid to an alternative in cases of intolerable toxicity.[108] As already noted, at one centre in Canada, switching opioids increased from 21% of patients in 1988–89 to 41% in 1991–92. In the UK, however, the incidence of switching is much lower, about 7% (Kirk & Twycross 1996, data on file).

Indications Generally speaking, switching opioids is recommended in cases of opioid-induced cognitive failure and of opioid-induced hyperexcitability. Switching is also appropriate in patients with an isolated toxic manifestation such as hallucinations, myoclonus or pruritus which does not remit with small-to-moderate doses of haloperidol, clonazepam or an antihistamine. For example, a 41 year-old woman with breast cancer experienced myoclonus when receiving hydromorphone 200mg/h by SC infusion. When switched to morphine 200mg/h, the myoclonus resolved without other measures in less than 24h. It is important to note that despite a 7–8 fold decrease in the dose of 'morphine equivalents', the patient did not experience any breakthrough pain.

In another case, a 19 year-old woman with a gliosarcoma, IV morphine 20gram/24h was replaced by diazepam 20–30mg daily and 'as needed' methadone tablets. For the last month of her life, she required only *methadone 5–10mg once every 2–3 days*. With very high doses of morphine or hydromorphone, the ability to maintain or improve pain control with a much reduced dose of 'morphine equivalents' is one of the phenomena associated with opioid rotation. It is sometimes explained in terms of 'incomplete cross-tolerance'.[108] This murky concept, however, is not really helpful. Opioid hyperexcitability is caused primarily by the cumulation of toxic non-analgesic metabolites (eg morphine-3-glucuronide) and secondarily by exceptionally high concentrations of the parent opioid itself. Switching from a high dose of one opioid to an alternative means switching from an opioid which is being partly antagonized by its own metabolite(s) and possibly also by the parent opioid itself to an opioid for which there is no such antagonism. In these circumstances, it is inevitable that a lower equivalent dose will be efficacious – often much lower.

Methadone and   In relation to a switch to methadone or levorphanol,
levorphanol   other factors play a part. Whereas morphine, hydromorphone, oxycodone and fentanyl are essentially mu-receptor agonists, methadone and levorphanol are mu-delta agonists. Methadone also manifests NMDA antagonism.[109] Thus, patients wtih nociceptive pain who fail to respond satisfactorily to a combination of a NSAID and a mu agonist, may obtain good relief when methadone or levorphanol is substituted for the latter.[110, 111] Thus regular methadone is 5–10 times more potent than high doses of regular morphine compared with a near unitary relative potency when given IM post-operatively.[111] NMDA antagonism may also mean that methadone is more effective in neuropathic pain than other strong opioids. To date, however, this postulate means untested.

As already noted, the incidence of opioid switching is much greater in parts of North America than in the UK. One reason for this is that megadoses of morphine such as 68gram/24h[110] are not used in palliative care centres in the UK. It is possible that, generally, a more multimodal approach to cancer pain management is practised in the UK. For example, perhaps more readily combining physical with psychological strategies, nondrug with drug treatments, analgesics with co-analgesics, and resorting to 'broad-spectrum' spinal analgesia with morphine and bupivacaine and clonidine at an earlier stage in patients with otherwise intractable pain.

LOOKING AHEAD

The amount of new laboratory and clinical data published about analgesics is overwhelming. New clinical developments are just around the corner.[101]

NMDA antagonists   Several opioids are now known to demonstrate NMDA receptor antagonism, notably methadone and dextropropoxyphene.[68, 102] In contrast, codeine, morphine, fentanyl and etorphine are devoid of NMDA antagonists activity.[69] Other drugs including amitriptyline, amantidine and memantine manifest

NMDA receptor antagonism.[70] This raises exciting questions about the analgesic action of amitriptyline.

COX-II inhibitors Equally exciting are advances in our understanding of NSAIDs[103] which inhibit cyclo-oxygenase (COX) and diminish prostaglandin synthesis. Traditionally, this is considered to be the basis of their analgesic action but it is not the whole story, because the analgesic effects of NSAIDs are *not* proportional to in vitro COX inhibition.[104] COX inhibition is responsible for many of the adverse effects of NSAIDs but the importance of uncoupling of oxidative phosphorylation probably also contribute to the gastrointestinal damage.[105]

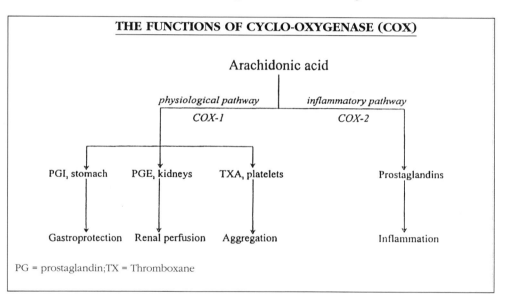

THE FUNCTIONS OF CYCLO-OXYGENASE (COX)

Arachidonic acid

physiological pathway COX-1 *inflammatory pathway* COX-2

PGI, stomach PGE, kidneys TXA, platelets Prostaglandins

Gastroprotection Renal perfusion Aggregation Inflammation

PG = prostaglandin; TX = Thromboxane

A major breakthrough has been made with the identification of two COX isoforms, COX-1 and COX-2. COX-1 is found in many tissues, including the stomach, kidneys and platelets, whereas COX-2 is found only after induction by endotoxin, or by certain cytokines, growth factors and mitogens.[106] The hope is that highly selective COX-2 inhibitors will cause little or no gastro-intestinal damage and have less impact on the kidneys. Efforts are now being made to develop highly selective COX-2 inhibitors.[103]

REFERENCES

1   World-Health-Organization. Cancer pain relief. Geneva: WHO, 1986.
2   World-Health-Organization. Cancer Pain Relief: with a guide to opioid availability. Geneva: WHO, 1996.
3   Jadad AR, Browman GP. The WHO analgesic ladder for cancer pain management. *Journal of the American Medical Association* 1995; 274: 1870–1873.
4   Reidenberg MM. Pain control and the WHO analgesic ladder. *Journal of the American Medical Association* 1996; 275: 835.
5   Twycross R, Lickiss N. Pain control and the WHO analgesic ladder. *Journal of the American Medical Association* 1996; 275: 835.
6   Ventafridda V, Stjernsward J. Pain control and the WHO analgesic ladder. *Journal of the American Medical Association* 1996; 275: 836.
7   Zech DFJ, Grond S, Lynch J, Hertel D, Lehmann KA. Validation of World Health Organization guidelines for cancer pain relief: a 10–year prospective study. *Pain* 1995; 63: 65–76.
8   Dickenson AH, Sullivan AF. Electrophysiological studies on the effects of intrathecal morphine on nociceptive neurones in the rat dorsal horn. *Pain* 1986; 24: 211–222.
9   Coderre T, Katz J, Vaccarino A, Melzack R. Contribution of central neuroplasticity to pathological pain: review of clinical and experimental evidence. *Pain* 1993; 52: 259–285.
10   Pace V. Use of nonsteroidal anti-inflammatory drugs in cancer. *Palliative Medicine* 1995; 9: 273–286.
11   Fallon MT, Welsh J. The role of ketamine in pain control. *European Journal of Palliative Care* 1996; 3: 143–146.
12   Twycross RG. Sympton Management in Advanced Cancer. Oxford: Radcliffe Medical Press, 1995.
13   Richtsmeier AJ, Barkin RL, Alexander M. Benzodiazepines for acute pain in children. *Journal of Pain and Symptom Management* 1992; 7: 492–495.
14   Consensus-Statement. Looking to the future. Oxford: CBC, 1997.
15   Hanks GW. Morphine sans Morpheus. *Lancet* 1995; 346: 652–653.
16   Vainio A, Ollila J, Matikainen E, Rosenberg P, Kalso E. Driving ability in cancer patients receiving longterm morphine analgesia. *Lancet* 1995; 346: 667–670.
17   O'Neill WM, Hanks GW, White L, Simpson P, Wesnes K. The cognitive and psychomotor effects of opioid analgesics: I. A randomized controlled trial of single doses of dextropropoxyphene, lorazepam and placebo in healthy subjects. *European Journal of Clinical Pharmacology* 1995; 48: 447–453.
18   Hanks GW, O'Neill WM, Simpson P, Wesnes K. The cognitive and psychomotor effects of opioid analgesics: II. A randomized controlled trial of single doses of morphine, lorazepam and placebo in healthy subjects. *European Journal of Clinical Pharmacology* 1995; 48: 455–460.
19   O'Neill WM. The cognitive and psychomotor effects of opioid drugs in cancer pain management. *Cancer Surveys* 1994; 21: 67–84.
20   Hanks GW, De-Conno F, Ripamonti C, Ventafridda V, Hanna M, McQuay HJ, Mercadante S, Meynadier J, Poulain P, Roca-i-Casas J, Sawe J, Twycross RG, Vainio A, Zech D. Morphine in cancer pain: modes of administration. *British Medical Journal* 1996; 312: 823–826.
21   Nelson KA, Glare PA, Walsh D, Groh ES. A prospective within-patient crossover study of continuous intravenous and subcutaneous morphine for chronic cancer pain. in press.
22   Hoskin PJ, Poulain P, Hanks GW. Controlled-release morphine in cancer pain: is a loading dose required when the formulation is changed? *Anaesthesia* 1989; 44: 897–901.
23   Kaiko RF, Healy W, Pav J, Thomas GB, Goldenheim PD. The comparative

bioavailability of MS Contin tablets (controlled release oral morphine) following rectal and oral administration. In: Twycross RG, editor. The Edinburgh Symposium on Pain Control and Medical Education. London: Royal Society of Med, 1989, pp. 235–241.

24   Kerr RO 1995. Clinical experience with 12–24 hourly Kapanol. Presented at: *Pain Control: Current Practice and New Developments*. Amsterdam, October 1995. *Conference*

25   Boisvert M, Cohen SR. Opioid use in advanced malignant disease: why do different centers use vastly different doses? A plea for standardized reporting. *Journal of Pain and Symptom Management* 1995; 10: 632–638.

26   Ferris FD, Kerr IG, DeAngelis C, Sone M, Hume S. Inpatient narcotic infusions for patients with cancer pain. *Journal of Palliative Care* 1990; 6: 51–59.

27   Schug SA, Zech D, Grond S, Jung H, Meuser T, Stobbe B. A long-term survey of morphine in cancer pain patients. *Journal of Pain and Symptom Management* 1992; 7: 259–266.

28   Bruera E, Schoeller T, Wenk R, MacEachern T, Marcelino S, Hanson J, Suarez-Almazor M. A prospective multicenter assessment of the Edmonton Staging System for cancer pain. *Journal of Pain and Symptom Management* 1995; 10: 348–355.

29   Berkowitz BA. The relationship of pharmacokinetics to pharmacological activity; morphine, methadone and naloxone. *Clinical Pharmacokinetics* 1976; 1: 219–230.

30   Sawe J. High dose morphine and methadone in cancer paitents: clinical pharmaco-kinetic consideration of oral treatment. *Clinical Pharmacology* 1986; 11: 87–106.

31   Bruera E, Schoeller T, Fainsinger R, Kastelan C. Custom made suppositories of methadone for severe cancer pain. *Journal of Pain and Symptom Management* 1992; 7: 372–374.

32   Weinberg D, Inturrisi C, Reidenberg B, al e. Sublingual administration of selected opioid analgesics. *Clinical Pharmacology and Therapeutics* 1988; 44: 335–342.

33   Shir Y, Shapira SS, Shenkman Z, Kaufman B, Magora F. Continuous epidural methadone treatment for cancer pain. *Clinical Journal of Pain* 1991; 7: 339–341.

34   Abramson FP. Methadone plasma protein binding: alterations in cancer and displacement from alpha 1–acid glycoprotein. *Clinical Pharmacology and Therapeutics* 1982; 32: 652–658.

35   Raistrick D, Hay A, Wolff K. Methadone maintenance and tuberculosis treatment. *British Medical Journal* 1996; 313: 925–926.

36   Sorkin E, Ogawa C. Cimetidine potentiation of narcotic action. *Drug Intelligence and Clinical Pharmacy* 1983; 17: 60–61.

37   Bruera E, Pereira J, Watanabe S, Belzile M, Kuehn N, Hanson J. Opioid rotation in patients with cancer pain. *Cancer* 1996; 78: 852–857.

38   Galer BS, Coyle N, Pasternak GW, Portenoy RK. Individual variability in the response to different opioids: report of five cases. *Pain* 1992; 49: 87–91.

39   Paix A, Coleman A, Lees J, Grigson J, Brooksbandk M, Thorne D, Ashby M. Subcutaneous fentanyl and sufentanil infusion substitution for morphine intolerance in cancer pain management. *Pain* 1995; 63: 263–269.

40   Fainsinger RL, Bruera E. How should we use transdermal fentanyl (TF) for pain management in palliative care patients? *Journal of Palliative Care* 1996; 12(1): 48–53.

41   Gourlay GK, Kowalski SL, Plummer JL, Cherry DA, Gaukroger P, Cousins MJ. The transdermal administration of fentanyl in the treatment of post-operative pain: pharmacokinetics and pharmacodynamic effects. *Pain* 1989; 37: 193–202.

42   Portenoy RK, Southam MA, Gupta SK, Lapin J, Layman M, Inturrisi CE, Foley KM. Transdermal fentanyl for cancer pain. *Anesthesiology* 1993; 78: 36–43.

43   Donner B, Zenz M. Transdermal fentanyl: a new step on the therapeutic ladder. *Anti-Cancer Drugs* 1995; 6(suppl 3): 39–43.

44   Himayakanthan S. Reducing multiple drug therapy. *Journal of Drug Development and Clinical Practice Case History Series* 1996; 3: 11–12.

45   Zenz M, Donner B, Strumpf M. Withdrawal symptoms during therapy with transdermal fentanyl. *Journal of Pain and Symptom Management* 1994; 9: 54–55.
46   Higgs CMB, Vella-Brincat J. Withdrawal with transdermal fentanyl. *Journal of Pain and Symptom Management* 1995; 10: 5.
47   Kirkham SR, Pugh R. Opioid analgesia in uraemic patients. *Lancet* 1995; 345:: 1185.
48   Lee C, McTavish D, Sorkin E. Tramadol: a preliminary review of its pharmacodynamic and pharmacokinetic properties, and therapeutic potential in acute and chronic pain states. *Drugs* 1993; 46: 313–340.
49   Raffa RB, Friderichs E, Reimann W, Shank RP, Codd EE, Vaught JL. Opioid and nonopioid components independently contribute to the mechanism of action of tramadol, an 'atypical' opioid analgesic. *Journal of Pharmacology and Therapeutics* 1992; 260: 275–285.
50   Vickers M, O'Flaherty D, Szekely S, Read M, Yoshizumi J. Tramadol: pain relief by an opioid without depression of respiration. *Anaesthesia* 1992; 47: 291–296.
51   Wilder-Smith C, Schimke J, Osterwalder B, Senn H-J. Oral tramadol and morphine for strong cancer-related pain. *Annals of Oncology* 1994; 5: 141–146.
52   Grond S, Zech D, Lynch J, Schug S, Lehmann KA. Tramadol: a weak opioid for relief of cancer pain. *The Pain Clinic* 1992; 5: 241–247.
53   Budd K. Tramadol – a step towards the ideal analgesic? *European Journal of Palliative Care* 1995; 2: 56–60.
54   Szekely S, Vickers M. A comparison of the effects of codeine and tramadol on laryngeal reactivity. *European Journal of Anaesthesiology* 1992; 9: 111–120.
55   Houmes R, Voets M, Verkaaik A, Erdmann W, Lachmann B. Efficacy and safety of tramadol versus morphine for moderate and severe postoperative pain with special regard to respiratory depression. *Anesthesia and Analgesia* 1992; 74: 510–514.
56   Preston K, Jasinski D, Testa M. Abuse potential and pharmacological comparison of tramadol and morphine. *Drug Alchol Dependency* 1991; 27: 7–18.
57   Vickers MD, Paravicini D. Comparison of tramadol with morphine for postoperative pain following abdominal surgery. *European Journal of Anaesthesiology* 1995; 12: 265–271.
58   Sykes N. Current management of constipation in cancer pain. *Progress in Palliative Care* 1996; 4: 170–177.
59   British-National-Formulary. Naloxone. In: British National Formulary (No. 32). London: British Medical Association and the Royal Pharmaceutical Society of Great Britain, 1996, pp. 22 & 533.
60   Korbon G, James D, Verlander J, DiFazio C, Rosenbaum S, Levy S, Perry P. Intramuscular naloxone reverses the side effects of epidural morphine while preserving analgesia. *Regional Anaesthesia* 1985; 10: 16–20.
61   Max MB, Payne R, (Co-chairs). Principles of analgesic use in the treatment of acute pain and cancer pain: American Pain Society, 1992.
62   Kanamaru T, Saeki S, Katsumata N, Mizuno K, Ogawa S, Suzuki H. Ketamine infusion for control of pain in patients with advanced cancer. *Masui* 1990; 39: 1368–1371.
63   Oshima E, Tei K, Kayazawa H, Urabe N. Continuous subcutaneous injection of ketamine for cancer pain. *Canadian Journal of Anaesthetics* 1990; 37: 385–392.
64   Luczak J, Dickenson AH, Kotlinska-Lemieszek A. The role of ketamine, an NMDA receptor antagonist, in the management of pain. *Progress in Palliative Care* 1995; 3: 127–134.
65   Clark JL, Kalan GE. Effective treatment of severe cancer pain of the head using low-dose ketamine in an opioid-tolerant patient. *Journal of Pain and Symptom Management* 1995; 10: 310–314.
66   Mercadante S, Lodi F, Sapio M, Calligara M, Serretta R. Long-term ketamine subcutaneous continuous infusion in neuropathic cancer pain. *Journal of Pain and Symptom Management* 1995; 10: 564–568.

67   Laird D, Lovel T. Paradoxical pain. *Lancet* 1993; 341: 241.
68   Ebert B, Andersen S, Krogsgaard-Larsen P. Ketobemidone, methadone and pethidine are noncompetitive N-methyl-D-aspartate (NMDA) antagonists in the rat cortex and spinal cord. *Neuroscience Letters* 1995; 187: 165–168.
69   Ebert B, Andersen S, Hjeds H, Dickenson AH. Opioid analgesics as non competitive NMDA antagonists. [in press]. 1996.
70   Kornhuber J, Weller M, Schoppmeyer K, Riederer P. Amantadine and memantine are NMDA receptor antagonists with neuroprotective properties. *Journal of Neural Transmission* 1994; 43: 91–104.
71   Eisenach J, Gebhart G. Intrathecal amitriptyline acts as an N-Methyl-D-Aspartate receptor antagonist in the presence of inflammatory hyperalgesia in rats. *Anesthesiology* 1995; 83: 1046.
72   Steinberg RB, Gilman DE, Johnson F. Acute toxic delirium in a patient using transdermal fentanyl. *Anesthesia and Analgesia* 1992; 75: 1014–1016.
73   Adair JC, El-Nachef A. Fentanyl neurotoxicity. *Annals of Emergency Medicine* 1994; 27: 791–792.
74   Olsen AK, Sjogren P. Neurotoxic effects of opioids. *European Journal of Palliative Care* 1996; 3: 139–142.
75   Leipzig RM, Goodman H, Gray G, Erle H, Reidenberg MM. Reversible, narcotic-associated mental status impairment in patients with metastatic cancer. *Pharmacology* 1987; 35: 47–54.
76   Caraceni A, Martini C, Conno FD, Ventafridda V. Organic brain syndromes and opioid administration for cancer pain. *Journal of Pain and Symptom Management* 1994; 9(8): 527–533.
77   Maddocks I, Somogyi A, Abbott F, Hayball P, Parker D. Attenuation of morphine-induced delirium in palliative Care by substitution with infusion of oxycodone. *Journal of Pain and Symptom Management* 1996; 12: 182–189.
78   Bruera E, Franco JJ, Maltoni M, Watanabe S, Suarez-Almazor M. Changing pattern of agitated impaired mental status in patients with advanced cancer: association with cognitive monitoring, hydration, and opioid rotation. *Journal of Pain and Symptom Management* 1995; 10: 287–291.
79   Bruera E, Schoeller T, Montejo G. Organic hallucinosis in patients receiving high doses of opiates for cancer pain. *Pain* 1992; 48: 397–399.
80   Stambaugh JE, Wainer IW, Sanstead JK, Hemphill DM. The clinical pharmacology of meperidine: comparison of routes of administration. *Journal of Clinical Pharmacology* 1976; 16: 245–256.
81   Szeto HH, Inturissi CE, Houde R, Saal S, Cheigh J, Reidenberg MM. Accumulation of normeperidine an active metabolite of meperidine in patients with renal failure or cancer. *Annals of Internal Medicine* 1977; 86: 738–741.
82   Kaiko RF, Foley KM, Grabinski PY, Heidrich G, Rogers AG, Inturrisi CE, Reidenberg MM. Central nervous system excitatory effects of meperidine in cancer patients. *Annals of Neurology* 1983; 13: 180–185.
83   Deneau GA, Nakai K. The toxicity of meperidine in the monkey as influenced by its rate of absorpion. *Bulletin Drug Addiction Narcotic Appendix* 1961; 6: 2460–2469.
84   Cowan A, Geller EB, Adler MW. Classification of opioids on the basis of change in seizure threshold in rats. *Science* 1979; 206: 465–467.
85   Eisendrath SJ, Goldman B, Douglas J, Dimatteo L, Van-Dyke C. Meperidine-induced delirium. *American Journal of Psychiatry* 1987; 144: 1062–1065.
86   Sjogren P, Jonsson T, Jensen NH, Drenck NE, Jensen TS. Hyperalgesia and myoclonus in terminal cancer patients treated with continuous intravenous morphine. *Pain* 1993; 55: 93–97.

87 Sjogren P, Jensen N-H, Jensen TS. Disappearance of morphine-induced hyperalgesia after discontinuing or substituting morphine with other opioid antagonists. *Pain* 1994; 59: 313–316.

88 Hagan N, Swanson R. Strychnine-like multifocal myoclonus and seizures in extremely high-dose opioid administration: treatment strategies. *Journal of Pain and Symptom Management* 1997; 14: 51–58.

89 Labella FS, Pinksy C, Havlicek V. Morphine derivatives with diminished opiate receptor potency show enhanced central excitatory activity. *Brain Research* 1979; 174: 263–271.

90 Smith GD, Smith MT. Morphine-3–glucuronide: evidence to support its putative role in the development of tolerance to the antinociceptive effects of morphine in the rat. *Pain* 1995; 62: 51–60.

91 Glare PA, Walsh TD, Pippenger CE. Normorphine, a neurotoxic metabolite. *Lancet* 1990; 335: 725–726.

92 MacDonald N, Der L, Allan S, Champion P. Opioid hyperexcitability: the application of alternate opioid therapy. *Pain* 1993; 53: 353–355.

93 Frenk H, Watkins LR, Mayer DJ. Differential behavioral effects induced by intrathecal microinjection of opiates: comparison of convulsive and cataleptic effects produced by morphine, methadone, and D-ala^2-methionine-enkephalinamide. *Brain Research* 1984; 299: 31–42.

94 De-Conno F, Caraceni A, Martini C, Spoldi E, Salvetti M, Ventafridda V. Hyperalgesia and myoclonus with intrathecal infusion of high dose morphine. *Pain* 1991; 47: 337–339.

95 Cherny NI, Chang V, Ingham JM, Tiseo PJ, Popp B, Portenoy RK, Foley KM 1993. The prevalence and outcome of sequential trials of opioid analgesics in the management of cancer pain. In: Abstracts of the American Pain Society 12th Annual Scientific Meeting. Orlando, FL: American Pain Society, 1993: A35. *Conference*

96 Gregory RE, Grossman S, Sheidler VR. Grand mal seizures associated with high-dose intravenous morphine infusions: incidence and possible etiology. *Pain* 1992; 51: 255–258.

97 Hoppe JO, Goble FC. The intravenous toxicity of sodium bisulfite. *Journal of Pharmacology and Experimental Therapeutics* 1951; 101: 101–105.

98 Halaby SF, Mattocks AM. Absorption of sodium bisulfite from peritoneal dialysis solutions. *Journal of Pharmaceutical Sciences* 1965; 54: 52–55.

99 Shih VE, Abroms IF, Johnson JL, et-al. Sulfite oxidase deficiency. *New England Journal of Medicine* 1977; 297: 1022–1028.

100 Boyd K, Quigley C. Morphine-induced myoclonus. *Palliative Medicine* 1992; 6: 167.

101 Parnham MJ, Dickenson AH. Developments and clinical leads in nonopioid analgesics. *Analgesia* 1996; 2: 43–56.

102 Andersen S, Dickenson AH, Kohn M, Reeve A, Rahman W, Ebert B. The opioid ketobemidone has a NMDA blocking effect. *Pain* 1996; 67: 369–374.

103 Hawkey CJ. Future treatments for arthritis: new NSAIDs, NO-NSAIDs or no NSAIDs? *Gastroenterology* 1995; 109: 614–616.

104 McCormack K. The spinal actions of nonsteroidal anti-inflammatory drugs and the dissociation between their anti-inflammatory and analgesic effects. *Drugs* 1994; 47(suppl 5): 28–45.

105 Somasundaran S, Hayllar H, Rafi S, Wrigglesworth JM, Macpherson AJS, Bjarnason I. The biochemical basis of nonsteroidal anti-inflammatory drug-induced damage to the gastro-intestinal tract: a review and a hypothesis. *Scandinavian Journal of Gastroenterology* 1995; 30: 289–299.

106 Hawkey CJ, Meade EA, Smith WL, DeWitt DL. Differential inhibition of prostaglandin endoperoxide synthase (cyclooxygenase) isozymes by aspirin and other nonsteroidal anti-inflammatory drugs. *Journal of Biological Chemistry* 1993; 268: 6610–6614.

107 Ahmedzai S, Brooks D. Transdermal fentanyl versus sustained-release oral morphine in cancer pain: preference, efficacy and quality of life. *Journal of Pain and Symptom Management* 1997; 13: 254–261.

108 Fallon M. Opioid rotation: does it have a role? *Palliative Medicine* 1997; 11: 177–178.

109 Gorman AL, Elliott KJ, Inturrisi CE. The d-and-1-isomers of methadone bind to the non-competitive site on the N-methyl-D-Aspartate (NMDA) receptor in rat forebrain and spinal cord. *Neuroscience Letters* 1997; 223: 5–8.

110 Hagan N, Swanson R. Strychnine-like-multifocal myoclonus and seizures in extremely high-dose opioid administration: treatment strategies. *Journal of Pain and Symptom Management* 1997; 14: 51–58.

111 Bruera E, Pereira J, Watanabe S, Belzile M, Kuehn N, Hanson J. (1996) Opioid rotation in patients with cancer pain. *Cancer*; 78: 852–857.

Chapter 6

Nerve Pain

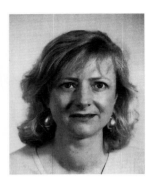

Dr Claire Sinnott
Claire Sinnott is Consultant and Senior Lecturer in Palliative Medicine at Guy's and St. Thomas' Hospital Trust. She moved into Palliative Medicine after completing a general medical hospital rotation and worked in a variety of teams and units. Neuropathic pain has been a particular interest for some time.

DEFINITIONS

- Nerve pain (neuropathic pain) results from damage to, or dysfunction of, the nervous system. The damage occurs to the system which carries and interprets pain messages.
- Nociceptive pain ('normal' pain) results from damage to any other body tissue. The pain message is carried by the intact nervous system.

N.B. In cancer pain both types of pain often coexist.

INTRODUCTION

Nerve pain is reliably diagnosed when there is **pain in an area of altered sensation**. However the diagnosis can be made even when no objective sensory change can be found. A series of 2118 cancer patients referred to a pain service showed 34% had neuropathic pains.[1]

In palliative care nerve pain is notoriously troublesome to control. There is a large amount of published research of nerve pain in non-malignant conditions. This information, plus anecdotal experience in cancer nerve pain, forms the basis for the management strategies in palliative care. Many questions however remain unanswered. It is not yet clear which is the most effective and least toxic therapeutic option for nerve pain in malignant disease.

PROBLEMS WITH THE EVIDENCE

- Despite the large literature there are relatively few satisfactory studies of many of the drugs used.
- Many different drugs have been looked at but useful comparisons are scarce.
- Different nerve pain models (eg post herpetic neuralgia, trigeminal neuralgia . . .) have been looked at, but it is unclear whether they all respond to treatment in the same way.
- Even if all nerve pains do respond to the same drugs, patients debilitated by advanced malignant disease may have increased susceptibility to drug toxicity and may need different strategies because of a short prognosis.

Diagnosis   Nerve (neuropathic) pains are distinguished from nociceptive (normal) pains by the characteristic description of the pain, the anatomical site and often by clinical evidence of nerve damage, (abnormal sensory signs).

Mixed pains, with components of nerve pain and nociceptive pain, are common.

Not all opioid-resistant pains are nerve pains. There are other types of difficult pain which may fail to respond to conventional analgesic strategies.

PATHOPHYSIOLOGY

Nervous system "plasticity"   The old fashioned "hard wiring" view of the nervous system has been undergoing radical review in the field of pain research.[2] The phenomenon of "plasticity", the ability of the nervous system to alter in structure and function in response to experience and injury, is now well recognised. Painful nerve damage sets up processes in the nervous system which are responsible for sustaining the pain. This explains why neuropathic pains are relatively unresponsive to surgical procedures designed to interrupt pain pathways. The characteristic of plasticity is of relevance to the development of new therapeutic strategies for managing difficult pain problems, including nerve pain (see later section on ketamine).

Sympathetically maintained pain

Damage to a peripheral nerve seems to induce a state of sensitivity to sympathetic activity. This can result in the classic syndrome of sympathetically maintained pain, causalgia: sustained burning pain, allodynia and hyperpathia after a traumatic nerve lesion, often combined with vasomotor and sudomotor dysfunction and later trophic changes. This full-blown syndrome is rarely seen in the palliative care setting, but an autonomic component to the pattern of neurological damage may be observed. This has relevance for therapeutic management options (see later section on sympathetic blocks).

CAUSES OF NERVE PAIN

- **Cancer**
  - Infiltration of nervous tissue
  - Compression of nervous tissue by tumour in contiguous soft tissues, lymphatics or bone
  - Paraneoplastic neuropathy (painful peripheral neuropathy remote from the anatomical sites of disease)

- **Treatment–Induced**
  - *Radiotherapy* (eg radiation fibrosis of the brachial plexus in breast cancer)
  - *Chemotherapy* (eg vinca alkaloids, platinum agents)
  - *Surgery* (eg post mastectomy pain)

- **Other conditions**
  - Post herpetic neuralgia (may be related to immunocompromise)
  - Trigeminal neuralgia
  - Diabetic neuropathy.

CLINICAL ASSESSMENT

History   The patient may find their pain difficult to describe. Terms such as: burning, tingling, pricking, shooting, stabbing, searing, raw, electric-shock like; will often be used in addition to more familiar terms like aching. Other neurological symptoms may be associated: numbness, pins and needles, weakness, hot or cold feeling of the affected area. Patients may complain of non painful stimuli being perceived as unpleasant; e.g. clothes feeling uncomfortable when in contact with the affected area of skin.

Examination   Look carefully for signs of **altered sensation** since this confirms nerve damage. Sensation may be reduced (most commonly to pin prick, temperature or touch) or increased, which may occur in various patterns:

- *allodynia*   – pain due to a stimulus which is not normally painful
- *hyperalgesia*   – increased pain due to a stimulus which is normally painful
- *hyperaesthesia* – increased sensitivity to stimulation
- *hyperpathia*   – painful reaction to a stimulus, especially a repetitive stimulus.

Autonomic changes may be visible (altered colouring and/or temperature of skin, sweat changes, piloerection, oedema). Look for signs of *motor damage* (muscle wasting, changes in muscle tone, weakness, altered reflexes). There may also be evidence of the cause of the nerve damage: primary or metastatic deposits palpable or there may be evidence of previous radiotherapy, chemotherapy, herpes zoster or advanced complications of diabetes mellitus.

Investigations   Imaging may be indicated to identify a tumour/metastatic mass causing the problem: X-rays, ultrasound examination, computerised axial tomography (CT), myelography, magnetic resonance imaging (MRI). Electrodiagnostic nerve studies are only required in exceptional cases.

Psycho-social Aspects

Nerve pains are often severe and particularly unpleasant. The patient may have been regarded strangely because of their unusual description of the pain. Several different analgesic strategies may already have been tried and failed. By the time of specialist referral the patient and carers, and indeed other health care professionals who have 'failed' to control the pain, may all be in desperate need of help.

The multi-disciplinary team can be of particular value in the psychosocial support of these patients and their carers, both personal and professional.

MANAGEMENT OPTIONS

Even successful anti-cancer therapies (in terms of tumour shrinkage) may not necessarily result in the control of the nerve pain. Early recognition of nerve pain and appropriate treatment is crucial to success.

Complete pain control may not be achievable. It is important for all those involved to acknowledge this and set realistic goals. Monitoring drug toxicity versus benefit is especially important. Treatment options include:

Treatment options

- Opioids
- Antidepressants
- Anticonvulsants
- Systemic local anaesthetics
- Corticosteroids
- Ketamine
- TENS
- Topical agents
- Epidural
- Nerve blocks
- Cordotomy

Opioids

The place of opioids in the management of nerve pain is an issue on which views have been polarised,[3] ranging from "nerve pain is defined by opioid insensitivity" to "nerve pains are fully opioid sensitive if you use enough of the right opioid". In fact opioid sensitivity is a spectrum. Nociceptive (normal) pains tend to be more fully opioid-sensitive, nerve pains tend to be less opioid-sensitive.

All patients with cancer nerve pain should receive a trial of opioids, beginning with a weak opioid, progressing to a strong opioid and titrating the dose against the pain in the usual fashion.

The views of individual clinicians differ as to how far the dose should be pressed before considering the use of adjuvant analgesics. Increasing signs of opioid toxicity, with inadequate pain control, suggest that other measures are required.

Opioids in nerve pain

A 51 year-old woman with locally recurrent cervical carcinoma, following incomplete primary surgical resection, presented with severe, intermittent, shooting, "exploding" pains which had been an increasing problem for several months. The pain radiated from the right groin down the anterior aspect of her right thigh. On examination she had an area of reduced sensation, to light touch and pin prick, over the anterior thigh corresponding to the cutaneous distribution of the femoral nerve. At presentation she was taking Co-proxamol as required, but had found this no help. She was commenced on sodium valproate 100mg bd. The pain responded partially to the valproate which was rapidly titrated up to 800mg/day. She was given morphine tablets, to use for breakthrough pain, and found that these provided additional analgesia. She began to reduce the dose of valproate, to which she attributed considerable nausea and vomiting, and morphine was given regularly and the dose titrated up. Eventually she opted to discontinue the sodium valproate because of toxicity problems. She continued on regular morphine, with breakthrough doses, which she found gave acceptable (though not complete) pain control with toxicity that she could tolerate.

Antidepressants

Classification of antidepressants

Antidepressants work by acting on monoamine neurotransmitters. The specificity of different antidepressants for particular monoamines (eg serotonin [5–HT], noradrenaline) may be relevant to their analgesic action in nerve pain[5]:

- **predominantly serotoninergic** (including selective serotonin re-uptake inhibitors (SSRIs)) e.g. clomipramine, trazodone, fluoxetine.
- **predominantly noradrenergic** eg desipramine, mianserin, maprotiline.
- **mixed** (drugs with both serotoninergic and noradrenergic actions): e.g. amitriptyline, imipramine, dothiepin, trimipramine.

Evidence in cancer nerve pain.

There have been no placebo controlled studies of antidepressants in cancer nerve pain specifically. The data which does exist often involves mixed groups of patients with nerve pain syndromes of mixed aetiologies, and/or combinations of drugs used as analgesics.

Evidence in non-cancer nerve pain[6]

There is an enormous amount of evidence for the use of mixed receptor activity tricyclics, in particular amitriptyline, in a wide variety of pain syndromes including nerve pain syndromes. A high proportion of this data is anecdotal or from uncontrolled studies but there is good data. Approximately two thirds of patients with post herpetic neuralgia experience significant pain relief from amitriptyline. Receptor-specific antidepressants have been less investigated. The evidence to date suggests that the predominantly serotoninergic drugs may be less effective than the older, mixed action drugs.

Mechanisms

Actions on descending noradrenaline and serotonin tracts may modulate pain signalling in the spinal cord. Many other views exist. It has been a common misunderstanding to assume that the antidepressants help pain only by altering mood. There is good evidence that antidepressants have a separate analgesic action.

EVIDENCE FOR ANALGESIC ACTION OF ANTIDEPRESSANTS

- Pain relief is often achieved at lower doses than antidepressant action
- Pain relief is more rapid
- Pain relief has been achieved in patients who were not depressed (by formal assessment)
- Pain relief has been achieved in the absence of an antidepressant response.

Dosing Start with low doses (especially in patients who are elderly or have multisystem debility). Doses equivalent to amitriptyline 25mg (or even 10mg) nocte should be used at the outset. Toxicity is the only impediment to rapid dosage titration. Sedative antidepressants should be given in a single nocte dose. Less toxic antidepressants (eg SSRIs) may be commenced in higher doses at the outset of treatment. Doses up to 150mg daily of amitriptyline (or equivalent) may be required, although toxicity may well be a limiting factor before this dose is achieved.

Plasma levels Plasma levels of these drugs and their metabolites vary widely between patients on the same doses. Blood levels of antidepressants are not easily available to most units and probably have little to offer over clinical criteria for altering doses/ regimes.

Adverse effects Mixed receptor action tricyclics have most toxicity (sedation, dry mouth, constipation, blurring of vision, confusion, hypotension and cardiac toxicity) and minor adverse reactions are common. The SSRIs (e.g. fluoxetine) have different side effects (gastrointestinal toxicity, agitation and insomnia).

Monoamine oxidase inhibitors have been shown to have analgesic properties, but they are not appropriate in palliative care because of problems with toxicity and drug interactions.

Antidepressants and anticonvulsants in nerve pain

A 66-year-old woman had had an adenocarcinoma of the lung diagnosed 4 years ago. She presented with a 6 week history of increasing pain in the left buttock and hip. The 'burning and bursting' painful sensation radiated down the lateral aspect of the left thigh. On examination the lumbar spine was tender to palpation but there were no neurological abnormalities detected. A bone scan showed metastatic lesions at L1 and L2. She had been commenced on morphine and was on a dose of MST 40mg BD when admitted with severe, persistent pain. Several additional doses of morphine elixir 15mg were given over 24 hours with no significant improvement. She was then given amitriptyline in a dose of 25mg nocte. The following morning her pain had almost completely resolved. 4 days later she remained well pain controlled but complained of an extremely dry mouth. Clonazepam 0.5mg nocte was substituted for the amitriptyline with no reduction in analgesic efficacy.

Anticonvulsants

Drugs: Carbamazepine, phenytoin, sodium valproate, clonazepam.

Evidence in cancer nerve pain

There have been no placebo controlled studies of these drugs in cancer nerve pain specifically. The only published data relate to anecdotal reports and trials involving a mixture of conditions and combinations of analgesics.

Evidence in non-cancer nerve pain

The classical pain model for which the anticonvulsants have been used is trigeminal neuralgia. A wide variety of nerve pains, mostly with a shooting or lancinating character of pain as common feature, have been studied. The most researched drug is carbamazepine which superseded phenytoin in the treatment of trigeminal neuralgia. Double blind studies support the use of carbamazepine and phenytoin; less evidence relates to the use of clonazepam and sodium valproate. In trigeminal neuralgia approximately 70% of patients experience significant pain relief with carbamazepine.

One study (which included 8 cases of "malignant neuropathy") investigated all 4 of these anticonvulsants.[7] 170 cases of lancinating pains of various aetiologies were reported retrospectively. All 4 of the above named anticonvulsants were used one by one, and interchanged if pain control was inadequate or unacceptable toxicity developed. 7 of 8 cases of malignant neuropathy were eventually "relieved". Clonazepam and carbamazepine were deemed "most effective" but the use of carbamazepine in particular was significantly limited by toxicity. The ineffectiveness of any one of the four agents was not a guide to the others.

Mechanisms of action   These drugs have widely differing receptor actions and there are many theories. The standard story relates to their shared property as membrane stabilisers, resulting in the diminution of abnormal neuronal hyperexcitability and the suppression of paroxysmal discharges.

Doses   In order to minimise toxicity start at a low dose and titrate up according to response and adverse effects.

ANTICONVULSANTS FOR NERVE PAIN[8]

Drug	Starting dose	Usual maintenance dosage (/day)
Carbamazepine	100mg BD	300–800mg
Clonazepam	0.5mg BD	1–4mg
Phenytoin	50mg BD	200–400mg
Sodium valproate	100–200mg BD	600–1200mg

Plasma levels   Plasma levels of anticonvulsants may occasionally be helpful, particularly when assessment of toxicity is difficult. The therapeutic ranges for analgesia are not well established but are probably towards the lower end of those for seizures.

Adverse effects   Toxic side-effects with these drugs are common (25–50%).[9] *Carbamazepine:* tolerance may develop to the common, milder toxicity problems (sedation, dizziness, nausea, anorexia). Haematological toxicity may limit its use in some vulnerable patients or necessitate monitoring of blood counts. Relevant drug interactions can occur with: propoxyphene, erythromycin, cimetidine, isoniazid.

Clonazepam: dose dependant sedation is the main problem. Reports of treatment-related depression may be particularly relevant in palliative care patients.

Sodium valproate: causes relatively few adverse effects. Nausea and anorexia can occur but the enteric-coated preparation offers reduced toxicity. Rarer problems include hepatotoxicity and thrombocytopoenia.

Phenytoin: has a narrow therapeutic range, so small increases in dose can precipitate toxicity.

Systemic local anaesthetics (Class I antiarrhythmics)

Drugs: parenteral (IV or SC) lignocaine, oral flecainide, oral mexiletine.

Evidence

In non-malignant nerve pain several good studies have confirmed the analgesic efficacy of this group of drugs.[10] In cancer nerve pain anecdotal reports of promising results with oral flecainide appeared to be supported by reports of 6 patients from a placebo controlled trial which was terminated prematurely.[11] Promising case reports of the use of lignocaine in cancer nerve pain, have also been published.[12] However no analgesic benefit was shown in a double blind cross-over study of IV lignocaine versus 0.9% saline in 10 cancer patients with cutaneous allodynia.[13]

Mechanisms

These are not fully elucidated. The drugs are certainly peripheral sodium channel blockers. Local analgesia occurs after injection into a peripheral nerve due to a non-depolarising block to the nerve impulse. There is also good evidence that they have central actions which result in analgesia when the drugs are administered systemically.

SYSTEMIC LOCAL ANAESTHETICS

	Usual Dose	Notes
Lignocaine[12]	IV 100mg over 30minutes S/C 100–160mg/hour	Can give test dose first
Mexiletine	200mg TDS (orally)	titrate from 150mg/day up to 10mg/kg/day[14]
Flecainide	100mg BD (orally)	range 50–200mg BD

Adverse effects Cardiac toxicity is a particular worry. However, with the exclusion of those at particular risk, this has not proved a problem in the palliative care population. Both CVS and CNS toxicity are directly related to plasma levels. CNS problems (e.g. dizziness) tend to develop at lower concentrations, thereby providing an early warning system of impending, more serious, toxicity.

Lignocaine has a narrow therapeutic range and there is a tendency for plasma levels to increase with time (because of reduced clearance).

Mexiletine has become the preferred oral drug in non malignant pain because serious adverse effects are uncommon.

Corticosteroids The use of steroids for predominantly nerve compression pain rests on the theory of the reduction of oedema and inflammation surrounding the compressing tumour mass. Clinically it is not entirely clear how a compressive versus an infiltrative process can be confidently distinguished. However there is evidence that steroids may act as analgesics by other mechanisms, including a direct influence on electrical activity in damaged nerves.

Steroids are probably most effective if used early in the history of the pain, before irreversible nerve damage has become established. "High" doses of steroids are advocated for nerve compression pains but there is no clear evidence to guide the choice of dose (usually starting at dexamethasone 16mg/day).

Of the wide range of potential toxicities associated with steroids oral candidiasis is the most commonly seen in cancer patients, although the use of higher doses increases the risks of more serious problems.

These drugs are best commenced for time-limited trials, with subsequent doses kept to the minimum necessary to sustain benefit.

Ketamine

Ketamine, commonly used as an anaesthetic agent, has potent analgesic properties at sub-anaesthetic doses. Ketamine analgesia seems to be mediated through inhibition of the NMDA (N-methyl-D-aspartate) receptor. The NMDA receptor is one of a group of excitatory amino acid receptors which are increasingly recognised as important in the CNS neuronal plastic changes initiated by nerve injury (see the section on pathophysiology above).

In theory blockade of the NMDA receptor may restore the opioid sensitivity of a relatively opioid resistant pain.

It is early days in terms of evidence for the use of ketamine in cancer nerve pain, but preliminary information looks promising.

The drug is usually given by continuous subcutaneous infusion, starting at 100–150mg/day and titrating up. As it may significantly potentiate the effects of opioids, it is recommended that the dose of opioid be reduced by half at the commencement of the ketamine infusion. The most significant adverse effects are psychomimetic (eg hallucinations, insomnia), but sedation and skin reactions at the infusion site are also common.[15]

Transcutaneous electrical nerve stimulation (TENS)

TENS is a relatively non-toxic therapeutic option which has been used successfully to treat nerve pains. In theory the electrical stimulation of large afferent nerve fibres activates local inhibitory circuits within the dorsal horn of the spinal cord which reduce pain perception. TENS may be most useful in focal nerve injuries, particularly if the nerve trunk can be stimulated proximal to the site of injury. It can only work if the patient can perceive the stimulus in the painful area. Such complications as exist are related to electrode application to the skin.

Topical agents

Various topical agents have been beneficial in nerve pain syndromes. They will be particularly relevant in patients with troublesome (and preferably small) areas of hyperalgesia and/or allodynia. Toxicity problems with systemic agents may justify a trial of one of these agents.

Capsaicin depletes peptide mediators of pain transmission (eg substance P) in small primary afferent neurones. It may be analgesic in nerve pain syndromes (e.g. post herpetic neuralgia). An initial (but sometimes more persistent) burning sensation on application can be a problem. In addition an "adequate trial" of the preparation may require 4 daily applications for 4 weeks! *Aspirin* – open studies of topical aspirin, in various delivery systems, show some promise in nerve pain syndromes. *Local anaesthetics* – EMLA cream has reduced pain in open studies.

Epidural

The epidural route for drug administration in cancer patients tends to be used only if intensive systemic strategies have been exhausted. In these circumstances epidural opioids alone are unlikely to be effective, particularly in nerve pain. The addition of epidural local anaesthetic (usually bupivicaine) does appear to increase the success rate in nerve pain, but toxicity, including lower limb paresis, may be a problem.[16] Epidural clonidine, in combination with morphine (or indeed a cocktail of morphine, clonidine and bupivicaine), may also have a useful role in nerve pain.

Nerve blocks and neurosurgery

One of the earliest defining characteristics of nerve pain was the poor response to neurolytic procedures. Apart from sympathetic blockade in selected cases, most of these procedures are considered only when all other options above have been fully explored.

Regional local anaesthetic blocks

Regional local anaesthetic blocks can relieve nerve injury pain, and the relief is sometimes much longer than the expected duration of nerve conduction block. The phenomenon may not predict a good response to neurolytic block.

Sympathetic blocks   A nerve pain which shows characteristics of sympathetic nerve dysfunction may respond to sympathetic blockade. This may involve: local limb perfusion with guanethidine; local anaesthetic blocks of the stellate ganglion or lumbar sympathetic chain (depending on the anatomical location of the pain). If relief is obtained then the pain is, by definition, "sympathetically maintained", and may respond to further sympathetic blockade, possibly including a neurolytic block.

Cordotomy   This procedure involves lesioning the spino-thalamic tract (anterolateral tractotomy) and can be performed via either an open or a percutaneous approach. If successful it results in loss of pain and temperature sensation on the opposite side of the body beginning 3–5 segments below the lesion. Percutaneous cordotomy (usually the more appropriate procedure for palliative care patients) is usually done at level C1 or C2. A unilateral cordotomy carries relatively low risk of morbidity, but is clearly only appropriate for unilateral pain below the level of the expected block. Bilateral cordotomy carries a significantly greater risk of serious complications.

Cordotomy for nerve pain

A 71 year old man presented with pain in the right shoulder. One year later a diagnosis of a Pancoast tumour of the right lung was made. 2 years later he was still suffering with pain in the right arm, shoulder and chest wall. On examination he had numbness and wasting of the right arm and allodynia and hyperaesthesia over an extensive area of the right chest wall. Almost every category of systemic analgesic mentioned in this chapter and TENS had been tried with, at best, very limited success. Eventually he requested sedation in an attempt to alleviate some of his suffering. Because his pain continued to extend in distribution, but remained unilateral, a percutaneous cordotomy was performed. He derived some pain relief from this procedure which enabled more successful pain control to be achieved with a combination of opioids and amitriptyline.

In a large series 78.4% with nerve pain had significant relief at discharge following the procedure, but only 50% of this group had *any* degree of relief at "post-discharge" follow up.[17]

DISCUSSION

Goals

Nerve pains are difficult to manage and, at best, only partial control may be achieved. Set achievable goals for yourself and the patient at the outset.

There is often a significant placebo effect demonstrated in clinical studies.

Trial of drugs

Try to keep a logical approach to the use of the many different drugs available. As far as possible give an adequate trial of one drug at a time.

Opioids

As a rule opioids will be the first choice, titrated in the usual way, but with a lower threshold for changing, or adding another drug, if toxicity or a lack of response are problems.

Steroids

In nerve pains which present early, where the clinical evidence suggests a compressing tumour mass, a short trial of high dose steroids may be worthwhile: e.g. dexamethasone 16mg daily for 5 days.

Antidepressants and anticonvulsants

The traditional view that burning pain should be managed with an antidepressant and shooting pain with an anticonvulsant is challenged by recent systematic reviews by McQuay et al.[6,9] They state that the evidence shows little to choose between these two classes of adjuvant analgesics. Choose the drug with the most advantageous therapeutic versus adverse effects profile for the individual patient.

Because of toxicity problems, and in line with the usual approach of titrating the dose of analgesia against a pain, both antidepressants and anticonvulsants need to be commenced in relatively low doses and titrated.

Many patients end up on both an antidepressant and an anticonvulsant. Whether this combination provides better pain relief than either component alone is another issue unanswered by the current evidence.

Systemic local anaesthetics

In general the systemic local anaesthetics will be used as second, or even third, line following failure of the antidepressants and/or the anticonvulsants.

Systemic local anaesthetics can have advantages (eg lower toxicity profile, speed of onset, available routes of administration – particularly parenteral lignocaine), which may make their earlier use appropriate in a particular case.

Very difficult cases

When a pain fails to respond to treatment then other factors (eg psycho-social or spiritual problems) should always be fully explored. Repeated re-assessment is essential. A new problem (eg pathological fracture, sepsis) may have occurred. For severe, uncontrolled pain a systematic trial of several drugs and gradual dose titration is too ponderous. Patients may have tried high doses of opioids, or have opioid toxicity and persistent pain. If the pain is neuropathic options include:

● Epidural route
● Trial of parenteral lignocaine
● Ketamine
● Percutaneous cordotomy.

The *epidural route* has the added advantage of resolving problems of accumulated systemic drug toxicity, but it requires technical expertise (as well as a suitable anatomical site).

REFERENCES

1. Zech DFJ, Grond S, Lynch J, Hertel D, Lehmann KA. Validation of World Health Organisation Guidelines for cancer pain relief: a 10–year prospective study. Pain 1995; 63: 65–76.
2. McQuay HJ, Dickenson AH. Implications of nervous system plasticity for pain management. Anaesthesia 1990: 45; 101–2.
3. Wall PD. Neuropathic pain. Pain 1990; 43: 267–8. An overview of the debate surrounding the use of opioids in neuropathic pain.
4. Monks R. Psychotropic drugs. In: Wall PD, Melzack R eds. Textbook of Pain, 3rd edition. London: Churchill Livingstone, 1994: 963–989.

5. Onghena P, Van Houdenhove B. Antidepressant-induced analgesia in chronic non-malignant pain: a meta-analysis of 39 placebo-controlled studies. Pain 1992; 49: 205–219.

6. McQuay HJ, Tramer M, Nye BA, Carroll D, Wiffen PJ and Moore RA. A systematic review of antidepressants in neuropathic pain. Pain 1996; 68: 217–227.

7. Swerdlow M, Cundill JG. Anticonvulsant drugs used in the treatment of lancinating pain. A comparison. Anaesthesia 1981; 36: 1129–32.

8. Swerdlow M. Anticonvulsants in the therapy of neuralgic pain. Pain Clinic 1986; 1(1): 9–19.

9. McQuay H, Carroll D, Jadad AR, Wiffen P, Moore A. Anticonvulsant drugs for management of pain: a systematic review. Br Med J 1995; 311: 1047–52.

10. Glazer S, Portenoy RK. Systemic local anesthetics in pain control. Journal of Pain and Symptom Management 1991; 6 (1): 30–39.

11. Dunlop RJ, Hockley JM, Tate T, Turner P. Flecainide in cancer nerve pain [letter]. Lancet 1991; 337: 1347.

12. Brose WG, Cousins MJ. Subcutaneous lidocaine for treatment of neuropathic cancer pain. Pain 1991; 45 (2): 145–8.

13. Ellemann K, Sjogren P, Banning A-M, Jensen TS, Smith T, Geertsen P. Trial of intravenous lidocaine on painful neuropathy in cancer patients. Clinical Journal of Pain 1989; 5: 291–4.

14. Dejgard A, Petersen P, Kastrup J. Mexiletine for treatment of chronic painful diabetic neuropathy. Lancet 1988; 1: 9–11.

15. Mercadante S. Ketamine in cancer pain: an update. Palliative Medicine 1996; 10: 225–230.

16. Hogan Q, Haddox JD, Abram S, Weissman D, Taylor ML, Janjan N. Epidural opiates and local anesthetics for the management of cancer pain. Pain 1991;46:271–279.

17 Tasker RR, Tsuda T, Hawrylyshyn P. Clinical neurophysiological Investigation of deafferentation pain. In: Bonica JJ et al eds. Advances in Pain Research and Therapy, Volume 5. New York: Raven Press 1983: 713–738.

Comments on the references

2. A relevant and accessible introduction to this immensely complex area.
4. This detailed chapter is an excellent reference text on the antidepressants and includes a section on possible mechanisms of action.
6. This is a rigorous review, incorporating only selected randomised controlled trials.
9. This is a rigorous review, incorporating only selected randomised controlled trials.
10. A thorough review of the subject.
16. This reference includes details of doses used.

Chapter 7

Update on Anti-emetics

Dr Philip Wilkins

Philip Wilkins is a Specialist Registrar in Palliative Medicine, based in Northamptonshire. He trained at Cambridge, then spent two years as a surgical SHO, mainly in London. He decided upon a career change from surgery to palliative care and spent a year in palliative medicine and oncology, in Birmingham. He then gained general medical experience, and passed the Diploma for the MRCP. He has a particular interest in controlling difficult symptoms, and always looks to new developments. He is married with a baby daughter and relaxes by painting in various media and has contributed work to several art exhibitions and publications.

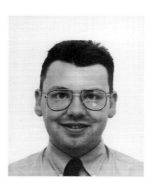

DEFINITIONS

- **Vomiting:** the forceful ejection of the contents of the stomach.

- **Nausea:** an unpleasant feeling of the need to vomit. It is often associated with autonomic symptoms, such as tachycardia, sweating, salivation, fear.

- **Retching:** the rhythmic, laboured spasmodic contractions of the diaphragm and abdominal muscles. It is essentially an effort to vomit that fails to expel the gastric contents. Nausea is usually present and retching often ends in vomiting.

INTRODUCTION

The purpose of the vomiting reflex

The vomiting reflex is a primitive mechanism designed to protect an animal from ingested toxins. Any noxious substances in the stomach are ejected. This has an obvious role in preventing further absorption of toxins. What is less clear is the role of vomiting in other circumstances. Why vomit, for instance, if the toxins are already within the blood? Why should extreme anxiety cause vomiting? One possible explanation comes from the fact that nausea is one of the most potent aversive stimuli known. Any activity associated with nausea is likely to be avoided in the future. The range of causes of nausea and vomiting is diverse. Unfortunately, in the palliative care setting, the emetic stimulus cannot usually be avoided, so the vomiting reflex must be interrupted by other means.

Prevalence

There is relatively little data on the prevalence of nausea and vomiting within the setting of palliative care. Studies that have been performed suggest that about 40% to 60% of patients with terminal cancer suffer from nausea.[1,2] Vomiting seems to be present in about 30% of such patients.

Nausea is more common in women. Certain cancers, such as breast, ovary, and stomach are associated with an increased incidence. It is less common in prostatic carcinoma. It is associated with hypercalcaemia and bowel obstruction. Many drugs commonly used in palliative care may cause nausea.

Unfortunately, despite the prevalence of nausea and vomiting, it is often undertreated. This is in spite of the widespread availability of potent treatment options.

The relief of nausea can also have considerable benefits in easing other symptoms and generally improving the quality of life in patients with terminal disease.

REVERSIBLE CAUSES OF VOMITING

Multifactorial causation

The causes of nausea and vomiting are often multifactorial, with several causes combining until a 'nausea threshold' is reached. The underlying disease itself is often a major factor, but not necessarily the only one. The treatment, including drugs to palliate other symptoms, can be a potent emetic stimulus. Nausea may also be due to indirect effects of the disease, such as paraneoplastic syndromes or infections. Lastly the nausea and vomiting may be due to a completely unrelated illness.

Reversible or potentially reversible causes of vomiting are always worth excluding. This might include metabolic causes, such as hypercalcaemia or certain causes of uraemia. Various drugs can cause nausea, both in standard dose and overdose. Palliative care patients are more susceptible to infection, due to relative immunodeficiency. Infections can often lead to nausea and need treating. Even infections outside the gastro-intestinal tract may cause nausea. Intestinal obstruction is dealt with elsewhere.

CAUSES OF VOMITING IN PALLIATIVE CARE

- Drugs (side-effect or overdosage)
- Chemotherapy
- Radiotherapy
- Brain metastases (increased intracranial pressure)
- Gastric irritation
- Squashed stomach syndrome
- Gastric outflow obstruction
- Bowel obstruction
- Constipation
- Hepatomegaly
- Ascites

- Hypercalcaemia
- Hyponatraemia
- Uraemia
- UTI (other infections)
- Septicaemia
- Oral thrush
- Cough
- Anxiety
- Pain

Opioid rotation

Morphine commonly causes nausea. Up to 35% of patients commenced on oral morphine will experience nausea in the first 48 hours. This is often transitory and will settle for most patients. However, it may persist and become more problematic than the pain the morphine is being used to treat. Until relatively recently, there were few alternatives and pain control was difficult for those unable to tolerate morphine. Various strong opiates are now available as analgesics in palliative care. This has introduced the concept of opioid rotation.[3,4] Alternative opiates available as oral preparations include hydromorphone, oxycodone and methadone. Methadone is available as an injection. Fentanyl is available as a transdermal patch. A trial of an alternative opioid should be considered when dose escalation with morphine produces intolerable side effects.

Vomiting due to morphine

A 68 year old woman with metastatic carcinoma of the breast presented with a painful metastasis in the neck of the right femur. X-ray excluded a fracture and she was commenced on oramorph 30mg as required. This improved the pain and she was eventually comfortable on 40mg of oramorph, 4-hourly. Unfortunately this coincided with gradually worsening nausea and vomiting. She was commenced on metoclopramide 10mg QDS with little effect. Cyclizine and haloperidol were also tried. The morphine was stopped and a 50mcg/hour fentanyl patch was applied. Adequate pain control was achieved with no associated nausea.

MECHANISMS OF VOMITING

Control centres

The vomiting reflex is poorly understood. The best model prevalent for a long time assumed the presence of a 'vomiting centre'. This was thought to lie in the lateral reticular formation of the medulla. There is little direct evidence for an anatomical centre, but this area has an important role in emesis. It is best regarded as a physiologically distinct area, which co-ordinates the vomiting process. Situated nearby is the area postrema, part of which was formerly known as the 'chemo-receptor trigger zone' (CTZ).

The cells that line the blood capillaries within the brain are joined together by endothelial occluding junctions. This is known as the 'blood-brain barrier'. There is also a similar 'cerebrospinal fluid-brain barrier'. These 'barriers' are relatively impermeable to polar molecules, including most drugs. This serves to protect the brain from noxious substances. The capillaries of the area postrema lack such occluding junctions and are relatively permeable to polar molecules. Hence blood-borne molecules can enter the area postrema and it can act as a chemoreceptor for toxins found in the blood or

CSF. At one stage it was suggested that all blood-borne emetic stimuli acted through this zone. The advent of new anti-emetics has shown that other mechanisms are equally as important in causing emesis from blood-borne stimuli. Hence there does not seem to be one distinct 'chemoreceptor trigger zone' and the term has been dropped.

Stimuli that cause vomiting

The 'vomiting centre' can receive a wide range of inputs to trigger the vomiting reflex. The important inputs arise from the vestibular apparatus, the vagus and other visceral afferents, higher centres and blood-borne stimuli. Each of these pathways seems to involve a slightly different set of neurotransmitters. Thus different receptor antagonists work on different pathways involved in vomiting. Consequently there is no one anti-emetic that can eradicate all nausea from all causes. Indeed, it has been suggested that the only thing capable of such an action is a general anaesthetic.

The identification of more receptors and neurotransmitters involved in the vomiting reflex makes the whole concept more and more complex. Our present understanding is best summarised as a diagram.

THE CAUSES OF VOMITING
(showing the receptors known to be important in the pathway.)

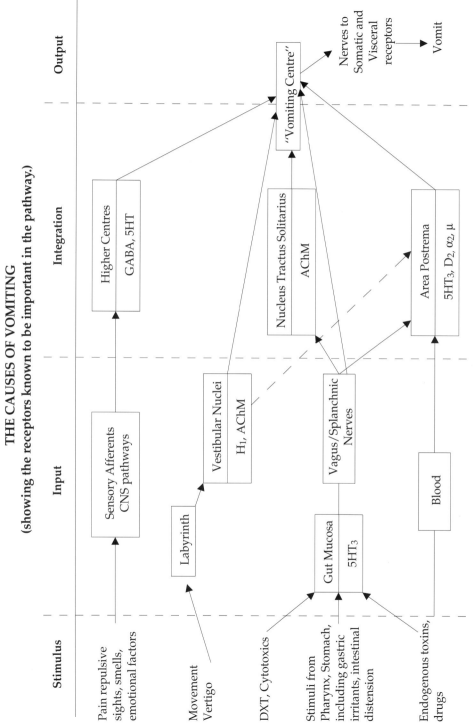

Key: GABA = Gamma Amino Butyric acid; 5HT = Serotonin; H_1 = Histamine; AChM = Muscarinic; D_2 = Dopamine; α_2 = a-adrenergic; μ = μ opioid

The efferent pathways are equally as complex. The vomiting paths seem reasonably well elucidated, though there are 2 main theories as to the precise routes. Less is known about the pathways involved in nausea.

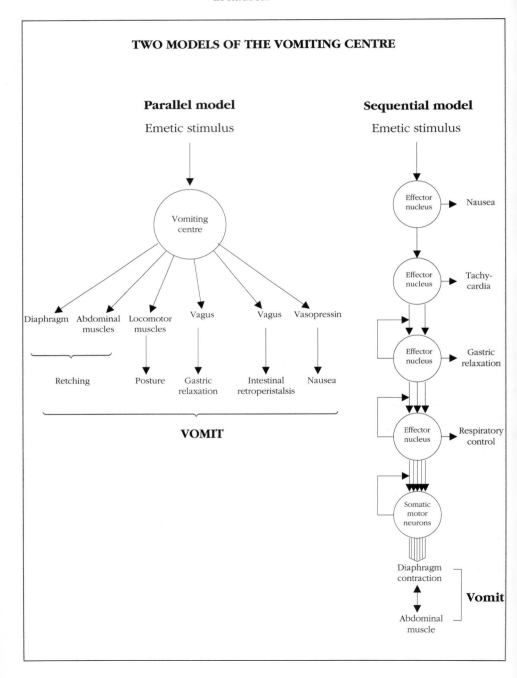

Receptors

Our understanding of the vomiting reflex has advanced tremendously with the identification of previously unrecognised neurotransmitter receptors. Antagonists at these receptors have been found to be potent anti-emetics. This area is still open to further discoveries. There are at least 15 different neurotransmitters found in medium to high concentrations in the area postrema.[5] There are almost 40 such neurotransmitters in the nucleus tractus solitarius. At least some of these chemicals are likely to be involved in the vomiting reflex.

Receptors tend to be named by the abreviation for the neurotransmitter that acts upon them. (Obvious exceptions include α and β adrenoreceptors and the opioid receptors). Research showed quite early on that there was not a simple relationship of one neurotransmitter to one receptor. Hence, receptors were subdivided – eg Dopamine receptors become D_1, D_2 receptors, etc.

Receptors for the vomiting reflex

Important receptors known to be involved in the vomiting reflex at present, with their sites, are as follows:

Dopamine, D_2 receptors – present in the area postrema. It is unclear where the dopamine comes from to stimulate these receptors.

Muscarinic receptors and **Histamine, H_1** receptors – in the vestibular nuclei. Probably also in the 'vomiting centre'. Histamine, H_2 receptors may be important, as selective H_1 antagonists do not completely abolish motion sickness.

Serotonin, 5–HT$_3$ receptors – in the gut, serotonin (derived from the enterochromaffin cells of the gut wall) causes release of acetylcholine from the myenteric plexus via these receptors. Almost 95% of serotonin in the body is found in the entero-chromaffin cells of the gut wall.[6] Blood-borne stimuli lead to the release of this serotonin, as well as direct noxious stimulation of the intestines. This path seems important for cytotoxic-induced vomiting. The receptors are also found in the area postrema.

Serotonin, 5–HT$_4$ receptors – in the gut, important for peristalsis. Possibly involved in the final efferent pathway in the vomiting reflex. It is agonists of $5HT_4$ receptors that are anti-emetic by being prokinetic.[4]

Adrenergic and **noradrenergic** receptors may be involved, but their role is unclear at present. Certainly, α_2 receptors seem important in the area postrema.

Neurokinin (such as **Substance P**) and **NK₁** receptors – these receptors may mediate the action of the vagus nerve in its central role in vomiting. New research is presently under way.[7]

RECEPTOR ACTIVITY OF ANTI-EMETICS

Drug	D_2	Mus	H_1	$5HT_3$	$5HT_4$
Hyoscine	−	+++	−	−	−
Cyclizine	−	+	+++	−	−
Promethazine	+	++	+++	−	−
Haloperidol	+++	−	−	−	−
Prochlorperazine	++	−	+	−	−
Chlorpromazine	++	+	++	−	−
Metoclopramide	++	−	−	+	++
Cisapride	−	−	−	−	+++
Domperidone	++	−	−	−	−
Ondansetron	−	−	−	+++	+
Methotrimeprazine	++	+	+	+	−

Key: D_2 = Dopamine D_2 receptor; Mus = Muscarinic acetylcholine receptor; H_1 = Histamine H_1 receptor; $5HT_3$ = Serotonin $5HT_3$ receptor; $5HT_4$ = Serotonin $5HT_4$ receptor.

N.B. All act as antagonists, except at $5HT_4$, where they are agonists.

DRUG PROFILES OF ANTI-EMETICS

Metoclopramide

Metoclopramide is useful for most causes of nausea and vomiting, except labyrinthine causes such as motion sickness. It is one of the most commonly used first-line anti-emetics in palliative care. In a survey of palliative care services in Australia, 82% of Units commonly used metoclopramide orally.[8] 41% commonly used metoclopramide subcutaneously.

METOCLOPRAMIDE

- Dopamine (D_2) antagonist
- Serotonin ($5-HT_3$) antagonist in high dose
- Serotonin ($5-HT_4$) agonist in the gut, hence gastrokinetic
- Extrapyramidal effects more common in the young; Hyperprolactinaemia is possible
- May cause hypertensive crises in phaeochromocytoma
- Plasma elimination half-life 4 hours
- Undergoes very variable hepatic first-pass metabolism
- Excreted in the urine
- 10–20mg as stat dose
- 30–100mg over 24 hours

Cyclizine Cyclizine is a useful first-line anti-emetic with a central action. It does not elevate prolactin levels, so may be particularly useful in patients with breast cancer. Cyclizine does seem clinically to be effective in drug-induced and post-operative emesis. The mechanism for this is unclear.

CYCLIZINE

- Histamine (H_1) antagonist
- Some anti-muscarinic activity
- Few clinically significant side-effects
- May enhance side-effects of anti-cholinergics
- Most effective if given before the onset of nausea
- Duration of action 4 hours, plasma half-life about 20 hours
- 50mg as stat dose
- 100–200mg over 24 hours

Haloperidol Haloperidol is particularly useful for drug-associated or metabolic nausea (such as that found in renal failure). Much lower doses are used than in psychiatric practice.

HALOPERIDOL

- Butyrophenone neuroleptic
- Dopamine (D$_2$) antagonist
- Sedating
- Extra-pyramidal side-effects
- Use with caution in epilepsy, liver disease, thyroid dysfunction
- Mean plasma elimination half-life 20–24 hours
- Undergoes first-pass metabolism
- 1.5–5mg as stat dose
- 1.5–10mg over 24 hours

Selecting the right anti-emetic

A 65 year old man with multiple myeloma was admitted under the haematologists with acute renal failure. His major symptom was nausea. This did not respond to oral or IM injections of metoclopramide or cyclizine. On the advice of the palliative care team, he was commenced on oral haloperidol 5mg at night, with considerable improvement in his symptoms.

Methotrimeprazine

Methotrimeprazine can be markedly sedating and cause postural hypotension, so should be used with caution in ambulant patients. It can be very effective in terminal care.[9] It is broad-acting and powerful. It is often kept as third line in the event of failure of other therapy, due to its side-effects. The biggest step forward in recent years has been the realisation that low dose methotrimeprazine (5–12.5mg) can be just as effective in treating nausea as high dose (50mg) and has fewer side-effects.

METHOTRIMEPRAZINE

- Phenothiazine – muscarinic and histamine (H_1) antagonist
- Has Dopamine (D_2) and 5–HT_3 antagonist properties
- Sedating
- Moderate extrapyramidal side-effects
- Risk of postural hypotension, particularly in the elderly
- Very variable plasma half-life
- 5–12.5mg as stat dose
- 12.5–50mg over 24 hours

5–HT₃ antagonists

The discovery of the 5–HT_3 antagonists has been one of the biggest advances in anti-emetic therapy in recent years. They are particularly useful for drug-induced nausea (particularly in association with cytotoxics). The three 5–HT_3 antagonists were reported preclinically to differ in their receptor binding, potency, dose response and duration. However, a recent review of clinical trials concluded that all three had almost identical anti-emetic efficacy and tolerability.[10] Tropisetron and granisetron are once-daily drugs.

5HT₃ ANTAGONISTS

- Ondansetron, granisetron and tropisetron available
- Few clinically significant side-effects
- May cause constipation
- Effectiveness enhanced by dexamethasone
- Metabolised in the liver – undergoes first-pass matabolism
- Elimination half-life about 3 hours for ondansetron

Prochlorperazine

Prochlorperazine is a useful anti-emetic. However, there is a risk of extreme dystonic reactions. They should be used with considerable caution in adolescents. There is also evidence that patients with AIDS may be more susceptible to these extra-pyramidal effects.[11] There is little information about blood levels, distribution and excretion in humans. Rate of metabolism and excretion decreases with age.

PROCHLORPERAZINE

- Phenothiazine – muscarinic and histamine (H_1) antagonist
- Duration of action 3–4 hours
- Extra-pyramidal side-effects
- Not suitable for sub-cutaneous infusion
- Available as a buccal preparation
- Postural hypotension possible
- Elimination half-life about 7 hours

Domperidone Domperidone does not cross the blood-brain barrier, so has fewer central side-effects. Extra-pyramidal effects are rarely reported, however.

DOMPERIDONE

- Dopamine (D_2) antagonist
- Gastrokinetic
- Not recommended for chronic use
- May cause hyperprolactinaemia
- Bioavailability 15% in fasting state, increased after food
- First-pass hepatic and intestinal metabolism
- Elimation half-life about 7.5 hours

Cisapride Cisapride is probably a fairly specific 5–HT_4 agonist. The action of serotonin in the myenteric plexus causes acetyl choline release. This results in a prokinetic effect throughout the whole GI tract. Cisapride is metabolised by the cytochrome P450 3A4 enzyme. Oral ketoconazole significantly inhibits this metabolism. This results in markedly increased levels of cisapride. This can lead to QT prolongation and ventricular arrhythmias.

CISAPRIDE

- 5–HT$_4$ agonist, hence gastrokinetic
- Effective in gastric stasis due to autonomic neuropathy
- Should be taken 15–30 minutes prior to a meal
- Metabolised in the liver and excreted in the urine
- Contra-indicated if the patient is on ketoconazole
- 20mg as stat dose
- 40mg over 24 hours

Steroids Steroids are widely used in palliative care. Their mode of action as anti-emetics may be via their inhibition of prostanoids from arachidonic acid. There is evidence that prostanoids act as emetogenic agents on the area postrema. For this reason, NSAIDs are also partially anti-emetic, though they are not effective enough and they also act as gastric irritants and actually induce vomiting.

CORTICOSTEROIDS

- Most often used in combination
  (eg chemotherapy regimes, obstruction)
- Can work as a single agent anti-emetic

Benzodiazepines The benzodiazepine most often used as an anti-emetic is lorazepam. This drug has the advantage of coming in a sublingual preparation, negating the need for the patient to swallow a tablet. Benzodiazepines are particularly useful for anticipatory vomiting.

BENZODIAZEPINES

- Sedative, anxiolytic, amnesic
- Main effect probably on input from higher centres
- Possible direct effect on medulla ('vomiting centre')
- Half-life of lorazepam 10–20 hours. Metabolised in liver

Cannabinoids   The use of cannabinoids as anti-emetics was proposed following the observation that smoking marijuana decreased the nausea and vomiting from cytotoxic drugs. They seem to work, but, at present, the side-effect profile make them too unsatisfactory to use. Interestingly, only 6% of American physicians that have used marijuana as an anti-emetic would prescribe it more frequently if there were no legal barriers.[12] Further work may find a purer compound that merely acts as an anti-emetic without the cortical problems.

CANNABINOIDS

- Probably act via the Area Postrema
- Anti-emetic effect blocked by naloxone
- Given orally (plasma half-life 2 hours,)
- Undergoes first-pass metabolism
- Metabolites excreted in urine and faeces,
- Side-effects common (drowsiness, dizziness, dry mouth, mood disturbances and postural hypotension)

ANTI-EMETICS FOR SPECIFIC SYNDROMES

	1st choice	2nd choice
Metabolic	Haloperidol	Ondansetron, Methotrimeprazine
Drug-induced	Haloperidol	Metoclopramide, Ondansetron
Radiotherapy, Chemotherapy	Ondansetron, Dexamethasone	Metoclopramide, Haloperidol
Raised intracranial Pressure	Cyclizine	Methotrimeprazine
Bowel Obstruction	Cyclizine, Hyoscine, Dexamethasone,	Octreotide, Ondansetron
Delayed Gastric Emptying	Metoclopramide	Cisapride, Domperidone

Note:
- Where ondansetron is mentioned, any 5–HT$_3$ antagonist may be used
- Dexamethasone potentiates effects of ondansetron and metoclopramide

SUGGESTED PROTOCOL FOR ANTI-EMETIC USAGE

Numerous attempts have been made to standardise anti-emetic regimes.[13] Unfortunately, since no universal anti-emetic exists, these are not as simple as the WHO Analgesic Ladder and can be laborious to use.

Different causes of vomiting require different forms of intervention. Hence, this symptom always necessitates an adequate assessment of the patient. A possible approach would be:

1. Assess the patient (history and examination).
2. Try to find a reversible cause (eg hypercalcaemia, intestinal obstruction or chemotherapy). The underlying cause may be open to treatment or self-limiting.
3. Always review the patient's medication. Consider stopping potentially emetogenic drugs.
4. Whilst the cause is being treated, specific anti-emetics are still appropriate (see table below).
5. If no reversible cause is obvious, it is still worth considering what is the most likely emetic stimulus. The concept of an anti-emetic for all causes of nausea is now questioned. As such, the choice of drug should be aimed at the most likely cause of nausea.
6. Give the chosen anti-emetic in adequate dosage and by the appropriate *route*. SC infusion is often needed initially to gain control. Oral anti-emetics are only effective for mild nausea or as prophylaxis.
7. Keep the patient under constant review. If the first choice of anti-emetic has failed, a second should be added or substituted. Again, this should be directed at the most likely cause of the nausea or vomiting.
8. A useful third-line anti-emetic, with actions on numerous receptors, is *methotrimeprazine*. Since it acts on many receptors, it has more side-effects than more specific drugs. Thus, it should not be used for first-line treatment.
9. Dexamethasone is a useful adjunct. As well as having intrinsic anti-emetic properties, dexamethasone enhances the properties of other drugs. It can be added if the vomiting persists.

A reversible cause for vomiting

A 50 year old gentleman with advanced carcinoma of the pancreas, presented with gradual onset of vomiting and constipation. His abdomen was soft and non-tender. He was unable to keep down tablets and so was commenced on an SC infusion of diamorphine, 40mg and haloperidol, 5mg per 24h. The diamorphine was thought to be exacerbating his constipation, so he was switched to a transdermal fentanyl patch. He continued to worsen. Bloods tests showed a calcium level of 3.99 mmol/l. This was treated with hydration and intravenous pamidronate, 60mg. Both his constipation and nausea gradually settled, such that his SC infusion with haloperidol could be stopped. (Note: hypercalcaemia is very unusual in pancreatic carcinoma.)

THE SUBCUTANEOUS ROUTE

Unfortunately, tablets can be a potent emetic stimulus. Persistent vomiting makes the oral route for medication inappropriate. Parenteral routes may need to be considered. It is often difficult to gain IV access in patients in a palliative care setting. The SC route is usually the kindest route. A way of avoiding recurrent injections in patients who often have fragile skin and poor tissue viability, is by SC infusion. This infusion may be temporary (if the nausea is likely to improve) or permanent.

INDICATIONS FOR SC INFUSIONS

- Persistent nausea and vomiting refractory to tablets
- Dysphagia
- Intestinal obstruction
- Semi-comatose or comatose states
- Profound weakness
- Poor absorption of drug in the G-I tract

When a subcutaneous infusion is required, it is usually necessary to include more than one drug. This is often an analgesic (typically diamorphine) and an anti-emetic. Unfortunately, there is very little data on the mixing of drugs in such infusions, partly due to the fact that many drugs are not actually licensed for this route. Local drug advisory units can usually furnish some guidelines.

Combinations of drugs in syringe drivers may result in precipitation. This is due to the reaction of soluble drugs, forming insoluble compounds. Attempts have been made to assess the use of combinations of drugs in syringe drivers. One such is the national survey of drug use in palliative care.[6] The experience of different palliative care units in Australia was assessed. Combinations of two or three drugs were preferred, though combinations of up to five drugs were used. A more recent study has tried to scientifically assess the compatibility and stability of diamorphine, cyclizine and haloperidol.[14]

The route of anti-emetics

A 68 year old lady presented with vomiting due to linitus plastica (secondary to breast cancer). She was only able to tolerate small amounts of clear fluids. Bone marrow infiltration, with thrombo-cytopaenia precluded surgical intervention. Various oral anti-emetics had been tried, including meto-clopramide, cisapride, methotrimeprazine and cyclizine. Oral steroids (up to dexamethasone 16mg) had had no benefit. She was admitted and commenced on an SC infusion of 16mg of dexamethasone. This had a remarkable effect and she was soon able to tolerate a liquidised diet. The improvement was maintained when the dose of SC dexamethasone was reduced to 8mg, but a trial back on oral steroids, dose 8mg, resulted in a return of the vomiting. The vomiting settled again on recommencing the SC infusion with dexamethasone 8mg, to which metoclopramide 40mg was added which controlled the persistent nausea.

Water for dilution   As a general guide, water for injection is the best diluent. The concentration of the drugs are important in determining their solubility and compatibility. As an example, cyclizine is renowned for crystallising in solution.

It is generally preferable to keep the volume of SC infusions to a minimum, although mixtures of drugs can be put into a 30cc syringe if necessary and can still be comfortably infused over 24 hours. It is useful to know the maximum concentrations of drugs that are unlikely to precipitate. The following is a guide for common combinations (adapted from references 14, 15):

MAXIMUM DRUG CONCENTRATIONS IN SC COMBINATIONS	
Drug	*Concentration (mg/ml)*
Cyclizine	25
Diamorphine	20
Haloperidol	2
Diamorphine	20
Metoclopramide	5
Diamorphine	50
Metoclopramide	5
Midazolam	5
Diamorphine	20
Cyclizine	20
Haloperidol	2

The following combinations are also commonly used:

● Diamorphine, cyclizine, midazolam
● Diamorphine, cyclizine, hyoscine
● Diamorphine, haloperidol, hyoscine
● Diamorphine, haloperidol, metoclopramide
● Diamorphine, haloperidol, midazolam
● Diamorphine, metoclopramide, midazolam
● Dexamethasone, midazolam, haloperidol.

There is little available data on maximum concentrations for these combinations.

There is also little data on the compatibility of methadone in syringe-drivers. 4-drug combinations are used in certain centres. Again there is little published information on this.

RELATIVE CONTRA-INDICATIONS TO SUBCUTANEOUS INFUSIONS

- Severe thrombocytopenia
- Systemic sclerosis
- Bullous disorders

CONCLUSION

The study of emesis, its causes and treatment is an area undergoing considerable research at present. It is one of the most distressing symptoms in terminal disease. Adequate treatment of nausea allows patients to eat some food and feel a little more 'normal'. As the actual neural pathways involved are better understood, so newer drugs should become available. The next type of drugs are likely to be NK_1 receptor antagonists.[7] These interfere with the action of the vagus nerve – central to the vomiting process. Hopefully, this will merely be the first of many advances.

References

1. Reuben DB, Mar V. Nausea and vomiting in terminal cancer patients. Archives of Internal Medicine 1983; 146: 2021–3.
2. Dunlop GM. A study of the relative frequency and importance of gastrointestinal symptoms and weakness in patients with far-advanced cancer. Palliative Medicine 1989; 4: 37–43.
3. Fallon M. Opioid rotation: does it have a role? Palliative Medicine 1997; 11: 177-8.
4. de Stoutz ND, Bruera E, Suarez-Almazor M. Opioid rotation for toxicity in terminal cancer patients. Journal of Pain and Symptom Management 1995; 10: 378-84.
5. Leslie RA and Reynolds DJM, Neurotransmitters and receptors in the emetic pathway. In: Andrews PLR and Sanger GJ, eds. Emesis in anti-cancer therapy. London, Chapman and Hall, 1993: 113–162.
6. Camilleri M, Von der Ohe MR. Drugs affecting serotonin receptors. Bailliere's Clinical Gastroenterology 1994; 8 (2): 301–319.

7. Bountra C, Gale JD, Gardner CJ, Jordan CC, Kilpatrick GJ, Twissell DJ, Ward P. Towards understanding the aetiology and pathophysiology of the emetic reflex: Novel approaches to antiemetic drugs. Oncology 1996; 53 (suppl 1): 102–109.

8. Drummond SH, Peterson GM, Galloway JG, Keefe PA. National survey of drug use in palliative care. Palliative Medicine 1996; 10: 119–124.

9. Twycross RG, Barkby GD, Hallwood PM. The use of low dose levomepromazine (methotrimeprazine) in the management of nausea and vomiting. Progress in Palliative Care 1997; 5 (2): 49–53

10. Roila F, Tonato M, Ballatori E, Del Favero A. Comparative studies of various antiemetic regimens. Supportive Care in Cancer 1996; 4 (4): 270–280.

11. Edelstein H, Knight RT. Severe parkinsonism in two AIDS patients taking prochlorperazine. Lancet 1987; 2: 1131–2.

12. Schwartz RH, Beveridge RA. Marijuana as an antiemetic drug: how useful is it today? Opinions from clinical oncologists. Journal of Addictive Diseases 1994; 13 (1): 53–65.

13. Regnard C. Nausea and vomiting – a flow diagram. Palliative Medicine 197; 1: 62–63

14. Grassby PF, Hutchings L. Drug combinations in syringe drivers: the compatibility and stability of diamorphine with cyclizine and haloperidol. Palliative Medicine 1997; 11: 217–224.

15. Bradley K. Swap data on drug compatibilities. Pharmacy in Practice 1996; March: 69–72.

Chapter 8

Anorexia & Weakness

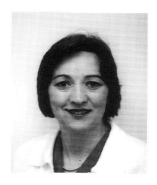

Dr Joanna Hocknell
Joanna Hocknell is Consultant in Palliative Medicine at the Nightingale Macmillan Unit, Derbyshire Royal Infirmary. Her research interests include the investigation and management of weakness in people with advanced cancer and the effects of exercise in overcoming functional disability.

INTRODUCTION

Anorexia and weakness are two of the commonest symptoms described by people with severe debilitating disease such as advanced cancer or AIDS. The two symptoms are often linked.

DEFINITIONS

- Anorexia is defined as loss of appetite
- "Weak" can have several meanings:
    - lacking physical strength (frail)
    - lacking mental strength (easily upset)
    - liable to complain ("I will be weak")
    - lacking in self-discipline ("being weak")

Anorexia Anorexia is suffered by up to 90% of patients with advanced cancer. It is an important symptom in terms of physical well-being and quality of life. Apart from the need for adequate nutrition much of our social activity is concerned with eating and drinking. A person's unwillingness or inability to eat can cause great distress to both the person and the informal carers. For someone to refuse food prepared by a carer may feel like personal rejection and may impinge on other aspects of the relationship. There may be the feeling that if only the person would eat (s)he would get better, and failure to eat is a sign of having given up. There are many possible causes of anorexia (and often several factors are present).

CAUSES OF ANOREXIA

Gastrointestinal
- Dry or sore mouth
- Coated tongue
- Oral candidiasis
- Poor dentition
- Altered taste
- Nausea
- Early satiety

Tumour related
- Cancer toxins
- Peptides produced by tumour
- e.g. bombesin, serotonin

Treatment related
- Drug-induced
- Post chemotherapy
- Post radiotherapy

Other Physical Problems
- Infection
- Weakness
- Pain
- Anxiety
- Depression

Environmental
- Poorly presented food
- Unfamiliar surroundings
- Unpleasant odours

Weakness

Weakness may result from physical or emotional problems or from cancer cachexia. Anxiety and clinical depression are probably still under-diagnosed in cancer patients and may present as generalised weakness. Weakness may be related to the cancer, but may be due to emotional factors, treatment or other disease processes.

CAUSES OF WEAKNESS	

• **Anxiety**
• **Depression**
• **Anaemia**
• **Infection**
• **Pain**
• **Arthritis**
• **Cardiovascular**
   – Angina
   – Postural hypotension
	• **Neurological**
	   – Spinal cord compression
	   – Hemiparesis
	   – Myopathy
	   – Neuropathy
	• **Drugs**
	   – Corticosteroids
	   – Anti-hypertensives
	   – Hypoglycaemics
	   – Diuretics

CANCER CACHEXIA

The syndrome of cancer cachexia consists of anorexia, weight loss and weakness. Studies have suggested that 50% of patients have some degree of cachexia at presentation whilst the majority develop cachexia at some point during their illness. It is the combination of poor nutrition and altered metabolism which leads to skeletal muscle breakdown and loss of body fat, causing weight loss and weakness.

Inadequate Nutrition

There are many factors which give rise to inadequate nutrition. Anorexia remains a major cause. Others include difficulties in swallowing (due to local tumour or bulbar muscle weakness), nausea, vomiting and malabsorption. There may also be physical problems with feeding including weakness, loss of function of upper limbs and social difficulties (such as being unable to shop for food or prepare sufficiently nourishing meals).

Metabolic Abnormalities in Cancer Cachexia.

The exact mechanism for cancer cachexia remains unclear. Animal and human studies confirm abnormalities in protein, carbohydrate and lipid metabolism.[1,2] Measurable abnormalities in cancer patients include raised triglyceride and cholesterol levels, reduced albumin and protein, glucose intolerance and raised lactic acid.

Increased metabolism

Resting energy expenditure is raised in many but not all cancer patients (opposite to other malnutrition states, where it is lowered). The tumour itself accounts for only a small percentage of the energy used. It appears to be the host response to the cancer which mediates the hypermetabolism. Coupled with low nutritional intake this leads to a negative energy balance and subsequent weight loss.

Carbohydrate metabolism

Abnormal carbohydrate metabolism has been observed. Insulin resistance is common leading to glucose intolerance. There is an increased rate of hepatic gluconeogenesis and abnormal peripheral utilisation of glucose. It has been demonstrated that there are increased levels of Cori cycle activity, an energy-inefficient pathway whereby lactate produced by anaerobic glycolysis is converted back to glucose in the liver. The body's normal ability to preserve skeletal muscle protein in chronic starvation states is lost. There is evidence for increased total body protein turnover and skeletal muscle proteins are broken down to release amino acids to be used for visceral protein synthesis. There is also evidence for increased conversion of alanine, an essential amino acid, to glucose in the liver. This altered metabolism leads to marked skeletal muscle loss and subsequent functional weakness.

Fat metabolism

Loss of body fat occurs due to both reduced lipid synthesis and increased lipolysis.

Increased plasma levels of glycerol and free fatty acids suggest increased fat mobilisation. Hypertriglyceridaemia is also noted and corresponds to reduced activity of lipoprotein lipase, the enzyme responsible for the movement of triglycerides from blood into adipocytes for lipid synthesis.

Humoral Factors

There is increasing evidence to support the role of circulating humoral factors in the mediation of the abnormal metabolism in cancer cachexia. Substances capable of producing cachexia are secreted by certain types of cancer but *most humoral factors are produced by the host* in response to the tumour.

Cytokines   Tumour necrosis factor (TNF) and interleukin-1 (IL-1) are cytokines produced by macrophages and lymphocytes in response to various stimuli including the presence of cancer cells.

TNF given to laboratory animals can cause anorexia and weight loss. Limited studies suggest that this effect is also seen in humans. In vitro studies show lipid depletion of adipocytes and increased glycogenesis in hepatocytes in the presence of TNF. These findings mimic those found in humans with cachexia. However, TNF levels in cachectic cancer patients are not consistently elevated, suggesting others factors are involved. Interleukin-1 (IL-1), is secreted by macrophages under the same conditions as TNF and acts synergistically with it. It appears that IL-1 has a role in the mediation of cancer cachexia. Animal studies also implicate interleukin-6 and interferon.

MANAGEMENT OF ANOREXIA AND WEAKNESS

Reversible causes   A clear history and careful examination of the patient is essential as there may be several reversible factors. Pain needs to be well controlled. Where appropriate to the patient's general condition anaemia and infection should be treated. Spinal cord compression should be excluded in a patient who complains of recent onset of weakness in the legs. There may be evidence of hemiparesis resulting from cerebral metastases which may respond to corticosteroid treatment and radiotherapy.

Depression   Depression can be easily overlooked in patients with advanced cancer. There is often overlap of symptoms such as tiredness, poor appetite and disturbed sleep pattern. Hopelessness, a feeling of worthlessness and persistent loss of enjoyment of any part of life may be the critical findings. Treatment of the depression will often allow for improved appetite and for the person to regain motivation, activity and strength.

Drug History

It is essential to review all drug therapy. Oral hypoglycaemics started at normal body weight may cause low blood sugar once the person has lost a significant amount of weight. Antihypertensives and diuretics may cause postural hypotension or hypokalaemia. Prolonged steroid usage may have led to proximal myopathy. Nausea and anorexia may be due to a number of drugs including digoxin and antibiotics. Consider stopping or reducing any drug which could be contributing to the person's weakness.

Treat any Gastrointestinal Symptoms
Mouthcare

Good mouth care is essential. Regular oral hygiene should be encouraged. A dry mouth may be eased by the regular use of mouth washes, chewing pineapple chunks, application of artificial saliva, sucking crushed ice or regular sips of water or fizzy drinks. A coated tongue may be scrubbed with a toothbrush or effervescent vitamin C may be left to loosen the debris.

Oral candida should be treated aggressively. Nystatin suspension or pastilles used four times daily may be difficult for patients to comply with. In these patients or those with oropharyngeal infection oral fluconazole, 50mg daily for 1 week, may be preferred. Regular cleaning of teeth and dentures is important and dentures should be soaked in Nystatin suspension overnight to prevent re-infection. Ill-fitting dentures can be easily relined.

Taste

Many patients find that their sense of taste and smell is altered, particularly a new dislike of cigarette smoke, tea and coffee. People may need encouragement to experiment with different types of food to identify which ones will now be enjoyed.

Pro-kinetic drugs

Early satiety is common with patients who have an enlarged liver squashing the stomach or ascites. This may be helped by agents that enhance gastric emptying such as metoclopramide, domperidone or cisapride.

Persistent nausea, the anticipation of vomiting and unrelieved constipation all play a large part in causing a person to be anorexic and feel generally lethargic. It may be hard to persuade patients to agree to bowel intervention when they feel too weak to be bothered sitting on a commode but judgement needs to be made about whether in the longer term the person will benefit.

Environmental effects on appetite

Presentation of food and the surroundings in which it is served have a big effect on appetite. Too much food piled on a plate may effectively turn off a patient's appetite. Small meals attractively arranged on a small plate are more likely to be enjoyed by an ill person. Soft or easily chewed and swallowed foods are preferable. People find it easier to eat sitting up at a table or well supported in bed than lying semi-recumbent.

Patients may be very sensitive to smells (even those which are not unpleasant to healthy people) and to the sight of food and meals may need to be served well away from the kitchen or ward area. For some patients, eg those who have had facial surgery or problems with excess saliva, it may be important to have privacy in which to eat.

Enhancing Nutrition

There are conflicting reports about the benefits of enteral tube feeding or total parenteral nutrition (TPN) in cancer patients.[3] Operative mortality and surgical complications in gastrointestinal cancer can be reduced but there is no evidence of improved tumour response or survival.

Weight gain was noted in patients being treated for small cell carcinoma of the lung after TPN but this consisted of fat and fluid rather than muscle bulk and patients lost weight more quickly than the control group when TPN was stopped. TPN or enteral tube feeding do not benefit cachectic patients in terms of weight gain, increased functional capacity or quality of life.

Active Patients with dysphagia

The exception to this is those patients with dysphagia due to head and neck cancers, oesophageal cancers or bulbar palsy who are still comparatively fit. They need feeding by NG tube or gastrostomy to prevent distressing symptoms of hunger and premature death from malnutrition.

However, for patients who are unable to utilise the increased calorie intake it seems doubtful whether their quality of life would be improved with time-consuming feeding regimes.

Dietician   The advice of a dietitian should be sought and will normally be welcomed by patients and families as many are uncertain as to which foods will be most beneficial. There are available a large range of high protein and calorie supplemental foods and the dietitian will be able to inform patients and staff about which will be suitable. The dietitian will also have expert knowledge about the cultural and psychological aspects of food and will be able to advise on alternative methods of feeding, where appropriate.

DRUG THERAPY

There have been several drugs suggested which may have an effect on appetite and weight but the only proven agents remain corticosteroids and progestogens.

Corticosteroids   Randomised placebo-controlled clinical trials have shown that corticosteroids improve appetite and sense of well-being in patients with advanced cancer. However this effect may only last for a few weeks and most studies show a significant placebo effect. Moertel et al.[4] randomised 116 patients to dexamethasone 3mg, 6mg or placebo. Patients on dexamethasone had significantly increased appetite although no weight gain or enhanced survival. There was a significant placebo response with 44% of patients in the placebo wing reporting increase in appetite.

Willox et al.[5] showed appetite and well being improved more on 15mg prednisolone as compared with placebo although again there was a placebo effect in 50% of patients.

A randomised, double-blind placebo-controlled crossover trial by Bruera et al[6] confirmed the appetite enhancing action of 32mg methylprednisolone. But the improvement at 2 weeks had disappeared by 4 weeks suggesting that the beneficial effect of steroids on appetite may be short-lived. There is no evidence that steroids have any effect on weight, performance status or clinical outcome. Steroids taken for a longer period of time may cause side-effects including oral candidiasis,

Timing of steroids

Mary was a 70 year old woman with carcinoma of the stomach and liver secondaries. She was referred to the outpatient clinic complaining of profound anorexia and weakness which she and her husband found intensely distressing. On more than one occasion they both voiced the feeling " If only Mary could eat more and have some energy they would be fine". She had no other symptoms and examination was unremarkable apart from a 5 cm palpable liver. After discussion she was started on dexamethasone 4 mg daily and was reviewed in the clinic 2 weeks later. There was a dramatic improvement in her appetite and she felt she had gained weight, possibly due to the fact that her face had filled out a little. She had much more energy and was able to go out for a meal with her husband for the first time for weeks. She remained well for another 5 weeks but then found that she was getting very weak and that her appetite was greatly reduced. She thought the dexamethasone was no longer helping her and asked to stop it, because she felt it was contributing to her swollen ankles. The dexamethasone was tailed off over the next 2 weeks and she died at home 3 weeks after that. Her husband commented that he was grateful to have had those few good weeks with her "as a bonus".

proximal myopathy, fluid retention and cushinoid facies.

Dose of steroids

The most effective corticosteroid and optimal dose for appetite stimulation is not known. Prednisolone 15mg daily or dexamethasone 2–4 mg daily are commonly used in practice. It would seem most beneficial to use steroids as a short term measure to improve appetite and to stop treatment after 4–6 weeks before major side-effects develop.

Progestogens

Megestrol acetate and medroxyprogesterone acetate cause weight gain in women with breast cancer. Several trials have shown that a proportion of patients with hormone insensitive tumours or

AIDS also have increased appetite and weight gain on progestogens.

Megestrol acetate   In a randomised study of 133 patients receiving 800mg megestrol acetate (median duration of 1.6 months) 16% gained 15lb or more compared with 2% of the placebo group.[7]

Another study treated 89 patients with 1600mg megestrol acetate or placebo for one month and found improved appetite in the megestrol group and a mean weight gain of 1.4kg compared with a mean weight loss of 0.2kg in the placebo group.[8]

Several authors have suggested that the weight gain is dose-dependent. The Tchekmedyian study[8] is disappointing in the relatively small weight gain seen for the large dose used compared with other studies. However, this study only lasted one month and it has been suggested that the effect of megestrol acetate is also *time-dependent*. Treatment may need to be sustained for at least 6–8 weeks before a definite improvement is seen. A proportion of patients may not respond but, at present, there does not seem to be any indicators of which patients will benefit.

A study of megestrol acetate varying from 160mg to 1280mg found a *dose related* response for improved appetite and a trend for weight gain. The optimal results were in patients treated with 800mg with no additional benefit from higher doses.[9] However, it is a relatively expensive drug and patients are less likely to comply with a large number of tablets, so it seems reasonable to start with a smaller dose.

A study of *body-composition* with megestrol acetate[10] showed the majority of the weight gain is body fat rather than fluid retention. There is no evidence that muscle strength is improved and there is the theoretical possibility that increasing a person's weight and not their muscle strength may reduce mobility. However, current studies suggest that this is probably not clinically significant.

The *side-effects* of megestrol acetate are minimal. Nausea has been reported although in Loprinzi's study nausea was more reported in the placebo group. Peripheral oedema and, less commonly, venous thrombosis have occurred but the vast majority of patients show no ill-effects.

Medroxyprogesterone Acetate

There have been fewer controlled trials using the progestogen medroxyprogesterone acetate. One study showed improved appetite but no weight gain using 300mg daily.[11] Higher doses are thought to have similar benefits and side-effects to megestrol acetate. The optimal dose is not yet clear but a suggested daily dose is 400–800mg daily.

Cyproheptadine

Cyproheptadine is a serotonin antagonist which has been used as an appetite stimulant in patients with anorexia nervosa and children with anorexia. Studies in cancer patients showed mild appetite stimulation but no weight gain and the overall benefit of this drug in cancer patients remains doubtful.[12]

Hydrazine

Hydrazine sulphate inhibits the action of the enzyme phosphoenol pyruvate carboxykinase which is responsible for the conversion of oxalo-acetate from the Krebs' cycle into the process of gluconeogenesis. This finding led to the hope that hydrazine might be beneficial in preventing some of the metabolic effects of cancer cachexia. However, despite some early studies with lung cancer patients who showed less protein breakdown than the placebo group, this has not yet been borne out in larger studies.[12]

Pentoxifylline

This is thought to inhibit TNF but studies have failed to confirm an appetite-enhancing effect.[12]

Cannabinoids

Cancer patients given dronabinol at doses higher than 2.5mg daily have shown elevation of mood and appetite enhancement but it is not known whether this is sustained and whether side-effects outweigh the benefits.

Beta-adrenergic Agonists

Clenbuterol can prevent muscle depletion in tumour-bearing rats receiving TPN. Both salbutamol[13] and clenbuterol[14] have been shown to increase voluntary muscle fibre strength in healthy men but it is not yet known whether these drugs have any effect in cachectic cancer patients.

Alcohol

There are no controlled studies to support the use of alcohol for appetite stimulation in the terminally ill, but anecdotally it is recognised that alcohol may improve appetite and may improve mood, sleep, and allow relaxation. Drinking alcohol is also an important social activity which may have been curtailed during the person's illness. This may be due to taste changes or to alcohol intolerance which seems to develop in certain people with some types of malignancy. Many patients have taken notice of the warning on the medication packaging advising them to avoid alcohol when taking potentially sedating drugs. Patients often need permission to drink alcohol with the explanation that if they are not driving or doing other activities needing absolute concentration they will not be adversely affected.

EXERCISE

Effects of immobility

It has been suggested that exercise may prevent or reverse the weakness of cachexia. Contractile activity increases muscle mass and protein content. Immobility in post-operative patients leads to reduced exercise tolerance and reduced aerobic capacity. One study gave healthy volunteers total parenteral nutrition (TPN) and randomised them to exercise or not.[3] Those in the non-exercise group showed a reduction in aerobic capacity whereas in the exercise group no such fall ocurred. This supports the theory that exercise is necessary for anabolic enhancement. Excercise also increases amino acid uptake in muscle and reduces protein turnover.

Comparison of exercise and reminiscence therapy

Exercise can improve function and quality of life in the elderly. In a study of 41 elderly people (mean age 81) in residential homes, randomised to twice weekly exercise or reminiscence therapy, the exercise group showed a mean improvement in grip strength, spinal flexion, chair-to-stand time and activities of daily living over 7 months, whereas the reminiscence group showed a deterioration. Both groups had reduced self-rated depression scores but the exercise group showed a significantly greater reduction[15]

Extrapolation from healthy people to those with cancer needs to be cautious, because of the underlying metabolic abnormalities. Cachectic patients may have great difficulty in complying with an exercise programme. The level of exercise needed to lead to benefits may be too strenuous for such patients.

Physiotherapy and Occupational Therapy

It is important that independence is maintained as long as possible. Early referral to an occupational therapist and physiotherapist allows appropriate advice and aids to be provided. Assess mobility, range of movement, muscle strength and daily functioning before designing a programme of rehabilitation. A home visit may be necessary to advise on the easiest way for the person to function at home. Bed, chair and toilet seat heights may need adjusting, stair rails may be fitted or the person may be advised to sleep downstairs. Walking aids or a wheelchair may help with mobility and confidence. People often find it hard to accept using these aids and they need to be introduced with sensitivity and careful explanation.

Diversional therapy

Diversional therapy is also important as boredom and social isolation will enhance symptoms. Attention needs to be given to exploring means by which people may be helped to continue with enjoyable social activities and hobbies and to take up new ones if they so wish.

PSYCHOSOCIAL SUPPORT

Treatments discussed in this chapter may improve weakness for a time, but it is often an inexorable process. Patients and their carers need help in understanding what is happening and that it is an integral part of the illness. They need to be encouraged to find ways of adapting to the change in life-style.

A great source of distress can be the change in roles within the family or partnership eg when a person can no longer manage the shopping or gardening or can no longer drive. Carers may feel they are

Appetite for life

Jim was 83 years and had a carcinoma of the lung. He complained angrily about being weak and not being able to eat properly. He had been prescribed steroids and anti-depressants for his appetite and mood but stopped taking them after a couple of weeks as "they weren't doing any good". His conversation was focused on his weakness and how no-one was doing anything for him. During one discussion he suddenly said "you're all no better than me!" When this was explored further he described how useless he was feeling and guilty that he could no longer look after his wife. He was concerned that she might need to go into a nursing home and felt that he had "let her down". He was encouraged to talk with his wife about his fears and it was arranged that they should both go into a nursing home together and that she would remain there after his death. At this point he appeared to take on a new lease of life, organising the move of some of their furniture to the nursing home and preparing to sell their own home. His appetite and mobility improved and for several weeks before his death he was able to play a very active part in the nursing home activities.

failing the patient if their role focuses on providing food. They need to be informed about the types of food which may be most palatable and to provide simple meals or snacks on a regular basis as most people will want to eat little and often. It may also ease their distress to be able to participate in other forms of care.

Patients may feel pressurised into eating larger quantities of food than they can face. They may need permission from professionals to eat less without feeling guilty and support in explaining this to relatives.

Both the patient and family may find it difficult to adapt to the patient needing to sleep downstairs or to the use of a wheelchair for outings. Patient and family members may accept change at a different pace, and fail to understand the hesitancy of the others.

A patient's complaint of weakness may be a way of expressing *emotional distress*. As the dictionary definitions quoted at the beginning of the chapter suggest weakness is not just a physical phenomenon. The fear of "giving way" or being "liable to break" is seen by many as being cowardly or inadequate and the patient may choose to express anger or fear in physical terms. It is important to spend time exploring these issues and to give patients the opportunity and permission to cry or be angry.

Assessment of quality of life

Quality of life is the important outcome in treatment of weakness and anorexia. Many clinicians in oncology and palliative care are now using Quality of Life measures to assess new treatments. There are a number of validated tools looking at aspects of quality of life:

- Hospital Anxiety and Depression scale
- Rotterdam Symptom Checklist
- EORTC QLQ-C30.

Bristol-Myers Instrument

Most of these were developed to assess a whole range of functions. A recent addition has been the development of Bristol-Myers Anorexia\Cachexia Recovery Instrument (BACRI) which is designed specifically to assess the impact of appetite stimulation and weight gain upon well-being, body image, health perceptions and global quality of life.

In a double-blind, randomised study of AIDS patients given either placebo or megestrol acetate (100mg, 400mg or 800mg) there was a significant improvement in weight with 400mg and 800mg of megestrol acetate as compared with the placebo and 100mg treatment group. Subjective recovery from anorexia\cachexia using a 7 item score (BACRI-7) and patient's perception of benefit using a one item score (BACRI-1) correlated with improvements in weight. [16] Further studies to assess the validity of using BACRI-1 and BACRI-7 with patients suffering from cancer-related anorexia and cachexia are on-going.

DISCUSSION AND SUMMARY

Anorexia and weakness occur frequently in patients with advanced malignant disease, due to physical, emotional, spiritual and social factors. Cachexia is largely irreversible with current knowledge and the focus of management should be to improve quality of life.

Assessment

The full multi-disciplinary team, including the patient and informal carers, should be involved. A detailed history is needed and careful examination and appropriate investigations should be performed to identify *treatable factors*. *Drug therapy* should be reviewed with the aim of reducing or stopping any drug which might be contributing to the symptoms. The patient's *emotional state* must be assessed and anti-depressants or anxiolytics prescribed as appropriate.

Attention needs to be paid to general measures such as the environment and *presentation of food*. The person's *daily functioning should be assessed* and advice and aids provided to maximise independence. The patient and family should be offered the opportunity to discuss the necessary changes in life-style and to explore and be supported in any emotional distress.

Increased nutrition will not improve survival but may improve quality of life. A few selected patients with mechanical difficulties in eating may benefit from enteral or parenteral nutrition but for the majority of patients with advanced cancer it is doubtful whether it would bestow benefit.

Drug treatment

Appetite stimulants can help. *Short term corticosteroids* will improve appetite and general well-being. If the prognosis is felt to be a few weeks, then dexamethasone 2–4mg daily or prednisolone 15mg daily can be prescribed and the patient carefully monitored for evidence of side-effects. After 4–6 weeks the steroid is unlikely to continue to be of benefit and should be stopped unless the patient needs steroids for other reasons. If the prognosis is longer than a few weeks then a *progestogen* such as megestrol acetate or medroxy-progesterone acetate should be considered. On current knowledge it would seem reasonable to prescribe megestrol acetate 320–480mg daily or medroxyprogesterone 400–800mg daily. Judging prognosis is difficult, so it may be pragmatic to combine these two approaches and prescribe both agents for a few weeks and then stop the corticosteroid. The patient may hopefully then gain the immediate benefit of the corticosteroid and the longer term benefit of the progestogen without the disadvantages of either drug.

Several other drugs have been suggested for reversing cancer cachexia, but more research needs to be done to establish or refute their effectiveness. There is no clear place for these agents outside clinical trials.

Exercise   *The role of exercise* in improving weakness in cancer cachexia is unproven. It may slow the catabolism of skeletal muscle or even help to strengthen muscle. In view of the improvement in depression scores and functioning seen in elderly patients who exercise regularly it would seem worthwhile encouraging a reasonable amount of activity in the hope of improving the patient's quality of life.

References

1. Langstein HN, Norton JA. Mechanisms of cancer cachexia. Haematol Oncol Clin North Am 1991; 5: 103–123
2. Keller U. Pathophysiology of cancer cachexia. Support Care Cancer 1993; 1:290–294
3. Ng E-H, Lowry SF. Nutritional support and cancer cachexia. Haematol Oncol Clin North Am 1991: 5: 161–184
4. Moertel CG, Schutt AJ, Reitemeier RJ, Hahn RG. Corticosteroid therapy of preterminal gastrointestinal cancer. Cancer 1974; 33: 1607–1609
5. Willox JC, Corr J, Shaw J, Richardson M, Calman KC, Drennan M. Prednisolone as an appetite stimulant in patients with cancer. Br Med J 1984; 288: 27
6. Bruera E. Current pharmacological management of anorexia in cancer patients. Oncology 1992; 6: 125–1307.
7. Loprinzi CL, Ellison NM, Schaid DJ, Krook JE, Athmann LM, Dose AM, Mailliard JA, Johnson PS, Ebbert LP, Geeraerts LH. Controlled trial of megestrol acetate for the treatment of cancer anorexia and cachexia. J Natl Cancer Inst 1990; 82: 1127–1132
8. Tchekmedyian SN, Hickman M, Siau J, Greco FA, Keller J, Browder H, Aisner J. Cancer 1992; 69: 1268–1274
9. Loprinzi CL, Bernath AM, Schaid DJ, Malliard JA, Athmann LM, Michalak JC, Tschetter LK, Hatfield AK, Morton RF. Phase 111 evaluation of 4 doses of megestrol acetate as therapy for patients with cancer anorexia and\or cachexia. Oncology 1994; 51 suppl 1: 2–7

10. Loprinzi CL, Schaid DJ, Dose AM, Burnham NL, Jensen MD. Body-composition changes in patients who gain weight while receiving megestrol acetate. J Clin Oncol 1993; 11: 152–154

11. Downer S, Joel S, Allbright A, Plant H, Stubbs L, Talbot D, Slevin M. A double blind placebo controlled trial of medroxyprogesterone acetate (MPA) in cancer cachexia. Br J Cancer 1993; 67: 1102–1105

12. Loprinzi CL. Management of cancer anorexia\cachexia. Support Care Cancer 1995; 3 (2): 120–122

13. Martineau L, Horan MA, Rothwell NJ, Little RA. Salbutamol,a beta-2–adrenoceptor agonist, increases skeletal muscle strength in young men. Clin Sci 1992; 83: 615–621

14. Maltin CA, Delday MI, Watson JS, Heys SD, Nevison IM, Ritchie IK, Gibson PH. Clenbuterol, a beta-2–adrenoceptor agonist, increases relative muscle strength in orthopaedic patients. Clin Sci 1993; 84: 651–654

15. McMurdo MET, Rennie L. A controlled trial of exercise by residents of old people's homes. Age Ageing 1993; 22: 11–15

16. Cella DF, Von Roenn J, Lloyd S, Browder HP. The Bristol-Myers Anorexia/Cachexia Recovery Instrument (BACRI): a brief assessment of patients' subjective response to treatment for anorexia/ cachexia. Qual Life Res 1995; 4: 221–231

Chapter 9

Intestinal Obstruction

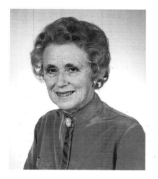

Dr Mary Baines
Mary Baines is a consultant physician at St Christopher's Hospice and has worked there since 1968. Her main interest is the control of symptoms in patients with advanced cancer and her research has been concerned with the management of malignant intestinal obstruction. In 1969 she was involved in setting up the first Hospice Home Care Department. She has written extensively, including chapters in the Oxford Textbooks of Medicine, Geriatric Medicine and Palliative Medicine. She has lectured widely and is especially interested in the development of Palliative Care services in the less developed world.

> "When thoust examinest a person who suffers from an obstruction in his abdomen and thou findest that it goes-and-comes under the fingers like oil-in-a-tube, then prepare for him: Fruit-of-the-Domplam, dissolved in Man's Semen. Crush, cook in Oil and Honey. To be eaten by the Patient for four mornings. Afterwards let him be smeared with dried, crushed, and pressed maqutgrain."
>
> (Ebers Papyrus, c.1500BC)

Intestinal obstruction has been recognized over 3000 years and some exotic remedies have obviously been tried. This chapter reviews our modern management.

INTRODUCTION

Intestinal obstruction is caused by an occlusion to the lumen of the bowel or a lack of normal propulsion, preventing or delaying intestinal contents from passing along the gastrointestinal tract. Obstruction may be the presenting symptom of cancer problem, but more commonly develops during the course of the disease. Any site in the bowel may be involved, from the gastroduodenal junction to the rectum and anus.

Until 20 years ago, most patients with advanced cancer who obstructed were sent for palliative surgery. The remainder, too ill for surgery, were managed with prolonged conservative treatment using IV fluids and a nasogastric tube. With the opening of hospices and the growth of Palliative Medicine as a specialty, a pharmacological approach to the problem was developed and described in 1985.[1] Since that time new drugs have become available which have improved the level of symptom control obtained. However, a proportion of patients with intestinal obstruction are still not well controlled with pharmacological measures alone and require some form of decompression. This is therefore an appropriate time for an update on the present situation.

PREVALENCE

There are only 2 patient groups in which the prevalence of intestinal obstruction has been studied. In patients with advanced cancer, admitted to a hospice, 3% developed intestinal obstruction during their terminal illness. The most common primary tumours were ovarian or large bowel (but many other primary tumours were, less frequently, involved.[2] In studies of patients with advanced ovarian cancer 25 - 42% developed obstruction.[3]

PATHOPHYSIOLOGY

Many different factors contribute to malignant obstruction in advanced abdominal or pelvic cancer. Primary tumours of the large bowel can occlude the lumen in a polypoid or annular fashion. Extramural compression is caused by tumour masses or malignant adhesions. Motility disorders, leading to a functional obstruction, can be due to tumour infiltration of intestinal muscle, mesentery or coeliac plexus. Frequently, these causes coexist and, in addition, the obstruction may be at several sites.

CLINICAL FEATURES

The symptoms and signs of intestinal obstruction will depend on the level at which it occurs.

SYMPTOMS AND SIGNS OF INTESTINAL OBSTRUCTION

	Pain	Vomiting	Distension	Bowel Sounds
Duodenum	None	Severe. Large with amounts undigested food	None	Succussion splash may be present
Small bowel	Upper to central abdominal colic	Moderate to severe	Moderate	Usually hyper-active with borborygmi
Large bowel	Central to lower abdominal colic	Develops late	Great	Borborygmi

Malignant obstruction may present acutely with sudden onset of colicky abdominal pain, vomiting and constipation. More often, however, the onset of obstruction is insidious, over weeks or months. Symptoms may gradually worsen and become continuous but, even without treatment, symptoms may be intermittent and the obstructive episodes resolve spontaneously, if temporarily.

The distinction is often made between complete and partial (subacute) obstruction, but this is far from easy in practice and, clinically, the obstruction may appear to alter from one type to the other on several occasions as the illness progresses.

DIFFERENTIAL DIAGNOSIS

Severe constipation occasionally presents with symptoms of intestinal obstruction. Differential diagnosis is usually possible following a careful history and examination. Sometimes abdominal X-rays are needed. Certain drugs, notably the opioids and those with anticholinergic effects reduce gut motility and increase the likelihood of severe constipation.

ASSESSMENT

History

Medical history must include records previous surgery and investigations. The presence and nature of pain should be noted, with specific questioning about colic which is often described as 'wind pain' or 'gripes'. The frequency, volume and composition of vomits is important; patients with faeculent vomiting will complain of its unpleasant taste and smell.

A careful history of bowel dysfunction will usually distinguish between constipation and obstruction. Constipation should be suspected if there is a history of infrequent defaecation with increasingly hard faeces. This contrasts with the situation in subacute obstruction when patients complain of colic and diarrhoea due to waves of peristalsis propelling bowel contents through a narrowing lumen. This precedes the development of a complete obstruction when there will be, of course, no passage of faeces or flatus.

Examination

Examination will show the patient's general condition and nutritional status. Abdominal examination will note distension, ascites, hepatomegaly, tumour or faecal masses and bowel sounds. A rectal examination must be done.

Investigations

Investigations should only be done if these will influence the treatment offered. In practice, there are two clinical situations where radiological and endoscopic investigations are of value. The first is to differentiate between severe constipation and malignant obstruction. The second is to confirm the obstruction and determine its site and nature in the patient who is being considered for surgery. In the patient with severe constipation abdominal X-rays show gross faecal retention throughout the colon and there may be associated gaseous distension and fluid levels.

Barium contrast studies and endoscopy will show the cause in the great majority of patients with duodenal obstruction. Erect and supine abdominal X-rays should be the first investigative procedures in patients with suspected small bowel obstruction. These show the size of bowel loops and the relative amounts of air and fluid within them. Dilation and fluid levels occur proximal to the site of obstruction. Anterograde and retrograde contrast studies using barium are occasionally needed to obtain information regarding the cause of obstruction.

If large bowel obstruction is suspected, abdominal X-rays should be taken with the patient in different positions, to outline different parts of the large bowel. These may be followed by a barium enema and sigmoidoscopy or colonoscopy.

Psychological factors

Psychological and social factors are extremely important in the decision about treatment options. The patient's age, emotional state, will to live and social support will all influence the decisions that are made about surgery, venting procedures and artificial hydration.

MANAGEMENT OPTIONS

Surgery

Surgery to restore continuity of the bowel should be considered for every patient with advanced cancer who develops intestinal obstruction. A proportion will have a non-malignant cause or an unrelated second primary tumour. Palliative surgery which can offer some individuals a long symptom free period, and should be considered in every case.

The decision to operate on a patient with advanced cancer is not easy and each case must be carefully and individually assessed. The situation is rarely an absolute emergency, so that time may be taken for investigations, if appropriate. The patient and family must be informed about the situation so that their wishes can be determined.

Poor prognostic factors for surgery include advanced age, poor general medical condition or nutritional status, ascites, abdominal masses and previous combination chemotherapy. Obstruction due to recurrent colorectal cancer has a better prognosis than tumours in ovary, endometrium, cervix or pancreas. Small bowel obstruction carriers a higher mortality and morbidity than large bowel obstruction. Emergency surgery increases the mortality threefold.

Surgical colleagues are becoming aware of the pharmacological approach to management, and no longer feel compelled to operate simply to prevent a distressing death from obstruction.

Controlling symptoms without surgery

Sarah, aged 63, had a transitional cell carcinoma of the bladder which had been treated, for 11 years, with repeated diathermy. When a large recurrence developed she had a total cystectomy and ileal conduit followed by pelvic irradiation. Unfortunately, 3 months later, she developed large bowel obstruction due to recurrent pelvic tumour. She was admitted to hospital complaining of lower abdominal pain, vomiting and constipation.

In addition to Sarah's malignancy, she had an above-knee amputation of the right leg, following an injury, and a left hemiplegia. The surgeon discussed the possibility of a colostomy with Sarah but said that, if she declined this, her symptoms could be controlled with drugs. After consideration, Sarah chose not to have surgery and she was started on a subcutaneous infusion of diamorphine and haloperidol. Until her death 16 days later, the pain and vomiting were controlled by an increase in diamorphine to 40mg/24 hours and a change to methotrimeprazine 50-100mg/24 hours as the anti-emetic. She had no bowel action for 5 weeks.

Gastrointestinal intubation

The insertion of a *nasogastric tube* is almost routinely done when an obstructed patient, with advanced cancer, is admitted to hospital. However, a review of the surgical literature shows that, sustained response to such treatment is very poor, being only 0-2%. Conservative treatment should be reserved for patients who are being considered for palliative surgery while investigations are performed and the patient's wishes elucidated.

If appropriate, surgery should be undertaken as soon as possible. There is no value in repeated hospital admissions for nasogastric intubation and IV fluids in a patient with advanced cancer in the hope that this treatment will resolve the obstruction. In the majority of cases, obstructive symptoms can be controlled pharmacologically without intubation. However a small group, mainly with gastroduodenal or jejunal obstruction, do require prolonged intubation or, possibly, a venting gastrostomy.

Venting gastrostomy

A venting gastrostomy or jejunostomy can be used to relieve intractable nausea and vomiting in patients with inoperable intestinal obstruction. It is more effective and more acceptable than prolonged nasogastric drainage. In most series, patients treated in this way were placed on a liquid diet, the gastrostomy tube being clamped at meals and for as long afterwards as could be tolerated. Good relief of nausea and vomiting was obtained and, in some, the gastrostomy output was reduced, presumably due to a remission of the obstruction.

Unfortunately, most authors describe the use of a venting gastrostomy as the primary treatment for inoperable bowel obstruction without first considering pharmacological treatment. It is probable that some patients could have been managed with medication, without recourse to surgery and tubes which inevitably add to the distress of terminal illness. Further studies are needed to define 'The small subgroup of patients who do not respond adequately to pharmacological measures and require some form of decompression or venting procedure.

PHARMACOLOGICAL TREATMENT

The opening of hospices and the development of the speciality of Palliative Medicine led to the search for pharmacological measures to relieve symptoms in patients with inoperable intestinal obstruction. This is because the majority of hospice patients are unfit for surgery or have already had a laparotomy at which no procedure was.possible.

The portable syringe driver was an important development and continuous subcutaneous infusion is the preferred route of drug administration. A combination of drugs can be given to control the symptoms (colic, continuous abdominal pain, nausea and vomiting) so the patient maintains mobility and independence. It is ideal for use in the home as it can be loaded every 24 hours by the visiting nurse. Other routes are less effective and are now, in developed countries, rarely used.

However, if a syringe driver is not available it is still possible to offer good symptom control; drugs can be given rectally or by bolus IV injections.

Analgesics

Diamorphine and morphine are equally effective in the management of continuous abdominal pain. They may relieve intestinal colic but often an anti-spasmodic is needed in addition. If diamorphine is available (as in the UK) it is preferred because of its greater solubility, The dose of opioid should be titrated against the response, increasing until pain relief is obtained.

Antispasmodics

Colic is caused by waves of increased peristalsis against the resistance of a mechanical or functional obstruction. Colic can sometimes be relieved with analgesic drugs alone but, more often, an anti-spasmodic is also needed. Hyoscine butylbromide (Buscopan) is most commonly used, it does not cross the blood-brain barrier and cause central side effects. This drug also reduces gastrointestinal secretions and has been shown to lessen the frequency and volume of vomits.

Antiemetics

The choice of an antiemetic to control obstructive vomiting and nausea is determined, to a

DRUGS USED TO RELIEVE SYMPTOMS IN INTESTINAL OBSTRUCTION

Symptom	Drug	Dose/24hrs (by subcutaneous infusion)	Comment
Intestinal colic	Diamorphine or morphine	As required	Antispasmodics is also needed
	Hyoscine butylbromide	60-300mg	Not sedating
Continuous abdominal pain	Diamorphine or morphine	As required	Antiemetic of choice
Nausea and Vomiting	Haloperidol	5-15mg	May crystallise in syringe driver
	Cyclizine	100-200mg	
	Hyoscine butylbromide	60-300mg	Reduces gastro-intestinal secretions
	Octreotide	0.3-0.6mg	Reduces gastro-intestinal secretions and motility
	Methotrimeprazine	50-150mg	Very effective antiemetic but sedating
	Metoclopramide	60-160mg	May increase colic
Diarrhoea (from subacute obstruction or faecal fistula)	Loperamide	6-16mg (orally)	
	Octreotide	0.3-0.6mg	Decreases secretions and peristalsis

considerable extent, by the possibility of giving it by SC infusion in the syringe driver. If prochloro-perazine or chlorpromazine are given by this method, painful swellings result that may take weeks to subside. Biopsy of these injection sites shows fat necrosis in the subcutaneous tissues.

Haloperidol and *cyclizine* are both used by different centres as initial treatment. Although they have quite different sites of action in the emetic process, there is probably little difference in their efficacy in this situation. However, cyclizine has a tendency to precipitate in the syringe driver when mixed with other drugs.

Methotrimeprazine

Methotrimeprazine is a phenothiazine with antiemetic and analgesic effects. It is of value in intractable vomiting but, as it causes sedation, it is mainly used for very ill patients. Subcutaneous irritation may occur necessitating changes of site every few days.

Prokinetic Antiemetics

Metoclopramide and cisapride one prokinetic antiemetics. Their place in the management of obstructive vomiting remains controversial. The early studies avoided these drugs as they had been found, on occasions, to increase colic and could lead to perforation or fistula formation if the obstruction was complete. In a study where metoclopramide was the antiemetic, the doses of morphine used were significantly higher than in a comparable study using haloperidol and hyoscine butylbromide.

However, many patients have partial obstruction and, theoretically, prokinetic antiemetics could be useful. In addition, metoclopramide, unlike many other antiemetics, is not sedating. Unfortunately, there will be little progress to help in the choice of antiemetic until controlled trials are done. For the moment, it is recommended that if metoclopramide is used, a 24 hour trial is given, stopping treatment if colic occurs.

Ondansetron

Ondansetron and granisetron have greatly improved the control of chemotherapy induced vomiting. Some verbal case reports suggest that they may be useful in patients with intractable obstructive vomiting. Ondansetron can be given by subcutaneous infusion, 8-16 mg/24 hours, but it is very expensive.

Octreotide

Octreotide is a synthetic stable analogue of somatostatin (which has a very short half-life and is not used therapeutically). Octreotide, has a half-life of about 1.5 hours with a duration of action of 12 hours. It is usually given by SC infusion and can be mixed with other drugs with no loss of efficacy.

Obstructed patients may still eat

Michael, aged 37, developed a carcinoma of the hepatic flexure of the colon and had a right hemicolectomy. He remained well for 10 months, then was admitted to hospital complaining of colicky abdominal pain, distension and vomiting. Abdominal X-rays indicated small bowel obstruction and a laparotomy was performed. Unfortunately, no procedure was possible as there was multiple malignant adhesions with adherence of the greater omentum to the peritoneum at many sites. He was discharged home but readmitted to hospital on three occasions during the next 4 months with symptoms of obstruction. On each occasion he was treated with intravenous fluids and naso-gastric suction. On hospice admission, he was complaining of colic, abdominal pain and vomiting, which was noted to be faeculent. A subcutaneous infusion using a syringe driver was started with cyclizine as the antiemetic, 150mg/24 hours. During the next weeks this was changed to methotrimeprazine, increasing the dose to 100mg/24 hours. On this regime, he vomited (usually once) on 15 out of 36 days. He was rarely nauseated and continued to eat small amounts. He remained alert until 2 days before his death. Post mortem examination showed multiple levels of obstruction with gross dilation of small and large bowel due to widespread malignant adhesions.

Somatostatin is a naturally occurring hormone, widely distributed in the body and having many physiological functions. Somatostatin causes a reduction in the volume of gastrointestinal secretions by increasing the absorbtion of water and electrolytes and inhibiting their secretion. It also decreases gut peristalsis, from the stomach to the large bowel. The role of octreotide in the symptomatic management of intestinal obstruction is due to its effect on gastrointestinal secretions and motility.

Octreotide has been used since 1992 to relieve obstructive vomiting and to reduce the diarrhoea caused by subacute obstruction and from entero-cutaneous or enterovaginal fistulae. Abdominal pain, colic and distension are often improved. Significant side effects have not been noticed in this patient group.

Unfortunately, octreotide is an expensive drug and, at this stage, probably it should be reserved for patients who have a high obstruction or whose vomiting is not controlled with antiemetics. Hyoscine butylbromide has similar effects in reducing gastrointestinal secretions and motility. A controlled clinical trial is planned to compare these two drugs.

The value of octreotide

Jane, aged 19, had developed a leiomyosarcoma of the ileum two years previously. She had been treated surgically on three occasions with debulking of the tumour and had received combination chemotherapy. On her last hospital admission, she was found to be in intestinal obstruction and X-rays showed this to be at 3 sites in the bowel. No further surgery was possible and she returned home. When she was first seen, she had no bowel action for ten days, she was vomiting every 2 or 3 hours and was unable to retain the MST tablets which had previously controlled her pain. A subcutaneous infusion of diamorphine 40mg, haloperidol 5mg and octreotide 300mg over 24-hours was started. An increase in octreotide to 600mg was needed to control her vomiting but, on this regime, she was able to drink well and eat the occasional meal (such as curry and rice) with her family. After having no bowel action for 30 days, she passed a large loose stool on 3 occasions. There was then no further bowel action until her death 14 days later. No vomiting occurred during the this time and the dose of octreotide remained at 600mg/24 hours.

Corticosteroids

Since the anti-inflammatory effect of corticosteroids causes reduction of peri-tumour inflammatory oedema, steroids have been used for some years in the management of obstructed patients with the expectation that they will cause an opening up of the obstruction and result in relief of symptoms.

Small groups of patients have been reported to have benefited but no clinical trials have been conducted. The intermittent nature of early obstructive symptoms makes it difficult to determine whether any improvement is due to the steroid treatment.

Laxatives

Stimulant laxatives, such as senna, are contra-indicated in obstructed patients. Faecal-softening laxatives, such as moderate doses of magnesium hydroxide and liquid paraffin or docusate, can be given to patients with a colonic or rectal obstruction. With the more usual small bowel obstruction, there is no role for laxatives.

Prescribing

In practice, the symptoms of colic, continuous abdominal pain and vomiting usually occur together and a typical prescription, when treatment is started, would be:

A TYPICAL PRESCRIPTION	
Diamorphine or morphine	30mg
Hyoscine butylbromide	60mg
Haloperidol	5mg
Given over 24 hours in the syringe driver.	

If continuous pain or colic are not controlled, the dose of diamorphine or hyoscine butylbromide should be increased. If vomiting is a problem, the dose of haloperidol can be increased, a trial of hyoscine butylbromide at a higher dose could be employed, or a change made to another antiemetic or to octreotide.

Gastroduodenal (high) Obstruction

This is much less common than intestinal obstruction and is usually caused by a primary tumour in the stomach or pancreas. Patients with pancreatic cancer are now usually treated with biliary stenting rather than by-pass surgery. Such surgery often included a gastroenterostomy, and this prevented the spread of tumour into the duodenum from causing a high obstruction. Pharmacological treatment is less useful than with intestinal obstruction but sometimes, if the obstruction is partial, a prokinetic antiemetic such as metoclopramide 60-240mg/day is effective. If there is no response, a trial of corticosteroids is suggested using dexamethasone 8mg/day by injection. Octreotide 0.3-0.6mg/day has sometimes proved very effective in controlling this type of vomiting.

If these methods do not give relief, a nasogastric tube should be inserted and a venting gastrostomy considered. Fluids should be given by hypodermoclysis or IV infusion unless the patient is in the terminal phase.

NUTRITION AND HYDRATION

With good control of nausea, most patients choose to eat small and mainly fluid meals. These are mostly absorbed in the proximal part of the gastrointestinal tract. With adequate oral fluids, thirst is rarely a problem. A dry mouth is treated with local measures such as providing crushed ice to suck. Occasionally, a patient is found who is attempting to eat too much, usually due to pressure from the family. It is then helpful to talk with them about the 'partial blockage' that exists and to remind them that a great deal of nourishment can be given in liquid form.

A small group of patients, mainly those with high obstruction, continue to vomit profusely in spite of medication. These may benefit from the insertion of a nasogastric tube or venting gastrostomy. Fluids have traditionally been given IV but, in this situation, hypodermoclysis (SC infusion) is recommended. This route avoids the problem of maintaining venous access, it can be given by any member of staff including a community nurse, and it can be used intermittently. Some patients receive hypodermoclysis overnight and it is removed during the day to allow normal mobility.

DISCUSSION

Anticipation of the problem

Some patients develop an obstruction unexpectedly but in many others with advanced, multifocal and especially ovarian disease this complication can be anticipated. This should mean that decisions about treatment can be planned beforehand.

In practice, this will mean that the oncologist or hospice doctor will have full records of previous surgery and relevant investigations. It may be helpful to monitor renal and hepatic function for, if these are deteriorating, the likelihood of successful surgery is small. It is important to know what each patient wants for his or her future. Direct questioning may not be appropriate but it is helpful to record phrases such as 'I could never cope with more surgery' or 'I'd give anything to get to her wedding this summer'.

If the patient is likely to obstruct and it is clear that surgery is not indicated it is important to have drugs written up and easily available.

When obstruction occurs

If there is any possibility that palliative surgery is an option, the patient should be admitted to hospital. Nasogastric suction and IV fluids will probably be given to decompress the bowel and maintain hydration and electrolyte balance. Relevant investigations will then be carried out to determine the site and nature of the obstruction before a decision about surgery is made. If this is indicated it should be carried out without delay.

If surgery is contraindicated there is no necessity to admit the patient to hospital or hospice. The syringe driver should be started with a combination of analgesics, antispasmodics and antiemetics appropriate to the symptoms. The same symptomatic treatment should be given to the patient who is in hospital receiving conservative treatment when a decision against surgery has been made. In most cases, as pain and vomiting are reduced it will be possible to withdraw the nasogastric tube and IV infusion.

However, any decision about the place to care must take into account the wishes of the patient and family, and the level of community support available. In some situations it will be right to admit the patient for a close monitoring of symptoms and for emotional support. Hopefully, as things improve, discharge will be possible.

Review regularly

It is almost certain that the drugs and doses will need changing over the course of the illness. Pain and colic may increase, stronger antiemetic may be needed, or a trial of octreotide or ondansetron.

If pharmacological treatment fails

Drug treatment is less successful in cases of high obstruction, though the use of octreotide has improved results considerably. If the patient continues to have frequent, large volume vomits in spite of medication, the decision about treatment will depend on the prognosis. If the patient is obviously within a day or two of death, it is appropriate to sedate. Methotrimeprazine is often used, and midazolam may be needed in addition. The aim is to keep the patient drowsy and comfortable.

If the prognosis is longer, the patient will need hospice or hospital admission for the insertion of a nasogastric tube and subcutaneous or IV fluids. This will often be followed by a referral for a venting gastrostomy.

The Future

When the original article on a medical management for obstruction was published it was dismissed by many surgical colleagues. Their understandable view was that a blockage must be cut out or bypassed. However, over the years things have changed; most surgeons now accept that a pharmacological approach is relevant for many with advanced cancer and is successful in controlling pain and vomiting. It is to be expected that this method will become more widely known and used.

There are now a considerable number of anti-emetics which are used for obstructive vomiting. It is essential that controlled trials are carried out comparing these drugs so that firm recommendations for treatment can be made. It is necessary to recognise, early in their obstructive illness, those for whom pharmacological treatment will be unsuccessful. This will enable them to be referred for a venting gastrotomy without delay. Finally, it would be helpful to conduct some quality of life studies on obstructed patients so that the use of pharmacological treatment compared with venting procedures could be evaluated.

References

1. Baines MJ, Oliver DJ, and Carter RL. Medical Management of intestinal obstruction in patients with advanced malignant disease: a clinical and pathological study. Lancet, 1985; ii: 990–993
2. Parker MC, and Baines MJ. Intestinal obstruction in patients with advanced malignant disease. British Journal of Surgery 1996; 83: 1–2
3. Beattie GJ, Leonard RCF, and Smyth JF. Bowel obstruction in ovarian cancer: a retrospective study and review of the literature. Palliative Medicine, 1989; 3: 275–280.
4. Ashby MA, et al. Percutaneous gastrostomy as a venting procedure in palliative care. Palliative Medicine 1991; 5: 147–150.
5. Baines MJ. The pathophysiology and management of malignant intestinal obstruction. In Doyle D, Hanks GWC, MacDonald N, eds Oxford Textbook of Palliative Medicine. Oxford: Oxford University Press, 1993: 311–16 (2nd Edition in Press)
6. Oliver DJ. Syringe drivers in palliative care: a review. Palliative Medicine 1988; 2: 21–26.
7. De Conno F, Caraceni A, Zecca E, Spoldi E, and Ventafridda V. The continuous subcutaneous infusion of hyoscine butylbromide reduces secretions in patients with gastrointestinal obstruction. Journal of Pain and Symptom Management 1991; 6: 484–6.
8. Isbister WH, Elder P, and Symonds L. Non-operative management of malignant intestinal obstruction. Journal of the Royal College of Surgeons, Edingburgh, 1990; 35: 369–372.
9. Ventafridda V, Ripamonti C, Caraceni A, Spoldi E, Messina L, and De Conno F. The management of inoperable gastrointestinal obstruction in terminal cancer patients. Tumori, 1990; 76: 389–393.
10. Mercadante S. Tolerability of continuous subcutaneous octreotide used in combination with other drugs. Journal of Palliative care 1995; 11: 4, 14–16.
11. Riley J, and Fallon MT. Octreotide in terminal malignant obstruction of the gastrointestinal tract. European Journal of Palliative Care 1994; 1: 23–5
12. Fainsinger RL, et al. The use of hypodermoclysis for rehydration in terminally ill cancer patients. Journal of Pain and Symptom Management 1994; 9: 298–302.

Chapter 10

Dysphagia

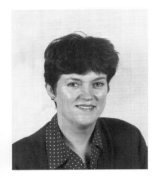

Dr C M Lewis-Jones
Cathy Lewis-Jones was born in Kenya and qualified from Liverpool University in 1981. She trained in General Medicine and General Practice before undertaking higher specialist training in Palliative Care. She took up a Consultant post in Palliative Care and Medical Director of St John's Hospice in Wirral in 1995.
As a consequence of her medical experience she has retained an interest in Palliative Gastro-enterological procedures.

INTRODUCTION

Eating performs two functions. It gives pleasure from a personal and a communal perspective and it results in hydration and nutrition. These should be achieved without difficulty and without risk of aspiration.[1] Dysphagia is distressing and generates anxiety in the patient and their carers.

DEFINITIONS

- **Dysphagia** is a subjective awareness of difficulty in swallowing. In its broadest sense it includes impairment of swallowing and also mastication (chewing).
- **Odynophagia** means painful swallowing.

Incidence

The incidence of dysphagia is increasing as more people are attentive to the diagnosis.[2] Dysphagia is a symptom of different underlying pathologies and the incidence can only accurately be described in relation to that primary diagnosis. In patients with advanced progressive disease, dysphagia is a common symptom and has been reported in approximately 10% of terminally ill patients.[3, 4]

Presentation The patient with dysphagia may present to a gastro-enterologist, a neurologist, an ENT surgeon, a facio-maxillary surgeon, a dentist, a dietician or a speech therapist. The recognition of its multi-professional nature has led to an increasing awareness of the problem and an increasing literature on dysphagia.

Patients may present with a mild disturbance in swallowing or symptoms of severe dysphagia.

CHARACTERISTICS OF SEVERE DYSPHAGIA

- Coughing whilst eating
- Dribbling
- Aspirational pneumonia
- Poor oral intake
- Hunger and thirst
- Weight loss and dehydration

PATHOPHYSIOLOGY OF DYSPHAGIA

Anatomy Swallowing is dependent upon the normal functioning of the buccal cavity, pharynx, upper oesophageal (crico-pharyngeal) sphincter, the body of oesophagus, lower sphincter of the oesophagus and the neurological pathways that supply them.

The muscles of the oro-pharynx and upper third of the oesophagus are skeletal muscle and are therefore influenced by disorders which affect skeletal muscle whereas the lower two thirds of the oesophagus are smooth muscle. There are principally three phases to swallowing.

3 PHASES OF SWALLOWING
• Oral
• Pharyngeal
• Oesophageal

Oral   *The oral phase* (1 second) involves the bolus of chewed food being transferred to the back of the mouth by the tongue, from where it is propelled into the oesophagus (a voluntary movement).

Pharyngeal   *The pharyngeal phase* (1 second) co-ordinates respiration and swallowing. The nasopharynx closes by elevation of the soft palate, (to prevent food from being directed into the nasal passageways) then the respiratory tract is closed by the epiglottis and the upper oesophageal sphincter relaxes allowing the transfer of food into the oesophagus as the pharynx contracts.

Oesophageal   *The oesophageal phase* (8–20 seconds) causes a peristaltic wave, synchronised with the pharyngeal contraction, to propel the bolus down the oeso- phagus. The lower oesophageal sphincter then relaxes to allow the passage of food into the stomach.

CAUSES OF DYSPHAGIA

Clinically there are two types of dysphagia which will be considered separately:

- Oro-pharyngeal when problems may arise as food or fluids are passed from the oropharynx into the oesophagus
- Oesophageal as food travels down the oesophagus into the stomach.

Causes   When delivering palliative care it is important to recognise all pathologies which may contribute to a problem. The tables of causes given here are not exhaustive. Many other causes of dysphagia are sited in individual case reports and have not been included. Dysphagia appears frequently in certain common conditions, for example, there is a 40% incidence of dysphagia in strokes.

Oropharyngeal dysphagia

Oropharyngeal dysphagia is most frequently caused by decreased saliva, painful oropharyngeal lesions or neuromuscular disorders, and less frequently by neoplasms and their treatment.

CAUSES OF ORO-PHARYNGEAL DYSPHAGIA

- **Mouth problems**
  - Dry mouth
  - Radiation induced mucositis

- **Infection**
  - Candidiasis
  - Herpes simplex
  - CMV
  - Pharyngeal abscess.

- **Neurological**
  - Cerebral tumour
  - MND
  - Multiple sclerosis
  - Huntington's Chorea
  - CVA
  - Parkinson's disease

- **Peripheral nerve**
  - Mononeuritis multiplex
  - Diabetic neuropathy

- **Myopathies**
  - Polymyositis
  - Dermatomyositis
  - Muscular dystrophies
  - Thyroid myopathy

- **Obstructive**
  - Oro-pharyngeal malignancies
  - Malignant lymphadenopathy
  - Surgical resection.

Oesophageal dysphagia

Oesophageal dysphagia is due to obstructive lesions in 85% of cases and 15% are due to motility disorders of the smooth muscle of the lower oesophagus. The commonest obstructive lesion is oesophageal cancer, with squamous cell cancer accounting for 95% of these.[5] Extrinsic compression from lymph node metastases (in particular from bronchial carcinoma) and strictures following radiotherapy or acid reflux may cause dysphagia.

Psychological factors may contribute. In a study of 50 hospice patients presenting with dysphagia, only 33 had clinical evidence of dysphagia and only 80% of these who underwent necropsy had locally obstructive lesions.[4]

CAUSES OF OESOPHAGEAL DYSPHAGIA

- **Neoplasms**
  - Oesophageal
  - Gastric
- **Oesophageal webs/rings**
- **Extrinsic compression**
  - Lymphadenopathy
  - Bronchial carcinoma.
- **Benign Stricture**
  - Radiation induced
  - Gastro oesophageal reflux
- **Neuromuscular**
  - Achalasia
  - Oesophageal spasm

  - Scleroderma
  - Nutcracker oesophagus
  - Thyroid dysfunction
  - Diabetes Mellitus

- **Inflammation**
  - Reflux oesophagitis
  - Radiation induced mucositis
  - NSAID
- **Infection**
  - Oesophageal candidiasis
  - Herpes simplex
  - CMV
- **Psychogenic**

Multiple causes

More than one factor may be responsible for dysphagia. Some may respond to treatment (eg oesophageal candidiasis) others may resolve with time (eg radiation-induced mucositis) and require symptomatic treatment in the interim. In malignancy, dysphagia may result from the tumour itself, from coincidental disease, (eg benign peptic stricture) be drug induced (e.g. xerostomia) or be exacerbated by other symptoms (e.g. nausea). Dysphagia is common in head and neck cancers but may be more closely related to interventions, in particular surgery, rather than the underlying cancer.

CLINICAL ASSESSMENT

The underlying diagnosis of a patient with dysphagia is usually known when they are referred for palliative care. Dysphagia, however, is a complex medical problem, often multifactoral in origin. Accurate clinical assessment is required to determine the relative contribution of each element. Treatable causes need to be identified. The characteristics of dysphagia, and its nutritional, psychosocial and respiratory consequences all require evaluation.

Team approach   The assessment and subsequent management of a patient with dysphagia is best performed through a *multiprofessional team*, including doctors, nurses, speech and language therapists, dieticians, physiotherapists and occupational therapists. Each has a specific role. The doctor assesses the medical and psychosocial needs of the patient and may orchestrate the team. Doctors are also required to re-evaluate the changing needs of the patient and their carers.

Therapists   The speech and language therapist assesses the swallowing mechanism and with videofluoroscopy helps to localise the physiological problem and to advise on oro-facial muscle exercises and (in consultation with the physiotherapist) will advise on the safest position for eating and drinking.

The physiotherapist can reduce the incidence of chest infections and assess and advise on mobility in these sometimes debilitated patients. The occupational therapist may advise on and provide appropriate feeding aids..

Dietician   The dietician can assess the nutritional requirements of a patient and advise on the feeding method and dietary composition. the appropriate texture, consistency and nutritional composition of the diet. They will also advise on nutritional supplementation, enteral and parenteral nutrition.

There must be close co-operation between all these health care professionals when managing individual patients.

History   The history will probably give the diagnosis in 80% of cases. Dysphagia must be recognised as the presenting complaint. Dysphagia causing regurgitation, due to oesophageal obstruction may be misinterpreted as vomiting without adequate history taking and observation.

Particularly relevant questions are whether the dysphagia is intermittent or daily, and whether it occurs with solids or liquids. Ask about the presence or absence (and timing) of associated symptoms of choking, coughing, regurgitation, changes in speech, heartburn or chest pain.[6]

> ### KEY QUESTIONS
>
> - Intermittent or daily?
> - Solids or liquids?
> - Choking or coughing?
> - Changes in speech?
> - Chest pain?
>
> *NB* Observe swallowing

Oro-pharyngeal dysphagia characteristically gives rise to dysphagia for liquids and may cause nasal regurgitation or coughing following aspiration.

Oesophageal obstruction tends to give the sensation of food sticking in the throat after swallowing solids (fluids being less of a problem). The patient's localisation of where the food sticks is not an accurate indicator of the site of the disorder. *Motility disorders* of the oesophagus cause dysphagia to liquids <u>and</u> solids and is intermittent initially.

A squeezing sensation is generally due to oesophageal spasm. *Painful swallowing* (odynophagia) often sharp in nature indicates ulcerative lesions.

Drug history

A careful drug history will identify those agents causing a dry mouth (such as opioids, anticholinergics, antihistamines, antidepressants, antihypertensives and diuretics.) Previous radiotherapy may also cause a dry mouth or if recent, a painful mucositis. Steroids and NSAID therapy may exacerbate dyspepsia. Steroids may also increase the susceptibility to oral candidiasis.

Clinical examination

The mouth should be examined for infection, inflammation and dryness. Evidence of a primary malignancy, regional lymphadenopathy or disseminated malignant disease should be sought. Examine the CNS and in particular the cranial nerves.

Observation of swallowing may provide valuable additional information. Drooling, failure to drink from a cup or to chew, and stasis of food within the oral cavity indicate a difficulty in the oral preparation of food. Gagging, choking or coughing suggest a disorder in the pharyngeal phase.

Malnutrition may be evident together with physical signs of aspiration.

Investigation

Investigative techniques include, cine or video-fluroscopy of swallowing, endoscopy, and intra-luminal pressure measurements (manometry).

As methods of investigation advance more anomalies are detected. However these methods of evaluation are tools and dysphagia is a symptom and we should aim to treat the symptom and not the results of investigation.[1] The yield from any examination is increased if the investigator is provided with accurate details of the history and examination.

Videofluroscopy

Videofluroscopy enable oral and pharyngeal aspects of swallowing (including possible aspiration) to be observed and recorded for analysis. Using barium-impregnated foodstuffs the consistency of foods causing aspiration and the characteristics of the swallowing patterns are noted. Referral for videofluroscopy is generally recom- mended by a speech and language therapist who in conjunction with the radiologist interpret the results. This examination may be helpful in planning suitable feeding regimes.[7] Assessment of nutritional status and pulmonary function may also be required.

PSYCHOSOCIAL ASPECTS

For most people eating is an important aspect of life. Sharing meals is an important social function and inability to participate can lead to social isolation. Self-feeding is an important aspect of self care. Insecurity about eating, especially in public, can be humiliating and the fear of choking can induce panic attacks. Adaptation to dysphagia is dependent upon previous experiences and beliefs as well as the professional and social support available.[8]

Rehabilitation in palliative care is a challenge. Patients with advancing disease may perceive that their clinical deterioration is all attributable to a poor nutritional intake which would reverse if they could be built up. Considerable discussion may be required for cachexia, (or in the case of MND muscle wasting) to be understood so that the expectations from improved nutrition are not unrealistic. Denial may prevent the development of adaptive strategies.

MANAGEMENT OF DYSPHAGIA IN PALLIATIVE CARE

Considerations   The care delivered should be appropriate to the needs of the patient, which may change as the patient passes through the palliative into the terminal phase of their illness. Treatment decisions are best undertaken by a multiprofessional team, taking into account the views of patients and their families.

Informed consent   Informed consent requires information, sensitively delivered, with respect to their disease, the clinical findings and expected outcomes. As decision makers we need to listen and converse and to avoid biased judgement. There are many factors which may influence decisions beyond clinical need, such as treatment availability, economic status, education, religious beliefs, ethnicity and age.

Artificial nutrition   Artificial nutrition must be appropriate to the needs of a patient with advanced disease. It can be a difficult decision and is best supported by considering the Guidelines on Artificial Nutrition versus Hydration in Terminal Cancer patients.[9]

PEG   Technological advances have greatly complicated the ethical decision (burden versus benefit) as to who should receive enteral nutrition.[10] The relative ease of placement of a Percutaneous Endoscopic Gastrostomy (PEG) and its subsequent management in the community means that, even patients debilitated by advanced disease may be thought suitable for PEG insertion.

Feeding via gastrostomy

John was a 65 year old divorcee who was found to have an inoperable carcinoma of the oropharynx following a presentation with progressive dysphagia. A Percutaneous Endoscopic Gastrostomy (PEG) was inserted following which he received palliative radiotherapy. Over the next 7 months he received all his nutrition, fluid and medication via his PEG. His sister was his principle carer at this time. Ultimately, he was admitted to the hospice for control of neuropathic facial pain, where he stayed until he died three weeks later. His treatment was rationalised as he entered the terminal phase by discontinuing his nutrition but maintaining his co-analgesic therapy of anticonvulsants and tricyclic antidepressant therapy until his death.

Objectives

The objectives of the treatment of dysphagia in the palliative phase must be clearly defined with the focus of care on enhancing the quality of life for patients. The objectives may vary with time but are essentially:-

1. To maintain a safe oral route for as long as possible.
2. To maintain adequate nutrition.
3. To rehabilitate patients with dysphagia to overcome social embarrassment.
4. To provide a route for medication and fluids.

Reversible causes

Reversible causes of dysphagia need to be sought rigorously and treated. Infection and ulceration may be apparent and specific treatment indicated. Empirical treatment may be necessary if there is suspicion of infection. Some conditions will resolve (eg radiation induced mucositis) but temporary enteral nutrition may be required until recovery has taken place.

Associated symptoms

Attention to other symptoms experienced by patients with advanced disease and applying the principles of palliative care can significantly contribute to an improvement in dysphagia.[3]

Radiotherapy,
chemotherapy and steroids

Although many patients may have already under-gone radiotherapy or chemotherapy done with a curative intent further treatment to relieve dysphagia may be possible. High dose steroid therapy may also be of value in reducing the pressure effects from the tumour.

Terminal phase

Just as it is necessary to rationalise treatments in the terminal phase (eg discontinuing hypoglycaemics, antihypertensives) it is also necessary to reassess nutrition. This may include the withdrawal of enteral nutrition when it is no longer appropriate. The withdrawal of enteral nutrition at this stage may be considered ethically the same as not starting it at that time.[10] However, the preservation of a route for medication and or fluids, may enhance symptom control.

Frequent communication and considerable support may be required at this stage to allow families and friends to come to terms with the disease progression.

FEEDING STRATEGIES IN THE DYSPHAGIC PATIENT

These apply principally in oro-pharyngeal dysphagia.

Rate of delivery of food

An unrushed atmosphere is essential as is the commitment from the carers of time and patience. The patient should be offered small volumes ($\frac{1}{2}$–1 teaspoon) at a pace they can manage, pausing for breaks as required. With liquids the rate of flow can be controlled using a feeder.

Preparation for eating

The patients mouth should be cleaned before food. This stimulates the flow of saliva and sensation and may improve taste. The patient should then be positioned at 60–90 degrees in the upright position, with the head flexed forward and in the mid line. Pillows at the low back may help to maintain this position. The person doing the feeding should sit at eye level or below to maintain neck flexion. Adaptation to drinking cups etc. can be made to allow for sustained flexion (eg cutting a nose hole out of a beaker and the use of straws). Various modifications of swallowing technique may assist swallowing according to the deficit present. Hand pressure may support the cheek when there is abnormal mandibular movement or poor buccal control. Following partial glossectomy, syringes or glossectomy spoons may assist in the transfer of food to the back of the mouth.

The mouth should be checked at the end of the meal to ensure no food is remaining on which the patient may aspirate. The patient should remain in the upright position after eating for 1–2 hours to reduce reflux and hence aspiration.[11]

Specialised utensils may help maintain self feeding and hence independence. Advice and support with respect to this may be offered by an occupational therapist

Food preparation

Several issues emerge in the dietary management of dysphagia. These include the food's taste, temperature, texture, consistency and potential to stimulate mucus production.

Taste

Strong flavours such as sweet, spicy, sour, or salty tastes may stimulate salivation, swallowing or mastication. Bland flavours should be avoided.

Temperature

Foods should be served at hot or cold temperatures, rather than at tepid or or at room temperature, to stimulate the swallowing response. Thermal stimulants may improve muscle tone and decrease transit time. Either hot or cold may be used but cold is probably safer. Iced liquids can be altered with semi-solid textures. Caution must be taken with patients with decreased oral sensation to avoid burning.

Texture

Avoid foods that are crumbly and fall apart in the mouth. Density and shape are important also. Jello slips down easily, however apple sauce may be difficult for some patients as it does not form a cohesive bolus.

Consistency

Purees and pastes are generally the safest texture since they do not require chewing, they readily form a bolus and do not spill into the trachea. Thin liquids are more difficult to hold in the back of the mouth without them spilling into the trachea. With limited fluid intake there is the risk of dehydration. Jelly like substances may alter to form a mixture of jelly and liquid which requires a double swallow. Evidence suggests that liquids and semisolids should be presented separately. Never use a fluid to wash the bolus down. Two different consistencies can send conflicting sensory stimuli. Medication may need to be crushed if possible, and placed in the puree. Liquid medication is thickened as necessary. Solid foods which require mastication should be avoided.

Saliva production

There may be excess or inadequate saliva production. Milk products are considered to increase saliva production and broth and meat juices may thin it. Many of the above issues may be addressed through the use of a standardised dysphagic diet, within which individual adjustments can be made. A four level dysphagic diet-plan which grades according to severity of dysphagia has been recommended.[12]

Management should be through the multi-disciplinary team with strategies of care tailored to meet the needs of the patient. With progressive disease it must be recognised that the needs of the patient will change with time.

Any strategies must be communicated to all concerned and take into account the views of patients and their families.

ENTERAL NUTRITION

Enteral nutrition needs to be considered in patients who are unable to maintain an adequate oral intake despite palliative treatment and conservative feeding strategies, and in whom nutritional support is appropriate.

The options most commonly employed are fine bore naso-gastric feeding tubes, surgically placed gastrostomies and percutaneous endoscopic gastrostomies (PEG).

NG tubes Naso-gastric tubes are cheap and simple to place, however, they have a tendency to block, become displaced, cause local ulceration and are not considered cosmetically acceptable. These complications make home care difficult. Surgically placed gastrostomies carry with them the risk of a general anaesthetic.

PEG A percutaneous endoscopic (PEG) is a safe and reliable method of delivering enteral nutrition. The procedure is brief and well tolerated even by those debilitated by their disease.[13] The incidence of reflux is less than with a naso-gastric tube and this mode of delivery facilitates home care. The PEG may be used to deliver nutrition when indicated and for the delivery of fluid and medication as a patients disease progresses. The insertion of a PEG may significantly improve a patients quality of life with little morbidity and at a low cost.

PALLIATIVE TREATMENTS IN SPECIFIC CONDITIONS

Head and neck malignancy Methods for treating head and neck malignancy have advanced but usually result in slowing of tumour advancement rather than cure. This may lead to a protracted palliative phase with difficult symptoms. Greater than 50% of patients die as a consequence of tumour expansion resulting in dysphagia, respiratory obstruction or brain displacement. The incidence of dysphagia may be as great as 38% in advanced head and neck malignancy.[14]

Dysphagia in head and neck malignancy may result from anatomical disruption after surgery, post radiation changes, tumour recurrence or peri-neural tumour infiltration causing neuropathic pain and dysfunction.

The approach to rehabilitation of a patient with dysphagia following treatment should be guided by a knowledge of the anatomy and physiology and an understanding of the patient's motivation and mental status. Tumour recurrence should always be considered in head and neck cancer if dysphagia occurs as a new symptom.[15] Management options are conservative feeding strategies to maintain an oral route or methods for delivering enteral nutrition.

Oesophageal malignancy

For patients with oesophageal malignancy surgery offers the only realistic hope of cure and should be considered in all cases. However for many, surgery is not an option because of advanced disease or associated medical conditions and alternative, palliative treatments are required.

The principle palliative treatments are:

- dilatation
- intubation/stents
- laser therapy
- radiotherapy
- gastrostomy.

Dilatation

Oesophageal dilatation may be used alone or in conjunction with other treatments. It is a relatively safe procedure although perforation may occur as a complication. Tapered polyvinyl or balloon dilators are passed over a guidewire at endoscopy. Dysphagia is inclined to recur at increasingly frequent intervals when dilatation is used as a single therapy but it may produce a temporary relief of dysphagia in those patients with a limited life expectancy.

Intubation

Oesophageal intubation with a rigid prosthesis produces a rapid and reliable relief of dysphagia. It is performed at endoscopy with IV sedation and topical pharyngeal anaesthesia. Relief of dysphagia is rapid but the quality of swallowing is poor. Perforation may occur at insertion and later complications include gastric reflux through the tube, which may be helped by a pro-kinetic agent or anti-secretory therapy. Tube displacement, obstruction or overgrowth by tumour can occur. Tumour overgrowth may be treated by laser therapy.[16]

Stents

Self-expanding metal stents have recently overcome some of the problems associated with semi-rigid prostheses. Their insertion is less traumatic as the diameter of the delivery catheters is only 8–12mm which reduces the need for oesophageal dilatation. The lumen achieved is larger and there is a lower risk of tube migration. They may be inserted as a one step outpatient procedure and the flexibility of the stent should improve swallowing further. The principle problem is tumour blockage. This has to some degree been overcome by a silicone covering which can also help overcome the problem of oesophago-tracheal fistulae but may increase the risk of stent migration (which in turn may be reduced by the stent being barbed). There are a variety of metal stents available each with their own individual properties. Depending on their construction, they are classified as Z, meshed, knitted-coat-of-mail, or coil stents. Expansion can be achieved either with a stable length (Z type) or with shortening (other types). Despite their considerably higher cost, the metal stents prove cost effective because of the decreased complication rate and shorter hospital stay. The development of expandable metal stents has been a definite advance in the palliative treatment of dysphagia.[18]

Laser   Thermal laser therapy of oesophageal malignancy (high-power neodymium yttrium-aluminium-garnet laser) alone or with other therapies is effective in palliating dysphagia. Patients should ideally be treated initially at 2–3 day intervals, until a lumen is achieved which relieves the dysphagia. Re-treatment at 4–6 week intervals maintains the response. The quality of swallowing obtained is variable but laser therapy has been shown to significantly improve the quality of life for patients with malignant dysphagia.[17] If laser therapy ceases to offer useful palliation, an endoprosthesis can be inserted.

Radiotherapy   External irradiation offers the potential of treating all the tumour but the relief of dysphagia is delayed. Immediately following radiotherapy, dysphagia may even be exacerbated. As a single therapy it is therefore limited but in multimodal regimes it may be of value.

Brachytherapy   Brachytherapy has the potential to control local tumour growth but in view of the fall off in dose with distance from the source it does not irradiate the whole tumour. The response is more rapid than with external beam irradiation and it is more effective at relieving the dysphagia (but oesophagitis and ulceration can occur). Combining the two irradiation techniques offer the potential to prolong survival and relieve dysphagia.[16]

Gastrostomy

A percutaneous gastrostomy tube may provide adequate nutrition in partial dysphagia, and the patient can also continue to eat some food normally, giving a sense of normality.

Enteral nutrition may improve quality of life. If nutritional intake is inadequate consider placement of a percutaneous endoscopic gastrostomy (PEG) before absolute dysphagia occurs. This ensures that a route for the delivery of fluid and medication is available up to the terminal phase.

Motor neurone disease

Motor neurone disease causes complex physical and psychosocial needs and often require specialist palliative care. The incidence of dysphagia in this group may be as high as 76%.[19] The severity of dysphagia varies widely and may involve the oral or pharyngeal phases of swallowing or both.

The progressive dysphagia may result from a bulbar palsy (lower motor neuron loss), a pseudobulbar palsy (upper motor neuron loss) or a combination of the two.

Bulbar palsy

Bulbar palsy causes lower motor neurone signs such as weakness and wasting of the involved muscles of the face, tongue and pharynx, and decreased gag and jaw reflexes.

Pseudobulbar palsy

Pseudobulbar palsy is characterised by weakness without wasting and hyperactive brain stem reflexes. In addition to muscle weakness, there is often a striking slowness and incoordination of voluntary side to side movement of the tongue. Discrepancy between involuntary and voluntary motor functions may be blatant, with exaggerated rise of the soft palate as part of the gag reflex yet no movement during attempted phonation.[20] Also present is the associated dysarthria.

Dysphagia may predominantly relate to difficulty in initiating swallowing, because of impairment of voluntary control (with relative preservation of reflex activity). Emotional lability is associated with pseudobulbar palsy.

Patient Choice

Ray is a 42 year old father of two teenage girls who, developed a progressive neurological deficit over 2 years period following a diagnosis of Multiple System atrophy. His initial presentation was with a 6 month history of deterioration in his gait. The subsequent rapid deterioration in his condition left him totally dependent, with a spastic quadraplegia, mute and with progressive dysphagia. His only movement and hence means of communication was one blink for yes and two for no.

Despite his severe disability, his wife continued to care for him at home supported by the Primary Health Care Team and the Community Dysphagic Team, comprised of the speech and language therapist, the dietician, the physiotherapist and the occupational therapist. Ray was reluctant to consider nutritional support via a Percutaneous Endoscopic Gastrostomy (PEG) feeding tube despite his increasing dysphagia being complicated by episodes of aspiration and recurrent urinary tract infections, attributed to poor fluid intake. Feeding became a continuous process, demanding considerable time, energy and patience. Meal times however, were an opportunity to communicate through touch and eye contact. Modified feeding techniques were employed, of head support to reduce his neck flexion and the timing of food insertion for when his jaw was not locked in spasm. He received a semisolid diet, with as high a water content as was possible without running the risk of aspiration. The option of enteral nutrition was frequently reviewed but declined.

Many dysphagic MND patients fear that they may choke to death. This frightening concept has not been observed and death usually results from a progressive respiratory failure. Pneumonia resulting from aspiration may be a contributing factor.[21].

Conservative strategies include modifications to eating and drinking to maximise intake. Enteral nutrition may be required, especially in patients who develop early bulbar symptoms. Survival in patients who have tube feeding is no different to those who have been managed conservatively.[18]

AIDS

Candidiasis is the commonest cause of difficult or painful swallowing in AIDS and is an AIDS-defining diagnosis. It can be treated empirically with a systemic azole. The second most frequent cause is cytomegalovirus (CMV), which produces either diffuse oesophagitis or discrete ulceration. The aetiology of these lesions can be confirmed by biopsy of the centre of ulcerated areas.

DYSPHAGIA IN AIDS

- Candida
- CMV
- Herpes simplex
- HIV

Oesophagoscopy occasionally reveals vesicles typical of herpes simplex oesophagitis, diagnosed either by biopsy or smears from brushings showing typical giant cells. 10% of oesophageal ulcers leading to dysphagia are idiopathic, possible causes being unknown opportunistic viruses or HIV itself. These ulcers may respond to thalidomide.[22]

CONCLUSION

The instinct to eat is essential for survival and is retained often into advanced disease. Dysphagia therefore, generates anxiety in patients and in those to whom they are important. We need to care for both the nutritional needs and also the social aspects of eating.

Treatment decisions should be based on the consensus view of the multi-professional team with the relevant expertise which has taken into consideration the views of patients and their carers.

Individual treatment   Each patient requires individualised treatment for their dysphagia. Treatment may be specific to the underlying cause or may be supportive, focusing on feeding strategies or adaptive equipment. When a patient is unable to safely maintain adequate nutrition by mouth then tube feeding may be required.

REFERENCES

1   Buchholz DW. What is Dysphagia? *Dysphagia.* 1996; 11:23–24
2   Kuhlemeier. KV Epidemiology and Dysphagia. *Dysphagia* 1994; 9:209–217.
3   Wilkes E. Dying Now. *Lancet.* 1984; 950–952.
4   Sykes NP,Baines M, Carter RL. Terminal Care. *Lancet* 1988; 1:8383:726–728.
5   Gilbody JS. Errors of Deglutination – real or imagined; or, don't forget the psyche. *J. of Laryngology and Otology* 1991; 105:807–811.
6   Hendrix TR Art and Science of History Taking in the Patient with Difficulty Swallowing. *Dysphagia* 1993; 73:69–73
7   Ott DJ, Pikna LA. Clinical and videofluropscopic evaluation of swallowing disorders. *Am J Roentgenol* 1993; 161:507–13.
8   Gustafsson B, Theorell T. Adaptedness and Coping in Dysphagic Students. *Dysphagia* 1995; 92:86–92.
9   Bozzetti F et al. Guidelines on Artificial Nutrition Versus Hydration in Terminal Cancer Patients. *Nutrition* 1996; 12:163–167.
10 McCamish MA, Crocker NJ. Enteral and Parenteral Nutritional Support of Terminally Ill Patients: Practical and Ethical Perspectives. *The Hospice J* 1993; 9:2/3:107–129.
11 Layne KA. Feeding Strategies for the Dysphagic Patient : A nursing perspective. *Dysphagia* 1990; 5:84–88.
12 Martin AW. Dietary Management of Swallowing Disorders. *Dysphagia* 1991; 6:129–134.
13 Moran BJ. Taylor MB, Johnson CD. Percutaneous endoscopic gastrostomy. *Br.J. Surg* 1990; 77:858–862.
14 Aird DW, Bihari J, Smith C. Clinical problems in the continuing care of Head and Neck Cancer Patients. *Ear Nose and Throat J.*1993; 62:230–243.
15 Kroenberger MB, Myers AD. Dysphagia following Head and Neck Cancer Surgery *Dysphagia* 1994; 9:236–244.
16 Sturgess R, Krasner N. Oesophageal Carcinoma treatment: palliative modalities. *Europ J Gastroenterol and Hepatol.* 1994; 6:8:684–691.
17 Lewis-Jones CM Laser Therapy in the Palliation of Dysphagia in Oesophageal Malignancy *Palliat Med* 1995; 4:52–53. .
18 Sturgess RP, Morris A I. Metal stents in the oesophagus. *Gut* 1995; 37:593–594.
19 Scott A., Heughan A. A review of dysphagia in four cases of motor neurone disease. *Palliat Med.* 1993; 7: (suppl 2):41–47.
20 Buchholz DW. Neurogenic Dysphagia: What is the cause when the cause is not obvious? *Dysphagia* 1994; 9:245–255.

21 O'Brien A., Kelly M., Saunders C. Motor Neurone Disease : A hospice perspective. *BMJ* 1992; 304:471–473.

22 Sharpstone D, Gazzard B. Gastrointestinal manifestations of HIV infection. *Lancet* 1996; 348:379–383.

Chapter 11

Dyspnoea

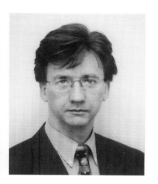

Dr Andrew Wilcock

Andrew Wilcock is Consultant in Palliative Medicine and Oncology, University of Nottingham, Hayward House Macmillan Palliative Care Unit and the department of Oncology, City Hospital NHS Trust, Nottingham

Note: This chapter considers dyspnoea in cancer patients.

DEFINITION

Breathlessness (dyspnoea) is a universal experience but is difficult to describe. A commonly used definition is an unpleasant or uncomfortable awareness of breathing or need to breathe. The overall experience includes the perception of difficult breathing and the response to it. It should not be confused with an increase in respiratory rate (tachypnoea) or ventilation (hyperpnoea).

Incidence and prevalence of breathlessness.

Breathlessness is less common than other symptoms, including pain, insomnia, general weakness, fatigue, anorexia, dry mouth, weight loss, constipation, sweating and nausea.

The largest surveys of patients with all types of cancer show an incidence in the last 6 weeks of life of 70%, with prevalence ranging from 24% for patients referred to a pain clinic to 64% in the last week of life.[1,2] The severity of breathlessness increases as death approaches, 16% of patients rated their breathlessness as severe or horrible at 6 weeks compared with 24% the week before death. Breathlessness is an independent indicator of prognosis, second only to performance status.[4]

Prevalence

The prevalence of breathlessness appears to be greater in patients with lung cancer. In 289 patients with non-small cell lung cancer 75% reported breathlessness at presentation (8% severe, 33% moderate and 34% mild). Only cough was more common (79%).[7] In 100 patients with lung cancer referred to a palliative care service the incidence of breathlessness was 70%, (47% severe or moderately so) and it was the second commonest symptom after pain (86% had pain).[8]

THE INCIDENCE AND PREVALENCE OF BREATHLESSNESS IN PATIENTS WITH ALL TYPES OF CANCER

Time of study	Number of patients	Incidence
Last 6 weeks of life[1]	1,400	70%
		Prevalence
At referral to pain clinic[2]	1,600	24%
At referral to palliative care service[3]	1,000	51%
Patients under palliative care service[4]	1,600	53%
On admission to hospice[5, 6]	6,700	51%
	1,100	27%
6 weeks prior to death[1]	900	49%
1 week prior to death[1]	1,400	64%

The normal control of breathing

The control of breathing can be involuntary, (controlled by oxygen delivery and acid-base balance) or voluntary (allowing activities such as talking, swallowing, coughing).

Involuntary control is due to the respiratory control centres in the brain stem producing a rhythmic breathing pattern, modulated by incoming sensory information. In voluntary control of breathing the brain stem centres are overridden by the thalamus and cerebral cortex.

Sensory inputs to the respiratory control centres come from: thalamus and cortex, central chemo-receptors, peripheral chemoreceptors, lung receptors and respiratory muscle receptors.

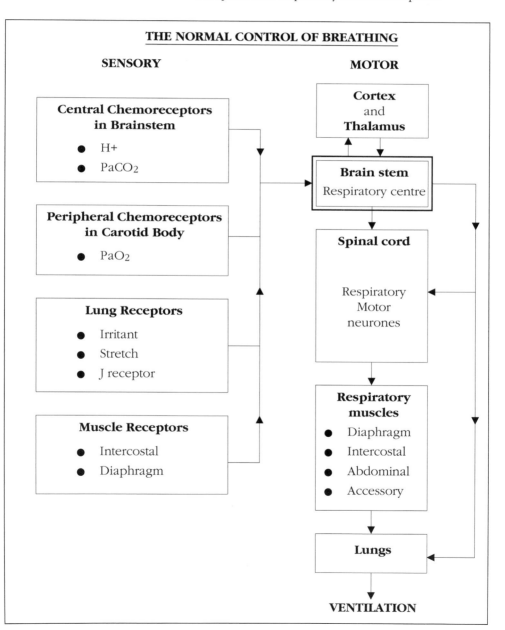

THE NORMAL CONTROL OF BREATHING

SENSORY

MOTOR

Central Chemoreceptors in Brainstem
- H^+
- $PaCO_2$

Peripheral Chemoreceptors in Carotid Body
- PaO_2

Lung Receptors
- Irritant
- Stretch
- J receptor

Muscle Receptors
- Intercostal
- Diaphragm

Cortex and **Thalamus**

Brain stem
Respiratory centre

Spinal cord

Respiratory Motor neurones

Respiratory muscles
- Diaphragm
- Intercostal
- Abdominal
- Accessory

Lungs

VENTILATION

NOTES ON THE CONTROL OF BREATHING

1. *The higher centers* (Thalamus and Cerebral Cortex.) can overide *The brain stem.*

2. *Central Chemoreceptors* (in the brain stem) respond to changes in hydrogen ion (H^+) concentration which mirrors arterial pressure of carbon dioxide (Pa CO_2).

3. *Peripheral Chemoreceptors* (carotid body) – respond to changes in arterial pressure of oxygen (PaO_2).

4. *Irritant receptors* the large airways respond to mechanical and chemical stimulation and are important in the cough reflex. *Stretch receptors* in the smooth muscle of the bronchi respond to lung expantion. They are slowly adapting and signal lung volume. *C-fibre (J receptors)* in the alveolar walls respond to vascular congestion and lung stiffness and chemical and mechanical stimulation.

5. *Muscle receptors* in the respiratory muscles (diaphragm and intercostals) are of 2 types: *Muscle spindles* detect changes in the length of the muscle and are mainly found in the chest wall. *Golgi tendon organs* detect changes in the tension of the muscle and mostly found in the diaphragm and regulate the force of diaphramatic contractions.

6. *Irritant receptors* in the bronchial epithelium of the large airways respond to mechanical and chemical stimulation and detect rate of change of lung volume. They are also involved in the cough reflex.

7. There are *motor nerves* to the airways especially through the parasympathetic branch of the autonomic nervous system via the vagus nerve.

Ventilation results in changes in thoracic displacement, PaCO_2 and PaO_2 which are detected by the sensors controlling the cycle.

The mechanisms involved in generating breathlessness are less well understood. In general terms, breathlessness appears to arise from discrepancies in the information between (1) Peripheral sensors in the lung, respiratory muscles and chemoreceptors; and (2) the conscious awareness of respiratory effort and (3) higher centres responsible for emotion.

A MODEL OF BREATHLESSNESS

Gift has described a model of breathlessness that integrates the physical and emotional elements and recognises 5 components of the symptom.[9]

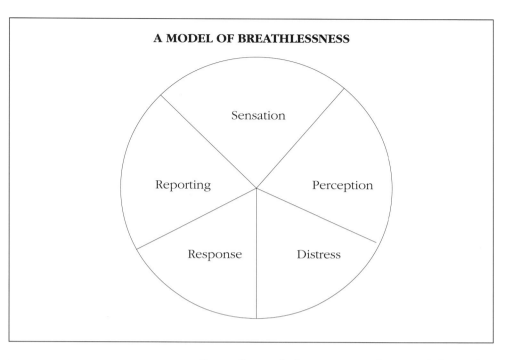

A MODEL OF BREATHLESSNESS

Sensation

Reporting

Perception

Response

Distress

Sensation of dyspnoea – Sensory information arriving at higher centres of the brain.

Perception of dyspnoea – the meaning of breathlessness depends on the individuals attitude to the seriousness of the situation in the light of previous experiences.

Distress of dyspnoea – the emotions caused by breathlessnessu will also colour how it is perceived.

Response to dyspnoea – Immediate and long term responses may differ. Responses may be problem-focused (eg adjust lifestyle) or emotion-focused (eg relaxation techniques) or both. Response may depend upon the coping style of the individual.

Reporting of dyspnoea – may vary with social norms, or ethnic background.

"Total breathlessness"   It is useful to apply the concept of total pain to breathlessness when considering these contributing factors, and for planning an holistic approach to its management. Breathlessness also has physical, psychological, social and spiritual dimensions.

CLINICAL CAUSES OF BREATHLESSNESS

A classification of the more common causes of breathlessness in patients with cancer based on *physiological considerations* is given in the table below. It is put forward as a simple guide designed to help the clinical assessment of the breathless patient rather than as a rigid classification or an exhaustive list. Some patients will have more than one cause. Previous classifications have considered causes due to the cancer, those due to debility, to treatment and to other conditions;[10] others have used speed of onset or anatomical-pathological correlations as a basis for classification.[11]

CAUSES OF BREATHLESSNESS

● **Delivery of air**
  – large airways obstruction
    – tumour, mediastinal lymphadenopathy
  – small airways obstruction
    – asthma, COPD

● **Lung function**
  – Pleural effusion
  – Pneumothorax
  – Infection (bacterial, viral, fungal)
  – Pulmonary infiltrates
    – tumour expansion, multiple secondaries
    – lymphangitis carcinomatosis
  – Pulmonary oedema
  – Anticancer therapy
    – surgery
    – radiotherapy
      – acute: pneumonitis
      – chronic: pulmonary fibrosis
    – chemotherapy
      – pneumonitis, (eg bleomycin, methotrexate)
      – fibrosis (eg cyclophosphamide, busulphan)

● **Chest wall function**
  – Muscle weakness
    – generalised cachexia
    – metabolic
    – neurological (e.g. phrenic nerve palsy)

(continued)

  - drug induced (eg corticosteroids)
  - endocrinopathy
- Restricted movement
    - splinting of the diaphragm
    - ascites, hepatomegaly
    - pain
    - chest wall deformity
    - obesity

- **Blood flow**
  - SVC obstruction
  - Anaemia
  - Congestive cardiac failure
  - Pulmonary embolism
  - Cardiac tamponade
  - Cardiac ischaemia
  - Cardiac arrhythmia

- **Psychological factors**
  - Anxiety
  - Fear
  - Isolation
  - Frustration
  - Anger
  - Depression

DIFFERENTIAL DIAGNOSIS

1. Are there any reversible causes?

Breathlessness is difficult to treat. It is important to identify any reversible causes. The table above indicates the commoner diagnoses to consider. Faced with a patient with increasing breathlessness it is important to consider non-malignant causes: congestive cardiac failure, infective exacerbation of COPD, acute onset of atrial fibrillation or pneumothorax. A recent survey of patients with lung cancer attending a chest clinic found that only 14% of those patients with coexistent COPD were receiving bronchodilator therapy, even though a high proportion of them complained of moderate or severe breathlessness. Subsequently, over 60% found that inhaled bronchodilator therapy help their breathlessness "quite a lot" or "a great deal".[12] Interestingly, for this group of patients at least, nebulized therapy was no more than a spacer device.

Depending upon the cause, patients should receive the most appropriate treatment or have their existing treatment optimised. The advice of colleagues should be sought if there is any doubt as to the best current treatment.

2. Can the cancer itself be modified?

Treatment that may modify the underlying disease process includes surgery, radiotherapy, chemotherapy or hormone therapy. Many patients may already be under the care of a specialist clinic and/or oncologist and their advice should be sought. However, it is still common to find patients who have never been seen by specialist oncology services. Unless you are completely aware of what options are available (which can vary locally and can rapidly change) obtain advice from your local oncology service.

3. Can the effects of the cancer be modified?

This includes the insertion of stents, the use of corticosteroids as anti-inflammatory agents and draining pleural or pericardial effusions or ascities.

4. Is the cause of breathlessness irreversible or not amenable to treatment?

With irreversible causes or patients whose general condition makes the above approaches inappropriate, the focus shifts to improving the symptom of dyspnoea as quickly as possible.

CLINICAL ASSESSMENT

Explore emotions

Assessment requires a thorough history and examination combined with appropriate investigation. It is important to explore the patients understanding about breathlessness and the emotions it produces (see psychosocial aspects). Patients often believe that they are causing further damage to their heart and lungs by becoming breathless during exertion. They are often frightened that they are going to die suddenly during an episode of breathlessness. It is important to stress that becoming breathless in itself is not dangerous.

Examination

Examination of the chest may reveal few clinical signs even in the presence of significant disease. A chest X-ray is often valuable. Even so, for a significant proportion of terminally ill patients (24% in one series[1]) breathlessness occurs in the absence of primary or secondary lung cancer or pre-existing cardiopulmonary disease. This may be due to generalised muscle weakness (which will include the respiratory muscles) resulting from cancer cachexia.

Observe the patient carrying out a task. This gives an immediate measure of performance and may reveal a tendency to hyperventilate which can be explained to the patient. Coping strategies already used by the patient can be reinforced. Speed of recovery can be noted. It also provides a baseline against which to monitor progress.

Anaemia

Anaemia can cause breathlessness. This is more likely when the haemoglobin is less than 8 g/dl but the speed at which the haemoglobin level has fallen is more important than the absolute level. In general, blood transfusions can be repeated as long as there continues to be symptomatic benefit from doing so.

Hyperventilation

If hyperventilation is suspected then asking the patient to hyperventilate to reproduce the symptoms is useful. This helps demonstrate the cause of the symptoms and allows the introduction of breathing/relaxation exercises that aim to give the patient a greater feeling of control over their breathing.

ASSESSMENT OF THE BREATHLESS PATIENT

● **History**
 — Speed of onset
 — Associated symptoms
  — e.g. pain, cough, haemoptysis, sputum, stridor, wheeze
 — Exacerbating and relieving factors
 — Symptoms suggestive of hyperventilation
  — poor relationship of dyspnoea to exertion
  — presence of hyperventilation attacks
  — breathlessness at rest
  — rapid fluctuations in breathlessness within minutes
  — *fear of sudden death during an attack*
  — breathlessness varying with social situations
 — Past medical history
  — e.g. history of cardiovascular disease
 — Drug history

(continued)

- e.g. drugs precipitating fluid retention or bronchospasm
- Symptoms of anxiety or depression
- Social circumstances
  - support networks
- Level of independence
  - ability to care for themselves
  - identify coping strategies
- Meaning
  - What does breathlessness mean to the patient?
  - How do they feel when breathless?

- **Examination**
  - A thorough examination is essential.
  - Observe the patient walking or carrying out specific task.
  - Does hyperventilation reproduce symptoms?

- **Routine Investigations**
  - Chest X-ray
  - Haemoglobin

- **Less commonly performed investigations**
  - Ultrasound scan – (differentiates between pleural effusion from solid tumour)
  - Oxygen saturation – (assessing value of oxygen)
  - Peak flow/spirometry – (assessing response to bronchodilators)
  - ECG/echocardiography (suspected heart failure)
  - Ventilation/perfusion scan (suspected emboli)

PSYCHOSOCIAL ASPECTS

Emotions such as fear, anxiety and anger can affect the pattern of breathing and can cause breathlessness. In several psychiatric disorders (e.g. depression, anxiety, phobias and mania) breathlessness, chest tightness and hyperventilation can occur in otherwise fit patients.

In patients with COPD anxiety and depression correlate better with severity of breathlessness than forced expiratory volume in one second (FEV_1). Reduction in anxiety or depression reduces breathlessness.[13–16] Hyperventilation is common in patients with breathlessness disproportionate to the severity of their pulmonary disease.

In patients with cancer, Hinton noted that anxiety is twice as common in patients with breathlessness compared to those with pain, nausea, vomiting or malaise.[17] Patients with lung cancer describe emotions such as anger, helplessness, depression, loss of strength, agitation, anxiety, fear of suffocating and nervousness during episodes of breathlessness.[18] Activities may be curtailed or avoided and many become socially isolated which can further exacerbate the situation.

MANAGEMENT OPTIONS

It is assumed that any reversible elements have been treated. Approaches can be specific or general. Specific treatments used in palliative medicine are discussed in 3 clinical settings:

● terminal
● at rest
● on exertion.

General supportive management is applicable to each of these situations (and is summarized in the section on dyspnoea on exertion).

TERMINAL DYSPNOEA (LAST DAYS OF LIFE)

Patients are often frightened of suffocating to death and it is useful to explore fears early on.

We should be positive about relief of terminal breathlessness to the patient, their family and to colleagues. Explanation is important, eg:

> "If the situation ever arose where you felt you were having to fight to get your breath even when resting – that is when we can help the most."

> "We can help relieve your breathlessness – but it may make you sleepy."

Most patients are happy to trade the risk of increased sleepiness for a relief of their distress. The family are often equally distressed observing their relative fighting for breath and are also prepared to accept this. Drowsiness is not the primary aim of therapy (unless there is overwhelming distress) and indeed some sedated patients become brighter with improvement of their symptoms.

However, as increasing drowsiness is usually a feature of their deteriorating clinical condition it is important to explain clearly to the relatives the aims of treatment and the gravity of the situation. In summary:

- No patient should die with distressing breathlessness.
- Failure to control breathlessness is a failure to utilise drug therapy correctly.
- Combination of opiate and sedative anxiolytic is very effective.

DRUGS FOR TERMINAL BREATHLESSNESS

Drug	Starting dose	Upper dose	Route given
Diamorphine	10mg per 24 hours (opiate naive)	Titrate according to efficacy and tolerability	SC infusion
Midazolam	10 – 30mg per 24 hours	200 – 260mg per 24 hours (maximum reported when used for restlessness)	SC infusion
Chlorpromazine*	12.5mg IV 4 hourly 25mg PR 8–12 hourly	300 – 900mg per 24 hours	IV or Rectal
Methotrimeprazine	25 – 50 mg per 24 hours	200 – 300 mg per 24 hours (maximum reported when used for restlessness)	SC infusion

(*See References 19, 20)

Relieving Terminal Dyspnoea

George a 70 year old man with advanced carcinoma of the lung was transferred to the hospice from a general medical ward for terminal care. On admission he was anxious, weary, had difficulty talking and was cyanosed. Despite receiving continuous oxygen and regular oral morphine (5mg 4 hourly) he felt he was fighting for each breath and was terrified of choking to death particularly at night. He knew he was dying. He was finding oral medication increasingly difficult. Following discussion with him and his wife together it was explained that we could relieve his breathlessness but that it may make him sleepy. They were both happy to accept this. A syringe driver was commenced delivering diamorphine 10mg and midazolam 10mg subcutaneously over 24 hours. He had the best night for some time. Over the following day he was comfortable and his breathing no longer distressed him. His condition continued to deteriorate and he died peacefully 3 days later with his family present. His wife could not understand why George did not receive such treatment earlier instead of having to struggle with his breathing.

My personal preference for terminal dyspnoea is a combination of diamorphine and midazolam.

Evidence for such an approach is largely anecdotal. Research is difficult to justify in the setting of a terminally ill patient. There has been one study: Continuous IV infusion of morphine produced good relief of terminal breathlessness in 6 patients with cancer, moderate relief in 1 and a poor response in 1.[21]

DYSPNOEA AT REST (WEEKS – MONTHS)

Treatments commonly used include:-

- opiates
- nebulized opiates
- oxygen
- benzodiazepines

Opiates   Morphine is seen as a standard treatment for breathlessness in the palliative care setting but there have been few studies looking at its use.

Studies of morphine for dyspnoea

- 20 patients breathless on continuous oxygen. 15 on opioids for pain. Given a stat subcutaneous injection of 2.5 x usual dose (mean

28 +/- 22mg) or 5mg morphine if opiate naive. Breathlessness reduced (Figure 3.), nausea and sedation occurred in 2 opioid naive patients.[22]

- 18 patients (16 opioids naive) given either (MST) 10mg bd (14 patients), or the equivalent 4 hourly oral morphine (2 patients) or a 30% increase in current morphine. Five withdrew, because of drowsiness or dizziness. Only 1 patient reported definite improvement.[23]

- 10 patients (all on opioids for pain) on continuous oxygen. Given 1.5 x usual 4 hourly dose of morphine or placebo subcutaneously. Breathlessness was reduced. 9 preferred morphine, 1 no preference.[24]

These studies highlight that whilst opiates are helpful for the relief of breathlessness at rest, they may be tolerated less well when used in patients without pain (at least initially). Following an initial bad experience with opiates (particularly when combined with pre-existing fears of opiates) it can be difficult for the patient to feel confident about trying opiates again. Therefore use small doses initially (e.g. 2.5mg oral morphine) and titrate the dose according to response and side effects. Doses above 15mg 4 hourly often causes unwanted side effects with little further symptomatic improvement.[10]

Morphine for Dyspnoea

Robert a 75 year old man developed carcinoma of the lung on the background of extensive fibrosing alveolitis. He was cyanosed, frightened and distressed by his breathlessness despite continuous oxygen even whilst resting. His breathlessness overwhelmed his day to day existence. He was unable to sleep at night. He found that oral morphine 2.5mg every 4 hours with 5mg at night made him more comfortable and gave him a sleepfull night. He was able to concentrate on other activities (e.g. reading the paper/watching television) and started to talk about his anxieties.

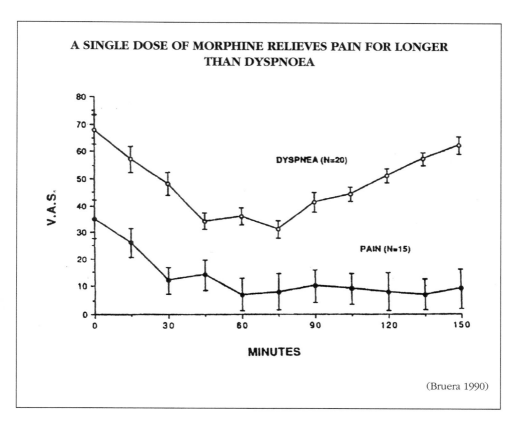

A SINGLE DOSE OF MORPHINE RELIEVES PAIN FOR LONGER THAN DYSPNOEA

(Bruera 1990)

Bruera found that duration of relief of dyspnoea was less (returning to baseline level after 2½ hours) than the relief of pain after a single dose of morphine in patients with cancer.[22]

> A single dose of morphine relieves pain for longer than dyspnoea.
>
> (Bruera 1990)

This suggests that the relief of breathlessness requires a higher concentration of morphine/ morphine metabolites compared to the relief if pain. This implies that for consistent relief of breathlessness either larger or more frequent doses of morphine would be necessary, but this may increase the risk of unwanted side effects. In my experience a continuous subcutaneous infusion of opiate can be tolerated better and be more effective for some patients – possibly by avoiding the peaks (with side effects) and troughs (with loss of effect) of oral medication.

Nebulized opioids

Nebulized opioids have recently received much attention. Opiates have been inhaled for at least 3,000 years and were suggested as a treatment for cough by Beigel in 1866.

> "He who expects wonders from that mode of treatment (nebulized drugs) will soon be disappointed: he who recommends it as an infallible one, will prove a false prophet: but an unprejudiced application of the atomizer will lead to a conviction that the invention . . . has been a most valuable addition to therapeutics.".[25]
>
> (Biegel, 1866)

Peak serum levels occur 10 minutes after nebulized morphine but bioavailability is only 2 – 8%.[26] It has therefore been postulated that relief of breathlessness may occur as a result of the opiate having a local effect on the lungs. A starting dose of morphine sulphate (for injection) 10–20mg is safe diluted to 5ml with normal saline, nebulized every 4 hours or as required. The dose can be increased up to 100mg 4 hourly if necessary.[27]

Nebulized diamorphine and fentanyl have also been suggested for the treatment of breathlessness.[11,27] As diamorphine and fentanyl are more lipophilic than morphine they demonstrate greater systemic absorption and reach initial peak plasma levels more quickly eg diamorphine (6 mins) and fentanyl (2 mins).

In summary however:-

● The initial impressive findings in a study of patients with COPD have not been replicated in later studies involving normal volunteers or patients with COPD or interstitial lung disease.

● Many of the published reports of its use in patients with cancer are anecdotal observation of its uncontrolled use.

● In the only randomised controlled trial in patients with cancer, nebulized morphine in single dose (5–50mg) was no better than saline although there was a trend towards benefit with higher doses. The maximal effect on breathlessness was seen one hour after the nebulization, which indicates a systemic rather than a local effect.[28]

● More information is required before it is seen as a standard treatment.

Much is unknown about the use of opioids for breathlessness. Research needs to address starting doses, dose scheduling (frequency, rate of dose escalation), route of administration and most effective opioid.

Oxygen There are no agreed guidelines for the use of oxygen. There undoubtedly can be a large placebo effect but it is probably underused in hospices. This may be due the practical difficulties rather than a lack of clinical benefit. (eg few hospices have piped oxygen – most rely on cylinders).

Studies of oxygen in patients with cancer

● 14 severely hypoxic patients already on oxygen. None with COPD. 5 l/min oxygen was compared to air over 5mins. 12/14 patients preferred oxygen.[29]

● 38 patients (6 hypoxic). None on oxygen. 13 with COPD. 4 l/min oxygen versus air over 15 mins. Both reduced breathlessness. 15 preferred oxygen, 11 air.[30]

The first study indicates that severely hypoxic patients are likely to benefit from oxygen. The second study illustrates the difficulty in identifying patients who are likely to benefit from an unselected group. Further work is needed.

Clinically oxygen can be given on a trial basis via nasal prongs. If available a pulse oximeter will help identify patients whose saturation is improved by oxygen therapy. Unfortunately, initial saturation can be a poor predictor of who may benefit. On review if the patient has persisted in using the oxygen and has found it useful it can be continued. If the patient has any doubts to its efficacy then it should be discontinued. If beneficial, oxygen can be delivered at home via cylinders or an oxygen concentrator. These are more convenient but can be limited by their maximal flow rate (4 l/min). If necessary tubing from two machines can be joined by a T-piece to deliver higher flow rates.

Benzodiazepines

Benzodiazepines are anecdotally useful, but there are no studies in patients with cancer. In patients with chronic lung disease they reduce in breathlessness *only if there is coexisting anxiety.* However, anxiety is common in breathless patients with cancer.[17] The oral benzodiazepine of choice is diazepam initially 2 – 5mg tid, reducing over several days (because levels of active metabolites rise) to a maintenance dose of 2–5mg at night. Oral or sublingual lorazepam 0.5 – 1mg (up to 4mg per day) can be useful for acute episodes of breathlessness. It is rapidly absorbed and relatively short-acting. The parenteral benzodiazepine of choice is midazolam initially 10–30mg per 24 hours by SC infusion. This dose is often sufficient when combined with an opiate. However, midazolam can worsen agitation or confusion, when it can be combined with haloperidol (5–10mg / 24 hours) or methotrimeprazine can be used instead.

Buspirone

Buspirone is valuable as a non-sedative anxiolytic. It is an azaspirodecanedione not a benzodiazepine. It is as effective as diazepam in the treatment of anxiety but does not depress ventilation. The starting dose is 5mg two to three times a day. This can be increased every 2 – 3 days. The usual therapeutic dose is 15 to 30 mg daily in divided doses with a maximum of 45mg daily in divided doses.

Phenothiazines

Anecdotally useful. No studies in patients with cancer. Their anxiolytic or sedative effects may be more important than a specific effect. The use of chlorpromazine for terminal breathlessness has already been described.

DYSPNOEA ON EXERTION (MONTHS – YEARS)

This type of dyspnoea is hardest to control. Often such patients have pre-existing cardiopulmonary

GENERAL MANAGEMENT OF DYSPNOEA

- Exploration of anxieties – (especially fear of sudden death)
- Explanation of symptoms and meaning
- Informing patient and family that breathlessness in itself is not dangerous
- What is/is not likely to happen ("you won't choke or suffocate to death")
- Help come to terms with deteriorating condition
- Exercise advice / use of aids for mobility
  - Enlist help of physiotherapist / occupational therapist
- Breathing control advice
  - Enlist help of physiotherapist – techniques vary. e.g. active cycle control.

> Slow their respiratory rate down (particularly by prolonging the expiratory phase) for several breaths and then allow to return to the rate that is comfortable for them for several breaths. The cycle is repeated until their respiratory rate is reduced. This demonstrates to the patient that they have control over their breathing and allows the patient to pace the reduction at a comfortable level.

- Relaxation techniques
- Use of fan / oxygen
- Plan of action for acute episodes for patient and family give simple written instructions of a step-by-step plan.
- Assessment of social support networks (patients often elderly, alone and socially isolated)
- Use of complementary therapies (beneficial for some patients.)

NB Increasing breathlessness (often as part of increasing weakness) is a clear sign of deterioration. The many issues this raises need to be looked for and addressed.

disease. Opioids are often poorly tolerated in this setting. More research is needed. General approaches become particularly important and required the involvement of the multidisciplinary team.

FACILITATING ADJUSTMENT TO DYSPNOEA

Dyspnoea clinic   Many of the aspects of general management described in the box above have been employed in the development of a nurse-led clinic to specifically

Dyspnoea due to Anxiety

Peggy, a 76 year old woman presented with increasing breathlessness due to multiple lung metastases from carcinoma of the breast 10 years after her original mastectomy. Her disease partially responded to hormone therapy and became static. However, she remained distressed by her persistent breathlessness on exertion (she also had COPD). This continued despite optimising her inhaled treatment. She lived alone and was becoming increasingly anxious and suffered frightening episodes of breathlessness. She started to attend the local hospice day centre. Over a matter of weeks she was transformed. Her complaints about her breathing gradually subsided without the need for further changes to her medication.

help patients cope with their breathlessness.[31] Initially, patients attend 4 weekly clinic sessions (each lasting one hour). The patients experience of breathlessness, its meaning to them and their feelings about it in the context of their understanding about their disease and prognosis are explored. Advice on managing breathlessness, breathing retraining, exertion, relaxation techniques and goal setting is given. Further follow-up sessions are offered. In a randomised controlled pilot study of this approach in patients with lung cancer breathlessness scores, distress caused by breathlessness, functional capacity and ability to perform activities of daily living were all improved. Anxiety and depression scores were unchanged. By contrast the control group scores remained static or worsened (Jessica Corner, personal communication).

DISCUSSION

Patients often fear breathlessness, and have the thoughts of suffocation or of choking to death. It is vital that these fears are explored. It should be explained that we can control distressing breathlessness at the end of life. We should not wait until the patient is terrified and exhausted before offering appropriate treatment. This continues to happen – almost as if patients have to earn their morphine.

We should give patients confidence that we can help improve breathlessness at rest and give patients a restful night by using morphine. Morphine can be less well tolerated in this setting and it should be used with care. The possible role of nebulized opiates awaits further clarification. The use of other agents (e.g. oxygen, anxiolytics and phenothiazines) needs to be tailored to the individual patient. Without the guidance of good research many will be given on an empirical basis. If after a predetermined trial period they are not helping they should be discontinued.

The general approach is important at all times but particularly so for patients breathless on exertion. It is common for the patient to fear that becoming breathless is dangerous and it is important to explore this. Breathlessness is a basic physiological response of the body to exertion and is impossible to prevent. Breathlessness becomes a problem when it occurs at a reduced level of exertion as it is then associated with the loss of ability to do things. It is an obvious marker of deterioration for the patient. In the absence of a reversible cause it becomes important to help guide the patient and family to adjust to the changing situation which is often punctuated by a series of such losses. The total care of the patient is important requiring all the skills of the multidisciplinary team. Support and respite provided by day care or inpatient facilities of palliative care units can be invaluable. It remains to be seen if nursing led clinics will develop on a wider scale.

It is only recently that the problem of breathlessness in patients with cancer has been formally addressed. To date, the number of published studies is disproportionate to the clinical significance of this distressing symptom which remains difficult to manage. Many basic questions remain unanswered about existing treatment options. The development of new therapies should be based on the results of good quality research rather than anecdote of their uncontrolled use. In view of the low recruitment and high attrition rate in patients with advanced cancer, the challenge for the future will be the development of greater multicentre collaboration for such research.

References

1. Reuben DB and Mor VM. Dyspnoea in terminally ill cancer patients. Chest 1986; 89 (2): 234–236.
2. Groud S, Zech D, Diefenbach C and Bischoff A. Prevalence and pattern of symptoms in patients with cancer pain: A prospective evaluation of 1635 cancer patients referred to a pain clinic. J Pain Symptom Manage 1994; 9: 372–382.
3. Donnelly, SM, Walsh, TD and Rybicki L. The symptoms of advanced cancer: Effects of age and gender on symptoms and survival in 1,000 patients. (Abstract) Pall Med 1995; 9(1): 71.
4. Reubin DB, Mor V and Hiris J. Clinical symptoms and length of survival in patients with terminal cancer. Arch Intern Med 1988; 148: 1586–1591.
5. Twycross RG and Lack S. Control of Alimentary symptoms in far advanced cancer. Edinburgh: Churchill Livingstone, 1986. p 6.
6. Brescia FJ, Adler D, Gray G, Ryan MA, Cimino J and Mamtani R. Hospitalized advanced cancer patients: a profile. J Pain Symptom Manage 1990; 5: 221–227.
7. Muers MF and Round CE. Palliation of symptoms in non-small cell lung cancer: a study by the Yorkshire Regional Cancer Organisation thoracic group. Thorax 1993; 48: 339–343.
8. Krech RL, Walsh D and Curtis EB. Symptoms of lung cancer. Pall Med 1992; 6: 309–315.
9. Gift GG. Dyspnoea. Nurs Clin North America 1990; 25 (4): 955–965.
10. Cowcher K and Hanks GW. Long term management of respiratory symptoms in advanced cancer. J Pain Symptom Manage 1990; 5: 320–330.
*11.Ahmedzai S. Palliation of respiratory symptoms. In: Doyle D, Hanks GWC and MacDonald N eds. Oxford textbook of palliative medicine. Oxford, Oxford University Press, 1993: 349–378.
12. Congelton J and Meurs MF. The incidence of airflow obstruction in bronchial carcinoma its relation to breathlessness, and response to bronchodilator therapy. Resp Med 1995;89: 291–296.
13. Burns BH and Howell JBL. Disproportionately severe breathlessness in chronic bronchitis. Q J Med 1969; 38: 277–294.
14. Light RW, Merrill EJ, Despars JA, Gordon GH and Mutalipassi LR. Prevalence of depression and anxiety in patients with COPD. Chest 1985; 87: 35–38.
15. Gift AG, Plaut SM and Jacox AK. Psychologic and physiologic factors related to dyspnea in subjects with chronic obstructive pulmonary disease. Heart and Lung 1986; 15: 595–601.
16. Kellner R, Samet J and Pathak D. Dyspnea, anxiety and depression in chronic respiratory impairment. Gen Hosp Psych 1992; 14: 20–28.
17. Hinton JM. Physical and mutual distress of the dying. Q J Med 1963; 32: 1–21.
18. Brown ML, Carrieri VK, Janson-Bjerklie S and Dodd M. Lung cancer and dyspnea: the patients perception. Oncol Nurs Forum 1986; 13:19–24.
19. Ventafridda V, Spoldi E and De Conno F. Control of dyspnoea in advanced cancer patients (letter). Chest 1990; 98(6): 1544–1545.
20. McIver B, Walsh D, Nelson K. The use of chlorpromazine for symptom control in dying cancer patients. J Pain Symptom Manage 1994; 9: 341–345.
21. Cohen MH, Anderson AJ, Krasnow SH, Spagnolo SV, Citron ML, Payne M and Fossieck BE. Continuous intravenous infusion of morphine for severe dyspnoea. South Med J 1991; 84: 229–234.

22. Bruera E, Macmillan K, Pither J and MacDonald RN. Effects of morphine on dyspnoea of terminal cancer patients. J Pain Symptom Manag 1990; 5(4): 83–93.
23. Boyd K and Kelly M. Oral morphine for dyspnoea in cancer patients? (abstract). Prog Pall Care 1994; 2(1): 10.
24. Bruera E, MacEachern T, Ripamonti C and Hanson J. Subcutaneous morphine for dyspnoea in cancer patients. Ann Intern Med 1993; 119: 906–907.
25. Beigel H. On inhalation, as a means of local treatment of the organs of respiration by atomized fluids and gases. London: Robert Hardwicke, 1866.
26. Masood AR and Thomas SHL. Systemic absorbtion of nebulised morphine compared to oral morphine in healthy subjects. Br J Clin Pharmacol 1996; 41: 250–252.
*27. Davis C. The role of nebulised drugs in palliating respiratory symptoms of malignant disease. Eur J Pall Care 1995; 2(1): 9–15.
28. Davis CL, Penn K, A'Hern R, Daniels J and Slevin M. Single dose randomised controlled trial of nebulised morphine in patients with cancer related breathlessness (abstract). Pall Med 1996; 10 (1): 64.
29. Bruera E, de Stoutz N, Velasco-Leiva A, Schoeller T and Hanson J. Effects of oxygen on dyspnoea in hypoxaemic terminal cancer patients. Lancet 1993; 342: 13–14.
30. Booth S, Kelly MJ, Cox NP, Adams L and Guz A. Does oxygen help dyspnoea in lung cancer. Int J Pall Nurs 1995; 1(1): 5–11.
31. Corner J, Plant H and Warner L. Developing a nursing approach to managing dyspnoea in lung cancer. Int J Pall Nurs 1995; 1(1): 5–11.

*Note: – Reference 11 is essential reading as a useful review of the subject. Reference 27 is an excellent review of the role of nebulized drugs.

Chapter 12

Constipation

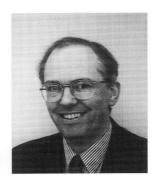

Dr Nigel Sykes
Nigel Sykes has been a Consultant in Palliative Medicine at St Christopher's Hospice, London, since 1991. He was previously Macmillan Lecturer in Palliative Medicine at Leeds.
Dr Sykes' research interests have centred on the management of gastrointestinal symptoms, particularly constipation, in terminally ill patients and he is the chapter author on constipation and diarrhoea in the Oxford Textbook of Palliative Medicine. *He is also co-editor, with Dame Cicely Saunders, of the latest edition of* The Management of Terminal Malignant Disease. *Dr Sykes has served as Treasurer and Executive Committee member of the Association for Palliative Medicine of Great Britain and Ireland, and is currently a member of the Association's ethics committee.*

WHAT IS CONSTIPATION?

Constipation means difficulty in passing stools. Objective measures (such as frequency of defaecation or amount of stool) can be quantified, but constipation is primary a symptom of difficulty defaecating. The success of treatment must be assessed in terms of the patients perception of difficulty. There is no set stool frequency to be achieved, but most people seem to become more uncomfortable in body and mind after two clear days without defaecation.

GUT MOTILITY

Food residues take 24–48 hours to travel through the bowel, with most of the time (90%) spent in the colon. In the small bowel motor activity every 90 minutes pushes the contents forward (the Migrating Motor Complex). This pattern is temporarily abolished by food intake, when irregular activity takes over (retaining food in the small bowel for mixing and absorbtion). The propulsive movement is mediated by the gut hormone Motilin.

Segmentation

The large bowel is just as active as the small bowel, but in a different way. Motility consists mostly of segmentation (alternating constriction and relaxation) which mixes gut contents (food and bacteria) and increases absorbtion of water.

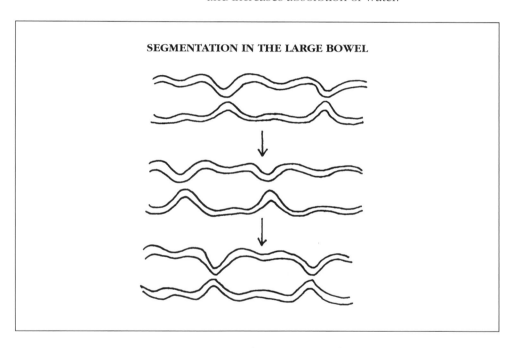

SEGMENTATION IN THE LARGE BOWEL

Forward movement of the large bowel contents only occurs about 6 times a day (mass movement) mainly during the daytime (stimulated by eating and physical activity, especially getting up in the morning.) This type of activity is perceived as borborygmi or an urge to defaecate, and is sometimes associated with defaecation itself.

The control of gut motility

In addition to co-ordinated motor activity, all regions of the gut respond to local distention, which causes a reflex peristalsis with contraction proximally and relaxation distally, resulting in propulsion of the mass along the lumen.

REFLEX PERISTALSIS IN THE GUT

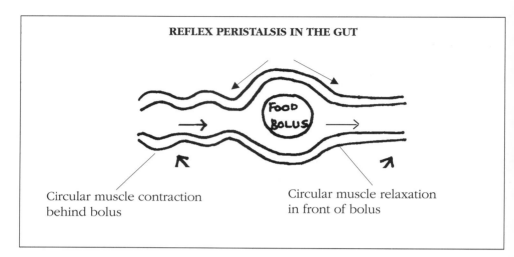

Circular muscle contraction behind bolus

Circular muscle relaxation in front of bolus

The gut has pacemaker cells (in the inner and outer circular muscle) which depolarize rhythmically. Contraction and relaxation are modulated by two distinct populations of neurones (see figure below).

Neuro-transmitters in peristalsis

One group of gut neurones causes muscle contraction via transmitters that include acetyl choline (ACh) and kinins such as Substance P. The other group produces muscle relaxation via transmitters that include vasoactive peptide (VIP), the enzyme that synthesises nitric oxide (NO), somatostatin, gamma amino butyric acid (GABA) and opioids. Endogenous opioids relax intestinal muscle and reduce peristalsis (the so called "ileal brake"). Fat or carbohydrate in the ilium also slow transit.

Central control of peristalsis

Gut motility is also controlled by the spinal cord, brain stem and cortex. Low cord transection or damage to the extrinsic pelvic nerves causes marked slowing of colonic transit. High cord transection produces little change in colonic activity but abolishes the gastrocolic reflex. Gut motility is affected by anxiety and increased by the anticipation of food.

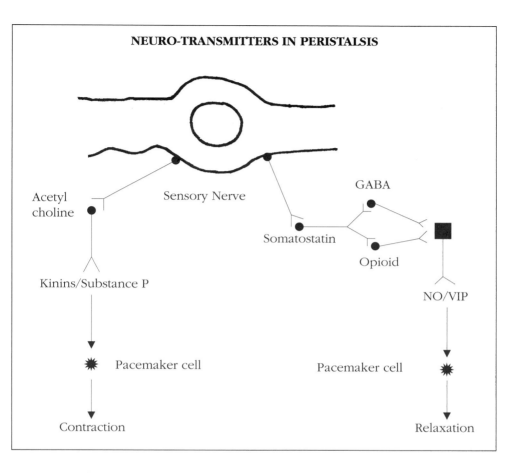

FLUID HANDLING

About 7 litres of fluid are secreted into the gut daily, with about 1.5 litres swallowed. All but 150 ml of this is re-absorbed. Water absorbtion is remarkably precise, the difference between constipation and diarrhoea in terms of fluid excretion being only about 100 ml per day. Most water is absorbed by the colon, with contributions from the jejunum and ileum.

The normal condition of gut epithelium is secretory. Adrenergic (alpha and beta sympathetic) efferents reduce secretion, cholinergic pathways stimulate it. Absorption is an active process under neuronal control. Both cholinergic and adrenergic systems are tonically active, and control normal bowel function.

CLINICAL CAUSES OF CONSTIPATION

Debility and reduced food and fluid intake can all predispose to constipation.

Reduced food intake

Reduced food intake reduces stimulation of the gastro-colic reflex and reduces distention of the colonic wall (with less reflex peristalsis.) People with poor appetites tend to prefer low fibre foods. *Debility (or poor symptom control)* reduce mobility and mass movements occur less frequently.

Anticholinergic drugs

Anticholinergic drugs (eg. amitriptyline, hyoscine, cyclizine) tend to worsen constipation. *Vincristine* causes constipation, due to a reversible autonomic dysfunction. *Hypercalcaemia* causes constipation because calcium is involved in nerve transmissions and muscular contraction.

OPIOIDS AND CONSTIPATION

Opioids are frequently blamed for constipation in palliative care. In fact they worsen an existing situation, rather than create a new one. In a sample of hospice in-patients on opioids, 87% on strong opioids required laxatives, 75% on weak opioids required laxatives *but 64% still required a laxative, (at a lower dose) even on no opioids.* The last figure is similar to that reported for elderly people without malignant disease in hospital, presumably reflecting factors related to debility and reduced food and fluid intake.

Morphine and other opioids act primarily on the colon to increase gut segmentation and reduce propulsive movements. It is not surprising that exogenous opioids cause constipation, because endogenous opioids are found in the neurones controlling gut motility.

Opioids increase sphincter tone at all gut levels, from stomach to anus. Rectal sensation diminishes with age and may be further reduced by morphine, increasing the likelihood of an elderly person developing faecal impaction. An opioid effect on intestinal fluid handling has not been demonstrated in man, but a reduction in bowel secretion occurs in some animals. In rodents morphine causes constipation centrally (via kappa receptors) as well as peripherally (chiefly mu receptors).

Studies in man suggest morphine acts primarily on the gut. Parenteral (non-oral) morphine does not avoid constipation, (although it might reduce its severity) because gut receptors are accessible via the blood stream as well as luminally.

Morphine dose

Does increasing the dose of morphine worsen constipation? It is often suggested that if opioid dose is increased, laxative dose should be increased. However, considerable variation occurs and performance status may be more important for predicting constipation than morphine dosage.[2] A study of 179 patients on strong opioids showed that as morphine dose increased laxative dose also increased in a hyperbolic curve, characteristic of a drug interaction with a receptor. This suggests that laxatives dose indicates the strength of opioid receptor affinity.[3] If so, higher doses of morphine would be relatively less constipating than lower doses, which may be a comfort to patients who fear that if their analgesia is increased further their constipation will worsen.

In a small study by the author of patients on morphine for 2 months stool frequencies were higher and laxative doses were no different to patients on morphine for shorter periods, suggesting that a degree to tollerance to opioid-induced constipation may occur.

Some opioids, such as *transdermal fentanyl*, are claimed to be less constipating than morphine. Whether this is due simply to its route of delivery or whether fentanyl differs from morphine in its relative affinity for receptors is not clear.

CLINICAL ASSESSMENT

History

Ask about frequency and difficulty of defaecation. Did constipation pre-date the present illness? What was the prior stool pattern? Longstanding constipation may justify wider investigations. Constipation can cause abdominal pain, bloating, flatulence, nausea, malaise, headache and halitosis. Constipation is thought to be a cause of nausea and vomiting by 90% of hospice nursing staff, but evidence for the true level of association is lacking. When persuaded to retain stool for over 48 hours, 1 in 4 normal volunteers complained of nausea.[4]

Nausea and malaise can be caused by packing the rectum with cotton or suppositories, and so is presumably a response to gut distension. However, the holder of what seems the record for delayed defaecation – 368 days – was able to work normally most of this time! In palliative care constipation should be excluded if there is a history of a recent onset of nausea and vomiting. Similarly, unexplained recent urinary incontinence or apparent "diarrhoea" and faecal incontinence in elderly patients may result from faecal impaction.

Examination

Abdominal examination and rectal examination are vital, and will help to avoid major mistakes in the diagnosis of constipation, such as faecal impaction, and intestinal obstruction.

Investigations

Investigations are rarely needed. Abdominal X-ray may distinguish between constipation and obstruction if there is persisting doubt. X-ray may show more constipation than does clinical assessment alone.[5]

An important principle is that constipation is a symptom, and the correlation between different degrees of faecal loading on an X-ray and physical discomfort has not been defined. Very rarely constipation may be due to another condition (hypercalcaemia, hypothyriodism). If clinically indicated, corrected calcium levels and thyroid function tests should be performed.

PREVENTION OF CONSTIPATION

Mobility should be encouraged, as much as physical limitations allow, because activity is a key stimulus to colonic peristalsis and defaecation. *Oral fluids* help because dehydration causes stools to have relatively low water content, rendering them hard and difficult to pass. *Dietary fibre* may help mild constipation in well people, but a study of radiotherapy patients showed that an intolerable 450% increase in dietary fibre was needed to achieve a 50% increase in stool frequency.[6] Thus fibre alone will not correct severe constipation.

Drugs which are likely to cause constipation should either be avoided or a laxative prescribed, simultaneously. *Lack of privacy* for defaecation and the use of bed pans are conducive to constipation. It should be a priority to allow patients privacy and the use of a lavatory, or a commode, for defaecation.

MANAGEMENT OF CONSTIPATION

Diet

Many people have their own remedies for constipation. Prunes, rhubarb and bananas, all contain laxative substances (some related to the active component of senna). Liquorice can be laxative, but is prone to cause hyperkalaemia. Coffee (both caffeinated and non-caffeinated) increases stool frequency. Some beers are potent laxatives.

Abdominal massage

Abdominal massage has been recommended as an extension of the principle of increasing activity. However, a controlled trial of abdominal massage failed to show benefit in either constipated patients or healthy volunteers.[7] Application of either heat or cold to the abdomen has been used in the management of constipation since Roman times, with no clear evidence of efficacy.

Laxatives

Aims of Treatment

The majority of patients with advanced cancer require laxatives. There is surprisingly little evidence to guide choice of laxative type or dosage. Most evidence comes from geriatric medicine. The aim of laxative therapy is comfortable defaecation, not increased frequency of evacuation. Even on regular laxatives, 40 – 60% of hospice patients also need rectal measures on a continuing basis, particularly if taking strong opioid analgesia. In a series of 100 hospice patients, 67 complained of constipation on admission and, despite considerable attention to the problem, 41 remained constipated at the end of their admission (although generally less severely).

No single laxative is adequate for everyone. Many patients need both rectal interventions and oral laxatives. Adequate dose titration can halve the requirement for rectal laxatives.[8] As with chronic pain, therapy should be regular, not intermittent.

Bulking agents

Bulking agents such as methyl cellulose or ispaghula are not appropriate for routine use in palliative care. They need to be taken with large volumes of water and are not effective for severe constipation.

Patient preference

In a study of healthy volunteers on loperamide (to mimic opioid-induced constipation) lactulose (predominantly softening), senna (predominantly stimulant) and codanthrusate (a combination laxative) all corrected bowel function. However, senna caused significantly more adverse effects than the other two and lactulose had to be used in excessive doses. Co-danthrusate was preferred for least adverse effects and medication burden.[9] This experimental evidence supports the clinical impression that a stimulant and softener used together are preferable to either used alone.

Action of laxatives

No drug acts purely to soften the stool or to stimulate gut peristalsis. Softeners also increases bulk (and thus reflexly stimulate peristalsis). Stimulants also enhance intestinal fluid secretion (and so soften the stool). Nonetheless, the predominant action does differ from drug to drug and can be used as a basis for choice.

Oral laxatives

Lactulose

Lactulose acts by osmotic retention of water in the small bowel, thereby increasing stool bulk. It is effective in opioid-induced constipation but large

PREDOMINANTLY SOFTENING LAXATIVES

	Mode of Action	Usual dose range	Comments
Lactulose	Osmotic agent: (retains water in gut lumen)	15–40 mls BD-TDS	Active principally in the small bowel. Latency of action 1–2 days
Docusate sodium	Surfactant agent (increases water penetration of the stool)	60–300 mg BD	Probably not very effective when used alone. Latency of action 1–3 days.
Magnesium sulphate	Osmotic agent	2–4 g daily	Act throughout the bowel and may have pronounced purgative effect, possible partly as a result of direct peristaltic stimulation. Latency of action 1–6 hr (dose dependent)
Poloxamer	Surfactant agent	–	Only available in combination with danthron.
Liquid paraffin	Lubricant	–	Only available in a 25% emulsion with magnesium hydroxide (Mil-Par).
Glycerine suppositories	Lubricant	1–2 PRN	May also have an irritant action that provokes expulsion of stools.

doses are required. It is degraded by bacteria in the colon so the osmotic effect does not extend throughout the colon. Flatulence is a problem for about 20% of patients and some dislike its sweet taste. *Sorbitol* has been reported to be as effective as lactulose, cheaper and less nauseating.

Docusate   Docusate alone is not widely used in British hospice practice. It increases water, sodium and chloride secretion in the jejunum and colon in addition to its surfactant action. In healthy volunteers it failed to increase colonic output of solids or water but was more effective than placebo in clinical trials in elderly and chronically ill patients.

Magnesium hydroxide and magnesium sulphate

Magnesium hydroxide and magnesium sulphate both increase intestinal water secretion and also stimulate peristalsis in addition to their osmotic effect. Latency of action (4–12 hours) is much shorter than the purely softening laxatives. Magnesium sulphate is the more potent and can produce an undesirably strong purgative action, but can be useful for resistant constipation.

Liquid paraffin and magnesium hydroxide emulsion

Liquid paraffin and magnesium hydroxide emulsion tends to be thought of as a combination of 2 softeners but it approaches the effcacy of a senna/lactulose combination. It is also much cheaper, but unfortunately tends to be less acceptable to patients.[3]

Senna

Senna Is an anthraquinone which acts directly on the bowel (its action can be abolished by local anaesthetic infiltration of the mucosa). It reduces absorption of water and electrolytes by the colon. It is almost inactive until colonic bacteria convert its glycosides into the active aglycone forms, so activity is limited to the colon. The aglycones are absorbed to a limited degree and secreted in the bile. This recirculation is more important for danthron and the polyphenolic agents (bisacodyl and sodium picosulphate) which undergo glucuronidation and are reconverted in the gut to active drug, prolonging the agents' action. Effective doses of stimulant laxatives show 4–8 fold variation between individuals. Equal proportions of senna liquid and lactulose are significantly more potent than standard codanthramer (danthron with poloxamer), but are probably less potent than higher strength Codanthramer.[8]

Bulk forming agents

Bulk forming agents, (methyl cellulose, psyllium or ispaghula) are not mentioned in the table as they should probably be avoided in palliative medicine. The volume of water they require (at least 200–300 ml) and their consistency are unacceptable to many ill patients, and if taken with inadequate water a viscous mass may form which can complete a partial malignant obstruction.

STIMULANT LAXATIVES

	Mode of Action	Dose range	Comments
Senna	All these stimulant laxatives have the same actions: * Stimulation of myenteric nerves * Increased gut mobility * Soften motion by reduced absorbtion of water from gut.	7.5 – 30mg bd	Anthraquinone family.
Danthron		50 – 450mg bd	Danthron only available in combination with docusate or poloxamer. Stains urine red/brown. Latency of action 6–12 hr
Bisacodyl Sodium picosulphate		10 – 20mg bd 5 – 50mg bd	Polyphenolic family Latency of action 6–12 hr.

COMBINATION LAXATIVES

	Constituents	Dose range	Comments
Codanthramer Suspension	Danthron 25mg Poloxamer 200mg per 5 ml	5–30ml BD	Latency of action for Danthron is around 8hrs.
Codanthramer strong Suspension	Danthron 75mg Poloxamer 1g per 5 ml	5–30ml BD	Danthron – containing laxatives have a limited license for patients with cardiac disease or terminal disease.
Codanthramer Capsule	Danthron 25mg Poloxamer 200mg	1–4 caps BD	
Codanthramer strong capsule	Danthron 37.5 Poloxamer 500mg	1–4 caps BD	
Codanthrusate	Docusate 60mg Danthron 50mg per 5ml or capsule	1–4 Caps BD	Capsule or suspension
Milpar	Emulsion magnesium hydroxide and liquid paraffin (3:1 ratio)	5–30ml BD	Liquid only. Latency of action 4–12 hours. Not as effective as a senna/ lactulose combination.

Rectal laxatives

Most patients prefer oral to rectal laxatives. Nevertheless enemas and suppositories are still frequently needed, often because oral laxative doses are too low. Rectal laxatives give a prompt and reliable result. Rectal laxatives all stimulate the ano-colonic reflex.

Bisacodyl suppositories

Bisacodyl suppositories cause colonic peristalsis. Their rapid action of 1 hour (in most patients) compared to oral bisacodyl is probably due to conversion to its active form by colonic flora in the rectum.

Glycerine

Glycerine softens stools by osmosis, is lubricant and may stimulate rectal muscles to provoke evacuation. *Surfactant agents* include docusate (which can be used as an enema) and the lauryl and alkyl forms of sodium sulphoacetate – both used in proprietary mini-enemas. Sodium phosphate and sodium citrate enemas have osmotic action and possibly also act like the saline laxatives.

Arachis oil

Arachis oil and olive oil are used as retention enemas overnight to soften hard faeces impacted in the rectum. Naturally their efficacy depends on the patient's ability to retain the oil.

Effectiveness of rectal measures

There is little data on the comparative efficacy of rectal laxatives. One study[10] monitored how many patients achieved defaecation within an hour of the rectal intervention:

EFFECTIVE WITHIN 1 HOUR	
phosphate enema	100%
mini-enemas, (Micralax)	95%,
bisacodyl suppository	66%,
glycerine suppository	38%

Phosphate and mini-enemas were equally effective. Biscodyl suppositories were more effective than over glycerine suppositories – confirming results from other studies.

One hospice survey of 164 patients showed rectal laxatives were used 337 times in 16 different combinations and doses, despite the existence of a

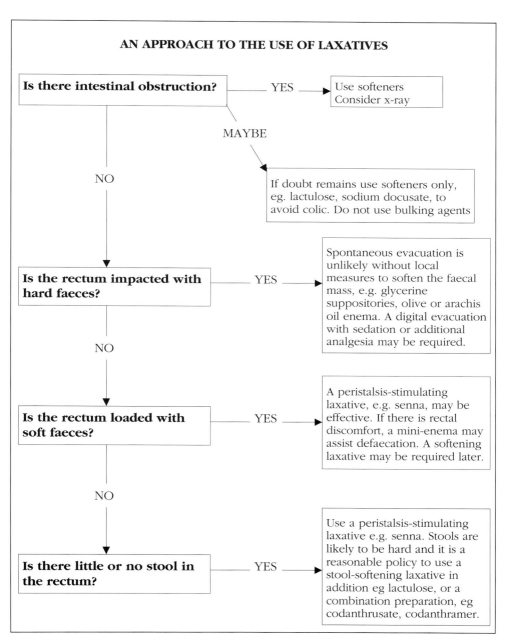

AN APPROACH TO THE USE OF LAXATIVES

Is there intestinal obstruction? — YES → Use softeners / Consider x-ray

MAYBE

If doubt remains use softeners only, eg. lactulose, sodium docusate, to avoid colic. Do not use bulking agents

NO

Is the rectum impacted with hard faeces? — YES → Spontaneous evacuation is unlikely without local measures to soften the faecal mass, e.g. glycerine suppositories, olive or arachis oil enema. A digital evacuation with sedation or additional analgesia may be required.

NO

Is the rectum loaded with soft faeces? — YES → A peristalsis-stimulating laxative, e.g. senna, may be effective. If there is rectal discomfort, a mini-enema may assist defaecation. A softening laxative may be required later.

NO

Is there little or no stool in the rectum? — YES → Use a peristalsis-stimulating laxative e.g. senna. Stools are likely to be hard and it is a reasonable policy to use a stool-softening laxative in addition eg lactulose, or a combination preparation, eg codanthrusate, codanthramer.

protocol, making it impossible to separate the effects of individual agents. Suppositories produced evacuation in 90% of cases, enemas in 86%. The median latency between administration and evacuation was 1hr for suppositories and 30 min for enemas.[3]

Rules for using laxatives

- give oral laxatives regularly
- Use a laxative favoured by the patient if possible
- keep a record of stool frequency
- have an approach to the choice between rectal and oral laxatives, and between softening and stimulant drugs.
- titrate laxative doses adequately, (avoiding colic or diarrhoea.)
- if diarrhoea effects occurs, stop laxatives for 24h and restart one dose step lower.
- check the patient's perception of their bowel function.

Obstruction or Constipation?

A lady of 62 with a 4 year history of endometrial carcinoma developed episodes of severe abdominal pain with constipation. She was found to have a large pelvic mass, possibly involving bowel, and intermittent bowel obstruction was diagnosed. She had, however, tended to be constipated over many years. In the hospice she continued to experience episodes of abdominal and rectal pain associated with distension, active bowel sounds and constipation. Evacuation of any stool in the rectum, with the aid of a mini-enema, relieved the rectal pain. Stimulant laxatives were suspended and lactulose used alone. This tended to give excessive wind and was changed to an emulsion of magnesium hydroxide and liquid paraffin (Mil-Par), gradually titrated upwards. It remained unclear whether her symptoms represented bowel obstruction by tumour or exacerbations of poorly controlled constipation, and so erect and supine abdominal X-rays were obtained. These showed extensive colonic faecal loading but no evidence of obstruction. Five grams of magnesium sulphate were given, with hyoscine butylbromide available in case of colic. This was repeated the following day and within 72h the abdominal distension had subsided following several large evacuations. Her laxative was changed to higher strength codanthramer and the dose titrated to 30 ml bd. This lady lived for a further three years and never developed intestinal obstruction despite gradual enlargement of her abdominal mass.

NEW DEVELOPMENTS AND ALTERNATIVE APPROACHES

Further work is needed on the comparative efficacy and palatability of current laxatives. However, several novel developments or alternative approaches are worth mentioning.

Cisapride

Cisapride is a prokinetic agents which increases gut motility and is better than placebo in treating idiopathic constipation.[12] It is a 5HT4 – agonist, enhancing acetylcholine release from myenteric neurones. Comparisons with other laxatives have not been reported. It may have value as a "co-laxative" which deserves investigation.

Metoclopramide

Metoclopramide increases gastrointestinal motility by interaction with gut 5HT4 receptors, Oral metoclopramide is less prokinetic than cisapride, but has been reported to be effective in the so-called "narcotic bowel syndrome" when given by continuous subcutaneous infusion.[13]

Erythromycin

Erythromycin causes diarrhoea on about 50% of occasions. Apart from altering the balance of the gut flora, erythromycin reduces transit time in the colon in healthy humans by stimulating motilin receptors.[14] This property is associated with the 14–carbon lactone ring. Non-antibacterial motilin agonists are being developed.

Vancomycin

Vancomycin has been used in chronic idiopathic constipation. Alteration of the gut flora apparently reduces symptoms of constipation.[15]

Misoprostol

Misoprostol may be a laxative, and in one placebo-controlled trial a patient with severe chronic idiopathic constipation had significantly improved stool frequency.[16] Misoprostol is a prostaglandin F analogue used to reduce gastric ulceration due to NSAIDs, so its value as a laxative in palliative care merits investigation.

Oral Naloxone

Oral Naloxone is an opioid antagonist and blocks the effect of morphine on the gut. It is an effective laxative experimentally in patients on strong opioids.[17] Oral naloxone has very low bio-availability of under 1%, (due to first pass hepatic metabolism,) and can counteract the constipation of morphine without reversing analgesia. The effective laxative dose is likely to be 20% or more of the prevailing morphine dose but the starting dose should not exceed 5mg. Early results with naloxone are encouraging but further work is needed. Opioid antagonists which do not cross the blood-brain barrier may be an alternative.

Polyethylene glycol

Polyethylene glycol is a dispersing and emulsifying agent used in ointments and lotions. It therefore has surfactant and lubricant properties, and has been shown to be a better than placebo in chronic constipation.[11] But the daily volumes of 500 ml renders it inappropriate for palliative care patients.

Loxiglumide

Loxiglumide is an oral cholecystokinin (CCK) antagonist, and accelerates colonic transit in healthy volunteers.[18] It presumably acts as an analogue of CCK which also increases colonic motor activity.

L-arginine

L-arginine opposes morphine-induced constipation in mice, possibly by releasing nitric oxide, a neuro-modulator in the gut.[19]

The last two agents are far from being clinically available therapies. Nonetheless, they illustrate that even in the apparently static world of of constipation, long left bobbing in the wake of medical progress, there are possibilities for the development of radically new agents.

CONCLUSION

The aim of therapy is an *easy* bowel action (not necessarily a daily one) without the need for enemas or suppositories.

Constipation occurs in most ill patients and in nearly all patients on strong analgesics. It can therefore be anticipated. It can present as diarrhoea (due to overflow), abdominal pain or nausea and vomiting. Hence a good history, with abdominal and rectal examination, is vital. Prophylaxis of constipation depends mainly on good general symptom control, maintenance of mobility and (as far as the patient can tolerate) a reasonable dietary fibre and fluid intake.

Most palliative care patients will need a laxative, often a combination of a stimulant and a softener. A laxative should always be started with opioid analgesics unless there has been a pre-existing problem with diarrhoea. Laxative doses need to be titrated against the response. Doses may have to be larger than normally used and given twice or even three times a day. There are prospects for new generations of laxative drugs in the future. Current ones could be used more effectively by careful attention to dosing and therapeutic response.

References

1. Maguire L C, Yon J L, Miller E. Prevention of narcotic-induced constipation. New England Journal of Medicine, 1981; 305:1651.
2. Fallon M T, Hanks G. Morphine, constipation and performance status in advanced cancer patients. Palliative Medicine (in press).
3. Sykes N P. Unpublished.
4. Donaldson A N. Experimental study of intestinal stasis. Journal of the American Medical Association, 1922; 78: 884–8.
5. Bruera E, Suarez-Almazor M, Velasco A, Bertolino M, MacDonald S M. The assessment of constipation in terminal cancer patients admitted to a palliative care unit: a retrospective review. Journal of Pain and Symptom Management, 1994; 9: 515–9.
6. Mumford S P. Can high fibre diets improve the bowel function in patients on a radiotherapy ward? Cited in: Twycross R G, Lack S A. *Control of alimentary symptoms in far advanced cancer.* Edinburgh: Churchill Livingstone, 1986: 183.
7. Klauser A G, Flaschentrager J, Gehrke A, Muller-Lissner S A. Abdominal wall massage: effect on colonic function in healthy volunteers and in patients with chronic constipation. Zeitschrift fur Gastroenterologie, 1992; 30: 247–51.
8. Sykes N P. A clinical comparison of laxatives in a hospice. Palliative Medicine, 1991; 5: 307–14.
9. Sykes N P. A volunteer model for the comparison of laxatives in opioid-related constipation. Journal of Pain and Symptom Management, 1996; Vol 2: 363–369.
10. Sweeney W J. The use of disposable microenema in obstetrical patients. Proceedings of a Symposium on the Clinical Evaluation of a new disposable microenema, New Brunswick, New Jersey, June 1963: 7–8.
11. Klauser A G, Muhldorfer B E, Voderholzer W A, Wenzel G, Muller-Lissner S A. Polyethylene glycol 4000 for slow transit constipation. Zeitschrift fur Gastroenterologie, 1995; 33: 5–8.
12. Muller-Lissner S A. Treatment of chronic constipation with cisapride and placebo. Gut, 1987; 28: 1033–8.
13. Bruera E, Brenneis C, Michand M, MacDonald N. Continuous subcutaneous infusion of metoclopramide for treatment of narcotic bowel syndrome. Cancer Treatment Reports, 1987; 71: 1121–2.

14. Hasler W, Heldsinger A, Soudah H, Owyang C. Erythromycin promotes colonic transit in humans; mediation via motilin receptors. Gastroenterology, 1990; 98: A358.
15. Celik A F, Tomlin J, Read N W. The effect of oral vancomycin on chronic idiopathic constipation. Alimemtary Pharmacology and Therapeutics, 1995; 9: 63–8.
16. Soffer E E, Metcalf A, Launspach J. Misoprostol is effective treatment for patients with severe constipation. Digestive Diseases and Sciences, 1994; 39: 929–33.
17. Sykes N P. An investigation of the ability of oral naloxone to correct opioid- related constipation in patients with advanced cancer. Palliative Medicine, 1996; Vol 10: 134–144.
18. Meyer B M, Werth B A, Beglinger C et al. Role of cystokinin in regulation of gastrointestinal motor functions. Lancet, 1989; ii: 12–15.
19. Calignano A, Moncada S, Di Rosa M. Endogenous nitric oxide modulates morphine-induced constipation. Biochemical and Biophysical Research Communications, 1991: 181: 889–893.

Chapter 13

Depression

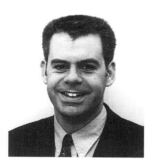

Dr Eoin Tiernan

Eoin Tiernan graduated from University College, Dublin in 1989. He completed a vocational training scheme in general practice in Cork and spend some time in radiotherapy/oncology before taking up his present post in 1994 as Registrar in Palliative Medicine in Our Lady's Hospice, Harold's Cross, Dublin. He has a special interest in education - as a member of the Irish College of General Practitioner's Task Group in Palliative Care, he is involved in the organisation and delivery of a Palliative Care Education Programme to it's members. His main research interest is the differentiation of sadness from depressive illness in the terminally ill, and he is engaged in a research programme funded by the Irish Hospice Foundation looking at this problem.

INTRODUCTION

Depressed mood is a frequent symptom in patients who present for palliative/terminal care, and is often a normal part of the distress of dying. The dilemma facing the physician is whether this depressed mood constitutes pathology requiring "medical" treatment, or whether the patient needs support alone, with no added benefit from pharmacotherapy or ECT.

2 schools of thought

There are 2 schools of thought: Those who focus exclusively on the psychological and existential aspects of terminal illness view the depressed state as a natural process which the person must pass through and experience (as, perhaps, with normal bereavement), and may be helped by supportive counselling. To medicate for this "reaction" might diminish it's importance. Others follow a purely biomedical model and argue that failure to recognise these patients as "clinically depressed" will deny them effective treatment, and worsen an already emotionally painful experience. Most of us would probably place ourselves at some point in the middle of these two extremes.

Screening tools

Unfortunately there are no research-based guidelines from a palliative/terminal care setting which help to identify those sad/depressed patients who would benefit from antidepressant therapy. There is little agreement even among the experts on the main determinants for the diagnosis of depressive illness in the context of palliative care. Individual palliative care physicians consider different criteria to be important, and there is little agreement in the way they rate severity of depression or prescribe anti-depressant in identical case scenarios (author's research).

Most diagnostic and screening tools available for depression have been developed in physically healthy populations. Tools developed for use in medically ill patients often contain items and language inappropriate to a palliative care setting. Context is the all-important determinant for the relative importance of any symptom. A specific set of diagnostic criteria are needed for palliative/terminal care, to reliably distinguish the subgroup of depressed patients who would benefit from antidepressant therapy.

This chapter presents an approach to the diagnosis and management of depression based on research in patients with cancer. Research will in time show whether these principles translate well into the palliative/terminal care setting.

PREVALENCE OF DEPRESSION

Karnofsky scale

Prevalence of depression in cancer patients shows a huge variation from 4.5–77%.[14, 15] This is due to different defining criteria and rating scales, and also reflect different populations of patients. Physical disease and functional capacity (as measured by the Karnofsky scale) bear a strong relationship to clinical depression. In one study 77% of patients with a Karnofsky score of 40 or less (the most severely disabled) met the criteria for major depression, but only 23% of those with scores above 60 had major depression.[15] Figures from the majority of studies concur and at least 25% of hospitalised patients with cancer meet the criteria for depression.

Thus, not all cancer patients are depressed, but a significant proportion might be, and so we need to assess prevalence by further research in the palliative care setting with properly validated diagnostic criteria.

WHAT DO WE MEAN BY "DEPRESSION"?

There is a problem of definition. Depression is a very broad term covering a range from sadness to depressive illness. This partly explains the wide spectrum of reported prevalence of depression, and why management strategies differ so much. For these reasons, it is important that we attempt a reliable definition of depression. The term "depression" has three different meanings.

● Depressed mood – normal
● Depressed mood – a symptom
● Depressive illness – a syndrome

Depressed mood may be normal and appropriate. In everyday language this would be synonymous with sadness, unhappiness, feeling low, miserable, or downhearted.

Depressed mood as a symptom can be a part of different syndromes, eg an adjustment reaction.

Depressive illness is a syndrome in which there is severe lowering of mood with a number of other features which constitute a recognisable pattern.

The distinction of these three meanings is not merely an academic exercise. It serves to differentiate depression requiring treatment with antidepressants from depression which does not. Of particular importance is the distinction of depressed mood as part of an adjustment reaction from depressed mood as part of a depressive illness. Studies have shown that depressive illness responds better to physical treatments that other syndromes. This chapter focuses mainly on the identification and treatment of depressive illness in the palliative/terminal care setting.

In the palliative/terminal care setting we need a definition which directs us towards the appropriate therapeutic option and highlights those patients who require antidepressant therapy.

DEFINING DEPRESSION

2 systems of classification

The World Health Organisation's most recent International Classification of Diseases (ICD 10) provides a widely used set of criteria for the diagnosis of depressive illness. The 4th edition of the Diagnostic and Statistical Manual of the American Psychiatric Association (DSM IV) provides another of the gold standard definitions of depressive illness (titled "major depressive episode" in DSM IV). Both these c;assifications are very similar. the DSM IV is used here.

CRITERIA FOR MAJOR DEPRESSIVE EPISODE (DSM IV)

1. Depressed mood most of the day, nearly every day.
2. Markedly diminished interest or pleasure in all, or almost all, activities most of the day, nearly *every day*.
3. Significant weight loss when not dieting or weight gain, or decrease or increase in appetite nearly everyday.
4. Insomnia or hypersomnia nearly every day.
5. Psychomotor agitation or retardation nearly every day.
6. Fatigue or loss of energy nearly every day.
7. Feelings of worthlessness or excessive or inappropriate guilt nearly every day.
8. Diminished ability to think or concentrate, or indecisiveness, nearly every day.
9. Recurrent thoughts of death (not just fear of dying), recurrent suicidal ideation without a specific plan, or a suicide attempt or a specific plan for committing suicide.

Either 1 or 2 plus 4 of the other symptoms present during the same 2–week period and representing a change from previous functioning.

The problem with these criteria is that they were developed in the context of the physically healthy general population, and 4 of the 9 criteria are somatic in basis. In the palliative/terminal care setting, some of these criteria lose their significance as they merge with the symptoms of the cancer itself eg weight loss, loss of energy.

Physical symptoms of depression

Using these criteria in cancer patients might lead to over-diagnosis of depression. However, physical features may indeed be pointers to a depressive illness, so it would be unwise to totally disregard physical symptoms when making an assessment, which might lead to an under-diagnosis of the disorder. The relevance of somatic symptoms should be assessed in the context of the physical illness. In other words, if loss of appetite or weight have developed in tandem with depressed mood, and out of synchronicity with the trajectory of the physical illness, then they are more likely to be significant features of the depression rather than the cancer. Endicott[2] suggests substituting some other features of depression for the physical symptoms.

ALTERNATIVES TO SOMATIC SYMPTOMS TO AID DIAGNOSIS

Somatic Symptom	Alternatives
● Change in appetite or weight	● Fearfulness or depressed appearance in face or body posture.
● Insomnia or hypersomnia	● Social withdrawal or decreased talkativeness.
● Loss of energy, fatigue	● Brooding, self-pity, or pessimism.
● Diminished concentration	● Cannot be cheered up, doesn't smile no good news or funny situations.

Depression in cancer patients

Other authors have suggested various distinctive features of depression in cancer/terminal patients[4].

Features of depression in cancer/patients

● Persistent tearfulness or irritability
● Hopelessness
● Loss of self-esteem, a sense of worthlessness or perceiving the illness as a punishment.
● A feeling of being a burden when this is obviously not the case.

- Chronic pain-resistant to treatment.
- Persistent panic attacks and anxiety.
- Desire for death – suicidal intent/actions, or, possibly, requests for euthanasia.

In practice we find these to be useful indicators of depressive illness in this setting.

Suicidal thoughts

Serious suicidal ideation, or attempts, are considered a strong indicator of clinical depression. In the terminally ill, this desire for death may manifest itself in requests for euthanasia. A recent study from Canada found that the prevalence of depressive syndromes was 58.8% among patients with a desire to die, but only 7.7% among patients without such a desire[5].

In the context of terminal care, a death wish may, to a certain extent, be understandable and not an indicator for depressive illness at all. This might be particularly so if associated with an appropriate fear of the future, eg patient with intractable pain where doctors have been unable to reassure them of relief. If not associated with such a fear but, rather associated with a sense that life is just not worth living for any reason, and where things are not as desperate as the patient feels them to be, then a serious death wish may be more likely to be an indicator of depressive illness.

Difficulties with diagnosis

Diagnostic criteria tend to emphasise the number of symptoms, but physicians are more likely to be influenced by the intensity of the symptoms rather than the absolute number.

Another drawback of existing psychiatric instruments is that they give equal weighting to various symptoms whereas, in reality, we often attach different significance to the presence for absence of certain symptoms, eg serious suicidal attempt may carry more weight in our opinion than serious appetite disturbance, but they are given equal importance in, for example, DSM 1V.

Quite often we simply "sense" a patient's depression – sometimes as a feeling of depression in ourselves after being with them. As yet we have no reliable criteria to predict depression which will respond to antidepressant therapy in this group of patients. The criteria chosen by any particular physician will depend on their personal "threshold" for treatment and beliefs about the potential benefits of treatment.

INSTRUMENTS FOR MEASURING DEPRESSION:

There are 4 main types of instruments used in psychiatry to define or measure depression.[6]

It is very important that all physicians involved in clinical practice, as well as those interested in research, are very clear about the indications for, and the limitations of the use of these various instruments. Inappropriate use will lead to inaccurate decision making, and possibly inappropriate treatment. The 4 types of instrument are:

MEASUREMENTS OF DEPRESSION

1. Diagnostic Instruments
   - Present State Examination
   - Structured Clinical Interview

2. Screening Instruments
   - Goldberg Health Questionnaire

3. Assessment scales
   - Beck Depression Inventory
   - Hospital Anxiety and Depression Scale

4. Predictive scales
   - Newcastle Rating Scale

---

1. Diagnostic　　These instruments are designed to aid differential diagnosis. They involve structured interviews, are time-consuming, and require special training. Examples are the Present State Examination (PSE)[7] and Structured Clinical Interview (SCI).

2. Screening　　Screening instruments identify probable psychiatric illness in need of more detailed assessment, eg., Goldberg's General Health Questionnaire (GHQ) to detect probable cases of depression presenting to GPs. Those with high scores should have a full psychiatric interview to determine diagnosis.[9]

3. Assessment　　Assessment Scales measure *severity* and are used *after* a specific diagnosis has been made. Examples include the Beck Depression Inventory (BDI) and the Hospital Anxiety and Depression Scale (HAD). They can be used to measure change over time eg response to treatment.

4. Predictive

Predictive scales measure the likelihood of response to therapy. The Newcastle Rating Scale (NRS) developed by Roth and colleagues in Newcastle provides a predictive index of response to ECT.[13]

The Hospital Anxiety and Depression Scale

The HAD Scale is a self-rating assessment scale designed to measure anxiety and depression in patients suffering from physical illness. It is probably the most commonly used rating scale for measuring depression in cancer patients. Moorey et al.[24] used it on 568 patients with cancer and concluded that "the HADS seems to be the best instrument for simple and rapid evaluation of psychological interventions in patients with physical illness".

Though originally designed to measure severity, studies have been done attempting to validate it's use as a screening instrument for depression in cancer patients.[12] Ravazi's study highlighted one of the drawbacks of using the HADS as a screening tool, ie they got a 22% false positive rate for depression and concluded that "self-reported distress is not always correlated with the presence of a given disorder". The opposite might also hold true. Cancer patients are often slow to admit negative feelings. These limitations of self-rating questionnaires should be kept in mind if one decides to base clinical decisions on their use.

Another drawback with the HADS is that items 2 and 8 are of dubious value in patients with poorer performance status (see Appendix). Some patients can appear depressed on item 2 ("I still enjoy the things I used to enjoy") because they are physically unable to do the things they used to and similarly item 8 ("I feel as if I am slowed down"). Patients might get a total of 6 for these two items. With a cut-off value of 11 recommended for the diagnosis of depression, this can give a false positive in a patient who is physically weak and yet not depressed.

Given these cautionary notes, the HADS is probably still the most useful instrument available in use in a palliative care setting, but should be interpreted with care, and in conjunction with some objective measure of mood.

DIFFERENTIAL DIAGNOSIS OF DEPRESSION

Adjustment disorder: An adjustment disorder is essentially a diagnosis of exclusion. The depressed mood develops within 3 months of the onset of a stressor(s), the distress is in excess of what would be expected, but does not meet the criteria of a major depression. The distinction is important as it separates depressed patients who require anti-depressant therapy from those who do not.

Depression due to a general medical condition: Depressed mood may be due to a general medical condition. If the condition is treatable the depression may resolve eg., hypercalcaemia. Depression due to certain medical conditions (eg hypothyroidism) may require anti-depressants despite correction of the underlying problem. Depression following a stroke almost always requires antidepressant therapy.

Thyroid disease Controversy exists surrounding the exact relationship between depression and thyroid function. "Biochemical hypothyroidism", in which thyroid-stimulating hormone (TSH) is raised in the presence of normal T4 concentrations, is associated with depression resistant to apparently adequate antidepressant treatment using drugs of any class. Administration of thyroid hormone at a dose sufficient to render the TSH concentration normal often converts such a treatment-resistant state to one of treatment responsiveness. The role of thyroxine in treatment-resistant depression in clinically and biochemically euthyroid patients is less clear, though some have reported responses.

Certain malignancies, (primary brain tumours and cerebral metastases) are also associated with psychiatric disturbances.

MEDICAL CONDITIONS CAUSING DEPRESSION

- **Neurological**
  - Parkinson's disease
- **Cerebrovascular**
  - Stroke
- **Metabolic**
  - hypercalcaemia
  - hypokalaemia
  - uraemia
  - hypo/hyper-glycaemia
  - hypoxia
  - vitamin B12 deficiency

- **Endocrine**
  - hypothyroidism,
  - hyperparathyroidism
  - Addison's disease
- **Autoimmune**
  - systemic lupus
  - erythematosus
- **Infections**
  - hepatitis
  - HIV
  - RTI
  - UTI

Mental testing

"Organic brain syndromes", cause cognitive impairment, with abnormalities of memory, concentration, orientation, and comprehension. A test of cognitive function such as the Abbreviated Mental Test Score (AMTS) is therefore an essential part of the assessment of a patient with depressed mood.[16] The AMTS is an abbreviated 10–question test derived from the Modified Roth Hopkins Mental Test. It is short, need not be self-administered and is well tolerated by patients and their families. The AMTS has been validated by comparison with more in-depth 37-item mental test score and by comparison with final clinical diagnoses.[25] Scores of less than or equal to 7 indicate mental impairment (see Appendix 2).

Substance-Induced depression

Depression may be due to drugs (either drugs of abuse, or medication). There may be features of cognitive impairment suggesting an organic brain syndrome.

Drugs associated with development of depression

- Vinca alkaloids (eg vincristine vinblastine)
- L-asparaginase
- Procarbazine
- Corticosteroids
- Sedatives, (benzodiazepines neuroleptics)
- Antihypertensives (alpha-methyldopa propanolol)
- H2 antagonists
- Anticonvulsants

"Pseudodementia"

Pseudodementia means a severe depression mimicking dementia. It describes a situation where an elderly patient with what appears to be a dementia improves when treated with anti-depressants – a "pseudodementia" masking a depressive illness.

In elderly individuals it is often difficult to determine whether cognitive symptoms (disorientation, apathy, difficulty concentrating, memory loss) are due to dementia or depression. The nature of the onset, temporal sequencing of depressive and cognitive symptoms, course of illness, and treatment response all aid differential diagnosis. In dementia, there is usually a steady decline in cognitive function, whereas in depression it is much more common to see an abrupt cognitive decline. A trial of anti-depressant is often the only means of distinguishing the two.

CLINICAL ASSESSMENT OF DEPRESSION

A careful history from both the patient, and a collateral history from close family or friends are essential. The physician should be mindful of known risk factors.

Risk factors for depression

- Past history
- Family history
- Prior suicide attempts
- Lack of social supports
- Recent stressful events
- Alcohol (or other substance) abuse
- Poorly controlled pain

Depression accompanying alcohol dependence largely remits with abstinence from alcohol, and antidepressant therapy may not be necessary.[17] Continued high alcohol intake blocks the effectiveness of anti-depressants.

Screening tools, such as Goldberg's General Health Questionnaire, in conjunction with a semi-structured interview based on a modified version of the DSM IV criteria can be helpful.

The HADS is the most commonly used tool used in cancer patients. It should be followed by a formal interview to make a definite diagnosis of depressive illness before initiating therapy. The observations of other members of ward staff (in the inpatient setting) may be invaluable if the patient persistently presents a bright "front" to the doctor. Physical and cognitive status should both be carefully assessed. Basic tests of haematology, biochemistry and thyroid function should be performed.

MANAGEMENT OPTIONS

The physician has 3 main options in terms of therapy:

● Psychological therapies
● Medication
● Electroconvulsive therapy

They are not mutually exclusive, and, in certain situations, may be more effective in combination.

Psychological Therapies

All sad/depressed patients benefit from consistent emotional and psychological support. Indeed this may be all that is required for many patients to "work through" their distress. Psychological therapies available for the management of depression include:

● Behaviour therapy
● Cognitive therapy
● Interpersonal therapy
● Brief dynamic psychotherapy

Reasons for choosing psychological therapies may include patient preferences for non-drug therapies, contra-indications to drugs, failure to respond to medication and non-compliance with anti-depressants. A helpful review of the various psychological treatments for depression is given by Scott in a recent article in the British Journal of Psychiatry.[18]

Behaviour Therapy

Behaviour Therapy (BT) is intended to control the symptoms of emotional disorders rather then deal with the original causes. There are a number of key elements in BT for depression: functional analysis (the complicated problems need to be broken down into manageable parts), daily monitoring and then planning of activities, managing aversive experiences and developing social skills. A graduated approach is used, with patients practising the treatment techniques in their own time. Examples of BT include relaxation training, self-control therapy, and social skills training.

Cognitive Therapy

Cognitive Therapy focuses on the negative thoughts depressed people often express about themselves, their world and their future. A cycle is set up in which low mood increases the intensity of negative thinking which increases affective, cognitive and behavioural disturbance. The acute symptoms of depression are tackled through the use of behavioural and verbal techniques aimed at identifying and challenging negative thoughts or cognitions. Later interventions are targeted at challenging dysfunctional beliefs to try to reduce vulnerability to future episodes.

Interpersonal Therapy

Interpersonal Therapy is based on the belief that interpersonal problems may be a cause or consequence of depression. This form of therapy aims to reduce the acute symptoms of depression and recognise and resolve associated role impairment in the following areas: prolonged grief reactions, role disputes, role transitions and interpersonal deficits.

Brief Dynamic Psychotherapy

Brief Dynamic Psychotherapy is based on psychoanalytic principles, and is intended to modify emotional reactions to other people. The depressed mood is viewed in terms of adaptive failure resulting from inner conflicts. Rather than targeting depressive symptoms per se, the goal is to use the therapeutic relationship to clarify and explore neurotic conflicts (such as problems of intimacy). This is often achieved by seeking connections between events in childhood or adolescence and the patients emotional reactions and other responses in the course of the treatment sessions.

Medication:

The choice of one particular antidepressant over another will depend on a number of factors. Trials of newer antidepressants have not shown increased efficacy over the older tricyclics, but they do have a more favourable side-effect profile. They are of particular use if tricyclic drugs cause side-effects, or fail to produce a response.

ANTIDEPRESSANTS AVAILABLE

- **Tricyclic antidepressants**
  - Amitryptyline
  - dothiepin
- **Monoamine Oxidase Inhibitors**
  - phenylzine
  - tranylcypromine
- **Selective Serotonin Uptake Inhibitor**
  - fluoxetine
  - paroxetine
  - sertraline

- **Other anti-depressants**
  - trazadone
  - mianserin
- **Psychostimulants**
  - dexamphetamine
  - methylphenidate
  - pimoline
- **Benzodiazepines**
  - alprazolam
- **Lithium salts**
  - lithium carbonate

Tricyclic Antidepressants

Tricyclics remain the drugs of first choice for the treatment of depression. They are the gold-standard against which all newer agents are compared, and, as yet, none of these agents have proved more effective. All antidepressants take 2–3 weeks to work. An adequate trial of treatment, therefore, involves perseverance on the part of the patient, but also adequate dosage by the physician. The dose required for antidepressant effect (75–150mg daily) is higher that used for their analgesic effect. In the elderly, and when initiating therapy, smaller doses should be used, with the dose being increased according to response, and conscious of side-effects. Response rates are lower in cancer patients than in the general population (40% vs. 80%). Treatment should be continued for 3–6 months after response to prevent relapse. Side effects of different tricyclics depend on affinity for various receptors (adrenergic, histaminergic, muscarinic, dopaminergic).

Note that tricyclics increase the bioavailability of morphine and potentiate its analgesic effect.

Side-effects of tricyclics
- Sedation
- Dry mouth, blurred vision, urinary hesitancy +/− retention, constipation.
- increased sweating
- Orthostatic hypotension, cardiac conduction defects (beware in heart block)
- Reduction in epileptic seizure threshold in at-risk patients

SIDE-EFFECTS OF DIFFERENT TRICYCLICS

	Sedation	Anticholinergic (dry mouth etc)	Hypotension
Amitryptyline	++++	++++	+++
Trimipramine	++++	+++	++
Imipramine	++	++	++
Dothiepin	+++	+	++

The sedative effects may be of benefit eg in insomnia. In this situation it may be useful to give the drug as a single night-time dosage.

Monoamine Oxidase Inhibitors: (MAOIS)

MAOIs have a limited role in palliative/terminal care because of side-effects dietary restrictions (hypertensive crises) and drug interactions. A washout period of 2 weeks is needed when switching from one to another drug of this type.

Foods containing tyramine can elevate blood pressure. MAOI drugs can potentiate this pressor effect by inhibiting the metabolism of tyramine.

FOODS CONTAINING TYRAMINE

- Cheese, pickled herrings, yeast
- Meat extracts (Marmite, Bovril)
- Chianti, beer, sherry
- Game, badly stored meat
- Broad bean pods

Drug interactions with MAOIs

Hypertensive crisis can occur with:

- ephedrine, phenylephrine and other nasal decongestants
- amphetamines
- phenypropanolamine
- levodopa
- Tricyclics
- SSRIs

Other drugs that interact with MAOIs.

- Pethidine and possibly other opioid analgesics – CNS excitation or depression (hypertension or hypotension, impaired consciousness)
- Insulin, metformin, sulphonureas – effects enhanced
- Carbamazepine – anticonvulsant effect antagonised
- Antihypertensives – hypotensive effect enhanced
- Antihistamines – increased antimuscarinic and sedative effects

Selective Serotonin Uptake Inhibitors (SSRIs)

The main advantage with this newer class of drugs is that they do not have the multiple receptor interactions typical of tricyclic drugs, causing anticholinergic effects.

Side-effects of SSRI's include nausea, diarrhoea, headaches, agitation and insomnia.

SELECTIVE SEROTONIN UPTAKE INHIBITORS (SSRIs)

		Main side-effect
Fluoextine (Prozac)	20–40 mg daily	anxiety
Fluvoxamine (Faverin)	100–200 mg daily	nausea, vomiting, diarrhoea
Paroxetine (Seroxat)	20–40 mg daily	sedation
Sertraline (Lustral)	50–100 mg daily	sedation

Drug interactions of SSRIs

- Anti-convulsants (levels reduced))
- Haloperidol (levels up by fluoxetine).
- Carbamazepine (levels up by fluoxetine).

Place in palliative care

It might be argued that the SSRIs might be first line antidepressants in patients with cancer because of their much lower side-effect profile. However, a recent meta-analysis of trials comparing the efficacy and acceptability of SSRIs with those of tricyclic antidepressants suggested that routine use of SSRIs as the first line treatment of depressive illness may greatly increase cost with only questionable benefit.[20] Studies comparing the two groups in the palliative/ terminal care population are required.

Psychostimulants

Psychostimulants are commonly used for terminally ill/hospice patients by physicians in North America.[21] Their main advantage is their rapid onset of action, ie., hours or days. Other benefits include improved appetite (unlike their appetite suppressing effect in healthy people), energy, and general sense of well-being. Studies by Bruera and co-workers suggest that psychostimulants enhance opioid analgesia and reduce opioid-related sedation.[22]

PSYCHOSTIMULANTS OR DEPRESSION	
Dextroamphetamine	2.5–10 mg bd
Methyphenidate	10 mg bd-tid
Pemoline	20 mg daily
N.B. Avoid giving second dose after midday	

There appears to be a reluctance to use psychostimulants for depression, perhaps because of their history as drugs of abuse, but also because they might increase anxiety levels in some patients. They should be used with caution, and perhaps not at all, in patients who are very anxious or with any borderline features of psychosis/paranoia. However, they may prove useful for the lethargic, retarded depressives, and are worth a trial.

Benzodiazepines:

Alprazolam is claimed by some authors to have antidepressant properties. It has been suggested as useful when other antidepressants are contraindicated or with milder depression mixed with anxiety. The evidence for this is still not certain.

Lithium Salts:

Lithium given alone is not a potent antidepressant. Addition of lithium to a tricyclic antidepressant will produce responses in more than 50% of patients resistant to the tricyclic alone. It is the drug of first choice for the management of bipolar depression. Its role is therefore limited in the management of depression in the palliative/terminal care setting.

Electroconvulsive Therapy

ECT is effective for the treatment of delusional and severe depression. It is not effective for patients with milder depression.

The most troublesome side-effect of ECT is short-term memory loss, (minimised by unilateral ECT on the nondominant hemisphere). Treatment usually consists of 3 treatments per week, with a total of 6–12 usually achieving a full response. The threshold for considering ECT in physically ill cancer patients is understandably higher than in the healthy population, but it is a useful therapeutic option which should be kept in mind for the more resistant depressions in patients who are severely handicapped because of the depression, and whose life expectancy may be only weeks.[23]

ELECTROCONVULSIVE THERAPY (ECT)

Indications	Contraindications
Life-threatening depression	Increased intracranial pressure
Refusal to eat/mutism	Space-occupying lesion*
Severe suicidal ideation	Recent myocardial infarction
Previous response to ECT	Contraindication to general anaesthesia
Antidepressants ineffective/intolerable	

*Space occupying lesion includes intracranial tumour, but also abscess etc.

DISCUSSION

Depression is a common symptom but confusion still exists as to how it should be treated. Failure to treat can increase physical and psychological distress. Severe depression may make general management and symptom control (eg. pain control) more difficult, may reduce compliance with recommended treatments, and cause death wishes, or requests for euthanasia.

Assessment

The use of an instrument, eg HADS to screen for depression should be considered in all patients entering care. Likely cases should then be assessed carefully with a full history from patient and family. Specific features suggestive of depressive illness should then be looked for using a semi-structured interview based on DSM IV with the addition of other likely symptoms (see the first two tables in this chapter).

Prescribing antidepressants

The reluctance to prescribe antidepressants in a palliative/terminal care setting is, to a certain degree, understandable. Many patients will already be suffering a number of uncomfortable physical symptoms, and will be on various medications, some of which may be adding to the list of unpleasant symptoms. Many physicians would consider the addition of an antidepressant with further potential side-effects unjustifiable. More accurate indicators of which patients will likely respond to antidepressants are needed.

In palliative care, formalised psychological therapies may prove to have a bigger role in the treatment of depressive illness than in other settings.

Many depressed patients in the palliative/terminal care setting would benefit from medication as well as psychological support. If tricyclics cause intolerable side-effects, the SSRIs should be considered. ECT is a worthwhile option when depression is severe, psychotic, or potentially life-threatening. When life-expectancy is relatively short, the use of amphetamines might be worth considering.

Future research

This discussion on depression has possibly provided more questions than answers. There are still many questions to be answered about the identification and management of depressive illness in a palliative/terminal care setting. Hopefully research will help us to identify this disabling problem more readily, and provide clearer directions as to which patients will most benefit from the various forms of therapies (psychological and pharmacological) that are available.

Anti-depressants can enable counselling

Mary, a 65 year old house-wife with advanced metastatic breast carcinoma, was admitted to the Palliative Care Unit on the recommendation of the Home-Care Team. Though breathlessness was her main physical complaint, depression and despair were, by her own admission, her main distress. She had been told by her medical oncologist 3 weeks earlier that her lungs were now affected, and that further active treatment would not be possible. However, her depressed mood had been present "for months", but now she could cope no longer. She had lost all interest in her usual hobbies, and could no longer concentrate long enough to read. Her husband had commented that while watching TV, her expression never changed, regardless of whether she was watching a comedy show or a serious documentary. Despite always having been a "fighter", she could not imagine being able to continue to live in her present debilitated state. Though she was able to speak quite openly about her distress, she continually referred to the fact that she "felt numb" – "I wish I could cry, but I just don't feel anything, just black". On another occasion she said "I've just been told I'm going to die, but I feel nothing. During the first 10 days of Mary's admission various members of staff tried to reach her in her distress, but nothing seemed to make a difference,and her family and carers were all feeling impotent and distressed themselves after spending time with her. Relaxation exercises and aroma-therapy helped somewhat, but Mary still pined for acceptance and peace of mind. Her poor concentration and fatigue precluded art therapy. It was decided to try an antidepressant, so Mary was commenced on paroxetine 20 mg mane. After about 10 days a slight improvement was noted. This continued over the next week. Though Mary remained sad, she no longer despaired and found it easier to spend time with and talk to her family. Despite her sadness, she was able to join in the cheerful banter with her guests. Mary felt able to concentrate enough to undergo some therapy in the form of guided imagery* which helped her to tap into some of her inner distress and pain. The terrible gloom that had surrounded her seemed to lift. Her family now recall a particular day when Mary spoke to each of her children and her husband, and made all her funeral arrangements – "She was in her best form that day.... she had found peace". Mary became increasingly weak over the next week, and died peacefully 7 days later. Looking at her in her last few days, it was obvious, as her family put it, that "all her pain had gone".

Comment: Mary remained sad to the end, a natural reaction to the great loss facing her. It is difficult to separate out the many factors which may have helped Mary. However, it seemed that the anti-depressant helped to lift her from the depths of a black depression, enough to give her the ability to deal more effectively with the hugh emotional trauma of what was happening to her. She was able to "feel" again and share the precious last few days with her loved ones.

*See "Further Reading" ("Mortally Wounded", by Michael Kearney) for an indepth account of the use of guided imagework/visualisation in similar situations.

Acknowledgements: The author would like to thank Professor Patricia Casey, Department of Adult Psychiatry, Mater Hospital/University College, Dublin, and Dr. Michael Kearney, Our Lady's Hospice, Harold's Cross, Dublin, for their helpful comments on the critical review of this chapter.

APPENDIX 1. The Hospital Anxiety and Depression Scale.

The HAD scale is probably the best validated and most commonly used screening instrument. However, it may over-estimate depression in cancer patients as they may score too high in questions 2 and 8 because they interpret them in terms of their physical weakness.

Scoring: < 7   "non cases"
             8–10   "doubtful cases"
             >11   "definite cases"

1. I feel tense or "wound up":   Anxiety

    most of the time   3
    a lot of the time   2
    from time to time, occasionally   1
    not at all   0

2. I still enjoy the things I used to enjoy: Depression

    definitely as much   0
    not quite so much   1
    only a little   2
    hardly at all   3

3. I get a sort of frightened feeling as if something
    awful is about to happen: Anxiety

    very definitely and quite badly   3
    yes, but not too badly   2
    a little, but it dosn,t worry me   1
    not at all   0

4. I can laugh and see the funny side of things: Depression

    as much as I always could   0
    not quite so much now   1
    definitely not so much now   2
    not at all   3

5. Worrying thoughts go through my mind: Anxiety

    a great deal of the time   3
    a lot of the time   2
    from time to time but not too often   1
    only occasionally   0

6. I feel cheerful: Depression

        not at all   3
        not often   2
        sometimes   1
        most of the time   0

7. I can sit at ease and feel relaxed: Anxiety

        definitely   0
        usually   1
        not often   2
        not at all   3

8. I feel as if I am slowed down: Depression

        nearly all the time   3
        very often   2
        sometimes   1
        not at all   0

9. I get a sort of frightened feeling like
    "butterflies" in my stomach: Anxiety

        not at all   0
        occasionally   1
        quite often   2
        very often   3

10. I have lost interest in my appearance: Depression

        definitely   3
        I don't take so much as I should   2
        I may not take quite as much care   1
        I take just as much care as ever   0

11. I feel restless as if I have to be on the move: Anxiety

        very much indeed   3
        quite a lot   2
        not very much   1
        not at all   0

12. I look forward with enjoyment to things: Depression

        as much as ever I did   0
        rather less than I used to   1
        definitely less than I used to   2
        hardly at all   3

13. <u>I get sudden feelings of panic</u>   Anxiety

       very often indeed   3
       quite often   2
       not very often   1
       not at all   0

14. <u>I can enjoy a good book or radio or TV programme:</u> Depression

       often   0
       sometimes   1
       not often   2
       very seldom   3

APPENDIX 2. Abbreviated mental test score

This 10-question test has been validated by comparison with a more in-depth 38-question test (modified Roth Hopkins test).

1	Age
2	Time (to nearest hour)
3	Address for recall at end of test – this should be repeated by the patient to ensure it has been heard correctly: 42 West Street
4	Year
5	Name of institution
6	Recognition of two people (doctor, nurse, etc)
7	Date of birth (day and month sufficient)
8	Year of first world war
9	Name of present monarch
10	Count backwards from 20 to 1

<u>Scoring</u>: Each correct answer scores 1

    0–3 severe impairment
    4–7 moderate impairment
    8–10 normal

FURTHER READING

Billings JA. Depression. Journal of Palliative Care. 1995; 11(1): 48–54.

Lynch ME. The assessment and prevalence of affective disorders in advanced cancer. Journal of Palliative Care. 1995; 11(1): 10–18.

Cody M. Depression and the use of antidepressants in patients with cancer. Palliative Medicine. 1990; 4: 271–278.

Peck DF, Shapiro CM, eds. Measuring Human Problems – A Practical Guide. Chichester. John Wiley & Sons, 1990.

Kearney M. Mortally Wounded – Stories of Soul Pain, Death and Healing. Dublin. Marino Books, 1996.

REFERENCES:

1. American Psychiatric Association (1994). Diagnostic and Statistical Manual of Mental Disorders (Fourth Edition), Washington D.C.
2. Endicott J. Measurement of depression in patients with cancer. Cancer. Supplement 1984; 53: 2243–2249.
3. World Health Organisation (1992). International Classification of Diseases, 10th Revision, World Health organisation, Geneva.
4. Casey P. Depression in the dying – disorder or distress? Progress in Palliative Care. 1994; 2: 1–3.
5. Chochinov HM, Wilson KG, Enns M, et al. Desire for death in the terminally ill. American Journal of Psychiatry. 1995; 152(8): 1185–1191.
6. Thompson C. Affective Disorders. In: Thompsom C, ed. The Instruments of Psychiatric Research. Chichester: John Wiley & Sons, 1989: 87–126.
7. Wing JK, Cooper JE, Sartorius N. The Measurement and Classification of Psychiatric Symptoms. Cambridge University Press, New York 1974.
8. Spitzer RL, Williams JB, Gibbon M. Structured Clinical Interview for DSM III- R. Biometrics Research Department, New York State Psychiatric Institute, New York, 1986.
9. Goldberg DP, Hillier VF. A Scaled Version of the General Health Questionnaire. Psychological Medicine 1979; 9: 139–145.
10. Beck AT, Ward CH, Mendelson M, Mock JE, Erbaugh J. An Inventory for Measuring Depression. Archives of General Psychiatry 1961; 4: 561–585.
11. Zigmond AS, Snaith RP. The Hospital Anxiety and Depression Scale. Acta Psychiatrica Scandinavia 1983; 67: 361–370.
12. Razavi D, Delvaux N, Farvacques C, Robaye E. Screening for Adjustment Disorders and Major Depressive Disorders in Cancer In-Patients. British Journal of Psychiatry 1990; 156: 79–83.
13. Roth M, Gurney C, Mountjoy CG. The Newcastle Rating Scales. Acta Psychiatr. Scand. 1983; Suppl. 310: 42–52.
14. Lansky SB, List MA, Herrmann CA, Ets-Hokin EG, DasGupta TK, Wilbanks GD, Hendrickson Fr. Absence of major depressive disorder in female cancer patients. Journal of Clinical Oncology. 1985; 3: 1553–1560.
15. Bukberg J, Penman D, Holland JC. Depression in hospitalised cancer patients. Psychosomatic Medicine. 1984; 46: 199–212.
16. Power D, Kelly S, Gilsenan J et al. Suitable tests for cognitive impairment and depression in the terminally ill – a prospective prevalence study. Palliative Medicine 1993; 7: 213–18.
17. Davidson K. Diagnosis of Depression in Alcohol Dependence: Changes in Prevalence with Drinking Status.
18. Scott J. Psychological treatments for depression. British Journal of Psychiatry. 1995; 167: 289–292.
19. Potter WZ, Rudorfer MV, Manji H. The pharmacologic treatment of depression. New England Journal of Medicine. 1991; 325: 633–642.

20. Song F, Freemantle N, Sheldon T, House A, Watson P, Long A, Mason J. Selective serotonin reuptake inhibitors: meta-analysis of efficacy and acceptability. British Medical Journal 1993; 306: 683–687.
21. Rosenberg PB, Ahmed I, Hurwitz S. Methylphenidate in depressed medically ill patients. Journal of Clinical Psychiatry. 1991; 52(6): 263–267.
22. Bruera E, Brenneis C, Paterson AH, MacDondald RN. Use of methylphenidate as an adjuvant to narcotic analgesics in patients with advanced cancer. Journal of Pain and Symptom Management 1989; 4: 3–6.
23. Bidder TG. Electroconvulsive therapy in the medically ill patient. Psychiatric Clinics of North America. 1981; 4: 391–405.
24. Moorey S, Greer S, Watson M, et al. The factor structure and factor stability of the Hospital Anxiety and Depression Scale in patients with cancer. Br J Psychiatry 1991; 158: 255–259.
25. Barrett J. Prescribing thyroid hormones. Prescribers' Journal 1996; 36(3): 176–7.
26. Jitapunkul S, Pillay I, Ebrahim S. The Abbreviated Mental Test; its use and validity. Age Ageing. 1991; 20: 332–36).

Chapter 14

The use of Steroids

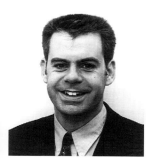

Dr Eoin Tiernan
Eoin Tiernan graduated from University College, Dublin in 1989. He completed a vocational training scheme in general practice in Cork and spend some time in radiotherapy/oncology before taking up his present post in 1994 as Registrar in Palliative Medicine in Our Lady's Hospice, Harold's Cross, Dublin. He has a special interest in education - as a member of the Irish College of General Practitioner's Task Group in Palliative Care, he is involved in the organisation and delivery of a Palliative Care Education Programme to it's members. His main research interest is the differentiation of sadness from depressive illness in the terminally ill, and he is engaged in a research programme funded by the Irish Hospice Foundation looking at this problem.

INTRODUCTION

Corticosteroids are widely used both in clinical oncology, e.g. treatment of lymphoproliferative disorders and breast cancer, and in palliating a wide range of symptoms in advanced cancer.[1,2] Patterns of usage varies considerably between centres, and there is great variability in the dosing schedules for corticosteroids used for the treatment of different conditions.

Several studies have been published on the effects of corticosteroids on symptoms in advanced cancer,[3,4] but there is a lack of controlled studies on the use of corticosteroids in many situations (eg lymphangitis carcinomatosis, malignant intestinal obstruction).

This chapter details the use of corticosteroids in various clinical situations, and highlights some of the potential risks.

CHOICE OF STEROID

Naturally occuring corticosteroids (produced in the adrenal cortex) have effects on many of the body's systems and metabolic pathways.

Action   Their chief uses are for replacement therapy, anti-inflammatory and immunosuppressive effects. They influence carbohydrate, protein, and lipid metabolism; electrolyte and water balance; the cardiovascular system, the kidney, skeletal muscle, the nervous system, and other organs and tissues.

Classification   It is on the basis of their varying effects on hepatic glycogen deposition and Na+ retention that corticosteroids have been traditionally classified into glucocorticoids and mineralocorticoids. A knowledge of the relative potency of individual agents with respect to these two effects is important in understanding therapeutic effects, and potential undesirable side-effects.[5]

PROPERTIES OF ADRENAL CORTICOSTEROIDS

	Equivalent dose (mg)	Relative anti-inflammatory (glucocorticoid) effect	Relative Sodium-retaining (mineralocorticoid) effect	Biological half-life (h)
Hydrocortisone	20	1.0	++	8–12
Prednisolone	5	4	+	18–36
Methylprednisolone	4	5	–	18–36
Triamcinolone	4	5	–	18–36
Dexamethasone	0.7–0.8	25–30	–	36–54
Betamethasone	0.7–0.8	25–30	–	36–54

Increasing anti-inflammatory activity is associated with more potent glucocorticoid effect. Mineralocorticoid effect causes Na+ and water retention. Thus *dexamethasone* is a suitable agent for high-dose anti-inflammatory therapy in conditions where water retention would be a disadvantage eg cerebral oedema. *Prednisolone* has dominantly glucocorticoid activity and is the corticosteroid most commonly used for longterm administration. *Hydrocortisone*'s mineralocorticoid activity is too high for it to be used on a long-term basis for inflammatory disease suppression, but it is used intravenously for the emergency management of certain conditions, e.g. anaphylactic shock, and it is the topical corticosteroid of first choice in the management of inflammatory skin conditions.

Prednisone and cortisone are now obsolete, as they are pro-drugs metabolised in the liver to prednisolone and hydrocortisone respectively.

The biological half-life reflects the duration of suppression of the hypothalmo-pituitary-adrenal axis after a single dose. Hydrocortisone (half-life 8–12 hrs) needs to be administered more than once daily. Prednisolone and dexamethasone, should be given in one single daily dose.

ADVERSE EFFECTS OF CORTICOSTEROIDS

Therapeutic usefulness of the corticosteroids is tempered by the risk side-effects.[6] These are best understood as exaggerations of the normal physiological actions of corticosteroids.

ADVERSE EFFECTS OF CORTICOSTEROIDS.

- **Mineralocorticoid effects**
  - Hypertension
  - Sodium and water retention and potassium loss
- **Glucocorticoid effects**
  - Diabetes
  - Osteoporosis/avascular necrosis of femoral head
  - Moonface, truncal obesity, striae, acne
  - Psychiatric disturbances e.g. depression/euphoria, paranoid psychosis.
  - Muscle wasting (proximal myopathy)
  - Peptic ulceration
  - Suppression of immune response (this may lead to opportunistic infection, eg candidiasis, and/or masking the signs of septicaemia)
  - Suppression of growth in children
  - Suppression of the hypothalmo-pituitary-adrenal axis

Toxic effects of corticosteroids occur after continued use of relatively large doses of the drugs.

In general, serious unwanted effects are unlikely if the daily dose is below the equivalent of hydro-cortisone 50mg or prednisolone 10mg.

Incidence of side-effects

A study by Hanks et al.[14] found oropharyngael candidiasis to be the most common side-effect, in nearly one-third of patients. Less than one-fifth developed oedema or cushingoid features. Dyspepsia, weight gain, neuro-psychological changes, and ecchymoses occurred in 5 to 10 per cent, and the incidence of other adverse effects, such as hyper-glycaemia, myopathy, and osteoporosis, was lower. In general, serious unwanted effects are unlikely if the daily dose is below the equivalent of hydro-cortisone 50mg or prednisolone 10mg. Choice of a particular corticosteroid may also influence the likelihood of developing certain side-effects. Animal studies suggest that fluorinated corti-costeroids, (dexamethasone) cause more atrophy and weakness than non-fluorinated corti-costeroids, (hydrocortisone and prednisolone).

The rapidity with which side-effects develop varies greatly between individuals. A retrospective study of 59 neuro-oncology patients found toxicity in 76% after receiving dexamethasone for more than 3 weeks, compared with 5% for shorter periods.[7] Patients receiving a total dose of dexamethasone greater than 400mg had an incidence of toxicity of 75% compared to 13% for total doses under 400mg. However, a significant number of patients (one-third) developed their first toxic event during the initial 3 weeks of therapy and having taken less than 400mg. This study also found that corti-costeroid toxicity was associated with hypoalbumi-naemia. Steroids are highly bound to serum albumin so that hypoalbuminaemia would allow for more unbound steroids and thus the potential for increased toxicity.

Onset of side-effects

Oropharyngeal candidiasis can develop within a few days. *Proximal myopathy* may occur after only 10 days, but the peak period of onset is usually in the third month of treatment. The myopathy associated with corticosteroid use seems to affect proximal muscles first, with the legs being affected before the arms. Women appear to be more susceptible than men. *Osteoporosis* is an unlikely occurrence in patients with advanced cancer, but a small group seem to be particularly sensitive to the osteoporotic effects of corticosteroids.[8] *Avascular bone necrosis* has been reported after relatively short courses of dexamethasone (3–4 weeks),[9] but symptoms usually take more than one year to develop. Most cases are bilateral involving the femoral head.

Peptic ulceration

The association between peptic ulceration and steroids appears to be significant primarily when NSAIDs are concomitantly prescribed (fourfold risk).[10,11.] Prophylaxis against gastrointestinal side-effects should be considered in patients on combination therapy who have other associated risk factors, viz. immunosuppression/advanced cancer itself, previous history of peptic ulceration, and a cumulative dose of dexamethasone >140mg. [12]

Psychiatric complications

Psychiatric complications which may occur include affective disorders, psychotic reactions, and global cognitive impairment.[13] Caution should be exercised when using corticosteroids in patients with anxious personalities or with previous psychiatric histories of affective or psychotic disorders.

Rarer side-effects

Other less common adverse effects include glaucoma (with prolonged use of eyedrops), posterior subcapsular lens cataract (risk if dose exceeds 10mg prednisolone/day or equivalent for more than one year), raised intracranial pressure and convulsions (i.e. pseudotumor cerebri), menstrual disorders, and pancreatitis.

Steroids – the pros and cons

A 69 year old man presented to Casualty following a grand mal seizure. On examination he had significant weakness of the right side of his body and dysphagia. Investigations revealed two lesions surrounded by a large amount of oedema in the left hemisphere consistent with brain metastases. A primary lung tumour was found. The weakness had been developing gradually at home over a 3 month

300 THE USE OF STEROIDS

period, but the man had not sought medical attention. He was a bachelor, living with his widower brother. In view of the site of the primary tumour (considered inoperable), and the degree of neurological disability, he was treated with steroids alone. The patient was discharged home after 10 days in hospital on 4mg of QDS. His brother was told that his prognosis was a matter of weeks, and that the general practitioner would follow-up. A referral was made to the Palliative Home Care Team. Their first visit was delayed for 6 weeks because the brother reported that they were managing well. When they eventually visited, they found a much improved patient. Still on a dose of dexamethasone 4mg QDS he had regained most of the power on his right side, and his speech was almost perfect. However, he had gained 3 stone in weight. His increased appetite and weight gain was viewed in a positive light by the brother as a sign of progress. He had signs consistent with a proximal myopathy, and wasn't sleeping well at night. A radiotherapy review was organised. In view of the dramatic response to steroids, the patient was treated with cranial radiotherapy. His dexamethasone was reduced over a 4 week period to a maintenance dose of 2mg daily and he maintained his clinical improvement. His appetite returned to a more normal level and he began to lose weight. His sleep improved, and the proximal muscle weakness showed signs of improving after about 6 weeks on the lower dose of steroids. His dexamethasone was further reduced to a maintenance dose of 1mg daily. He lived a further 6 months of good quality life before succumbing to advancing lung disease.

This case emphasises 3 points about steroids:-

1. Response to corticosteroids is an indicator of potential benefit from radiotherapy.
2. Patients should never be prescribed corticosteroids without a definite plan for close monitoring and follow-up.
3. Always be prepared to re-assess and readjust the therapeutic approach even if a decision about prognosis has apparently been carved in stone!

STOPPING STEROIDS

Adrenal suppression   High dose or prolonged steroid therapy, can suppress the hypothalamo-pituitary-adrenal axis, and abrupt withdrawal can then result in acute adrenal insufficiency with possible hypotension and death.

Corticosteroids should therefore be given for the shortest length of time at the lowest dose that is clinically effective. In patients requiring long-term corticosteroids, the dosage should be reduced as soon as possible to the lowest effective level that maintains therapeutic benefit. Moderate doses of corticosteroids (30mg daily of prednisolone or less) for less than one week can be safely stopped abruptly. Courses of corticosteroids at supra-physiological doses, ie >7.5mg prednisolone lasting longer than 3 weeks should be reduced gradually. During dose reduction corticosteroid cover may still be required in stressful situations. The table below relates to patients who still have a reasonably long prognosis. If symptoms of a medical disease are likely to recur on steroid withdrawal, then reduction is usually as gradual as possible, eg 1mg per month.

WITHDRAWAL OF CORTICOSTEROIDS

Change Dexamethasone to prednisolone, then:

Daily dose of Prednisolone

If <u>more than 3 weeks</u> treatment has been given	<u>Above 7.5mg</u>: reduce by 2.5mg every 2 weeks <u>Below 7.5mg</u>: reduce by 2.5mg every 4 weeks <u>Below 2.5mg</u>: reduce by 1mg month 0.5mg alternate days for 2 weeks, then STOP
If <u>less than 3 weeks</u> treatment has been given	<u>Above 7.5mg</u>: reduce by 2.5mg every 3–4 days <u>Below 7.5mg</u>: reduce by 2.5mg every week, then STOP

Steroid withdrawal syndrome   A characteristic corticosteroid withdrawal syndrome can occur if steroids are reduced too quickly and is often not recognised. It consists of fever, myalgia, arthralgia, and malaise (and less commonly include rhinitis, conjunctivitis and painful pruritic skin nodules).

Hypersensitivity   Corticosteroid hypersensitivity is a recognised occurrence. Reports exist of anaphylactic-type reactions with hydrocortisone and dexamethasone. Due to reported asthmatic attacks with hydrocortisone succinate injections in patients with a history of aspirin-induced asthma, it has been suggested that sodium phosphate salts of corticosteroids be used for injection in these patients.

Steroid card   Patients on corticosteroids need to be educated about the importance of compliance, and should always carry a steroid alert card. They must be aware that the dose of corticosteroid must be increased with intercurrent illness or under severe stress.

ANALGESIA

Effects on pain   Corticosteroids have been shown to reduce pain in various situations. There are a number of possible mechanisms for their analgesic activity:

- inhibition of prostaglandin synthesis leading to a reduction in inflammation
- a reduction in capillary permeability and peritumoral oedema
- a reduction in spontaneous discharge in injured nerves
- a reduction in injury-induced nerve sprouting
- a reduction in the calcitonin gene-related peptide and substance P content of sensory fibres possibly, a central effect related to improved mood.

These actions of corticosteroids may explain why they have been found useful as adjuvant analgesics in the management of bone pain, certain types of neuropathic pain, and in situations where the mechanism for the production of pain is due to a large tumour mass within a relatively confined space. Controlled studies of the use of corticosteroids as analgesics are rare in the literature, but a review of the major ones can be found in an article by Watanabe and Bruera.[15] The table below lists situations in which corticosteroids might be useful as co-analgesics.

PAINS POSSIBLY RESPONSIVE TO CORTICOSTEROIDS.

- Bone metastases
- Spinal cord compression
- Headache associated with raised intracranial pressure
- Nerve compression pain
- Reflex sympathetic dystrophy
- Pain associated with hepatomegaly
- Expanding tumour in confined space, e.g. pelvic tumour

Dosage High dose IV dexamethasone is favoured in some centres in the US[16] and Scandinavia[17] for the treatment of spinal cord compression, 96mg i.v./day tapering to zero in 14 days. However, an unacceptably high incidence of serious side-effects occurs with these regimes.[18]

A relatively safe and effective regime is recommended by Twycross.[6] 12mg orally at the time of diagnosis of cord compression, followed by 16 to 32mg/day during the initial phase of palliative radiotherapy. The dose is then reduced in the light of response to treatment, and adverse effects, aiming to achieve a dosage in single figures within 2 weeks.

Painful rib metastases may sometimes respond to a local injection of bupivicaine 0.5% and depot methylprednisolone. Epidural injection of corticosteroids is sometimes effective in relieving radicular pain.[19]

ANOREXIA AND CACHEXIA

Effect on appetite A number of trials published in the literature have reported a significant improvement in appetite in patients treated with corticosteroids.[20] This effect on appetite appears to be shortlived however, sometimes only for a few weeks, and they do not seem to improve caloric intake, nutritional status, or lead to any substantial nonfluid weight-gain in treated patients.[21] Progestational drugs, on the other hand, have been shown to increase caloric intake and nutritional status (with an increase in nonfluid weight gain) as well as improving appetite.[22] Results of trials using other agents, e.g. cyproheptadine, hydrazine suphate, pentoifylline, and cannabinoids have been disappointing.

BRAIN TUMOURS

Corticosteroids can lead to a reduction of neurologic signs and symptoms in more than two-thirds of patients with brain tumours. Their effect is mainly on peri-tumoral oedema and a reduction in cerebral blood flow. In some situations, they may also have a direct cytotoxic effect. Dexamethasone is most commonly used because of it's relatively lower mineralocorticoid activity. Dosing schedules vary between centres. A study of the effect of dexamethasone on Karnofsky performance in metatstatic brain tumours[23] concluded that 4mg of dexamethasone per day for brain tumour oedema resulted in the same degree of improvement as 16mg/day after one week of treatment.

Toxic effects were dose-dependent and more common in patients using 16mg/day for 4 weeks. All patients in this study were undergoing cranial irradiation. If larger doses are used in the initial stages of treatment (eg 16mg/day), this should be tapered over the course of 4 weeks eg 16mg/day for 4 days, 8mg/day for a further 4 days, then 4mg/day until the end of the course of radiotherapy.[24]

Ideally, the lowest maintenance dose possible which maintains neurological stability should be used. The maximum beneficial dosage is not known, but there appears to be a definite subgroup of patients who show improvement on further increases in dose when symptoms or signs recur or progress on a lower dose. Some authors have reported a benefit with as high a dose as 96mg/day.[25] These were in patients taking anticonvulsants concomitantly, and so would be equivalent to approximately half that dose in patients not on anticonvulsants. When considering increasing the dose at any time, but particularly beyond what might be considered the normal range (i.e. above 16mg/day), then the benefit versus the cost in terms of side-effects must be carefully weighed up in each individual case.

Steroids for cord compression

A 79 year old lady with Stage IV breast carcinoma and multiple bone metastases began to complain of weakness and "pins and needles" in both arms. 3 months earlier, she had been treated for threatened spinal cord compression with lower limb signs. She lived some distance from a radiotherapy centre, and was not keen to travel for further assessment and possible treatment. Her general condition was fragile with lung and liver metastases as well as widespread bone disease. Her maintenance dose of dexamethasone was increased from 2mg daily to 16mg daily for 5 days and, following complete resolution of her symptoms, it was reduced to a maintenance dose of 4mg over a 3 week period. She died 3 months later from bronchopneumonia, but retained her independence at home up until a short time before her death.

CYTOTOXIC EFFECT

Glucocorticoids are often included with other agents in combination chemotherapy for both acute and chronic lymphocytic leukaemias, Hodgkin's and non-Hodgkin's lymphomas, multiple myeloma and breast cancer.

Low dose dexamethasone (0.75mg BD) has been shown to produce symptomatic improvement and decreased PSA (Prostate Specific Antigen) levels (with associated radiographic evidence of disease regression) in patients with hormone-resistant prostate cancer.[26]

DYSPNOEA

Corticosteroids have a number of possible uses in the control of respiratory distress in patients with advanced cancer. As in the general medical setting, they have a role in the management of airway obstruction unresponsive, or incompletely responsive to bronchodilators and methylxanthines. The inhaled route is used for maintenance relief of symptoms, with the oral or parenteral routes more effective in relieving acute distress due to bronchospasm. Corticosteroids are also of use in the acute relief of SVC obstruction, relief of stridor due to tracheal obstruction, as an adjunct in the management of lymphangitis carcinomatosa, and in symptomatic relief of the dyspnoea associated with post-radiation pneumonitis.

HOLLOW ORGAN OBSTRUCTION

There is little evidence in the literature supporting a definite role for corticosteroids in relieving obstructions to hollow viscera. Due to their anti-inflammatory effect, corticosteroids might be expected to reduce inflammatory oedema around luminal or intraluminal tumour deposits, perhaps relieving the obstruction. Farr et al.[4] reported on nine patients with either a partial small bowel obstruction, an upper gastrointestinal obstruction, or a colonic obstruction. The patients were treated with parenteral corticosteroid (i.e. solu-medrol 50mg 8 hourly) for 2–3 days followed by oral prednisone 10mg TDS daily. 67% of patients had symptomatic improvement of the obstructive symptoms.

In that same review, the authors describe 3 patients with renal insufficiency which was presumed secondary to malignant obstructive uropathy, in whom there was an improvement in renal function and symptoms following either parenteral or oral prednisone. They add a cautionary note of risk of developing sepsis in patients given corticosteroids. Corticosteroids may also help to relieve stridor due to tumour compression of the trachea.

Relief of pyloric obstruction

A 52 year old man with gastric carcinoma presented with increasing nausea and vomiting over a 2 week period. The vomiting was worst after meals, and relieved the nausea. He had previously refused surgery. Cisapride 10mg TDS was commenced, which relieved the symptoms for only about 10 days. A clinical diagnosis of progressive pyloric obstruction secondary to encroaching tumour was made. He refused admission for assessment or consideration of a venting gastrostomy. Dexamethasone 8mg daily was commenced with relief of the vomiting after 48 hours. In combination with prokinetics, the dexamethasone maintained relief of the nausea and vomiting for a further 6 weeks, at which point symptoms returned. This coincided with a general deterioration in the man's condition, so that further invasive interventions were not appropriate. His symptoms were managed with subcutaneous cyclizine 150mg and octreotide 600mg in 24 hours. The patient died peacefully 4 days later.

HYPERCALCAEMIA

Bisphosphonates are the treatment of choice for hypercalcaemia associated with most solid tumours. Corticosteroids may still be effective for hypercalcaemia associated with myeloma, lymphoma, and breast cancer. Relatively high dose prednisolone (60–100mg/day) needs to be given for any effect.[27]

NAUSEA AND VOMITING

Anti-emetic action

Corticosteroids are often included in anti-emetic protocols for patients receiving highly emetogenic chemotherapeutic regimes.[28] They are most commonly given in combination with 5–HT₃ antagonists in this situation. A common practice is to give dexamethasone IV, eg 20mg, 30 minutes before administering chemotherapy.[29] The anti-emetic action of corticosteroids is poorly understood, but it may involve central inhibition of the synthesis of prostaglandins. Dexamethasone is also effective in relieving the vomiting associated with raised intracranial pressure.

REPLACEMENT THERAPY

In chronic primary adrenocortical insufficiency (Addison's disease), hydrocortisone orally is used (20–40mg total daily) in the lowest dose that maintains well-being and body weight, with two-thirds of the total dose in the morning and one-third in the evening to mimic the natural diurnal rhythm of secretion.

Fludrocortisone

Most patients also require the mineralocorticoid, fludrocortisone 0.1–0.2mg once daily. The patient should be advised to double the hydrocortisone dose and seek medical advice in the event of any complicating event, e.g. infection, severe stress and should carry a steroid card.

Addisonian Crisis

In the situation of an acute life-threatening Addisonian crisis, hydrocortisone sodium succinate 100mg IV should be given immediately it is suspected, with other appropriate supportive therapy. High dose IV therapy should be continued for a few days (ie 50–100mg i.v. 6–8 hourly × 24 hours, then 12 hourly), with oral therapy introduced once the condition has stabilised.

DRUG INTERACTIONS

Probably the most important interaction in the context of palliative care is with the anticonvulsants. Phenytoin, carbamazepine accelerate the metabolism of corticosteroids. When used concomitantly, the aniticipated dose of dexamethasone should be doubled.

Other drugs which accelerate corticosteroid metabolism include aminoglutethimide and rifampicin. Corticosteroids antagonise the effects of oral antihyperglycaemics, insulin, and antihypertensives. The risk of hypokalaemia associated with B2–adrenoceptor agonists and carbenoxolone is increased with concomitant corticosteroid use.

PRACTICAL USE OF CORTICOSTEROIDS

Dosage Starting dosage depends on clinical indication for their use. In acute, emergency situations, e.g. spinal cord compression, raised intracranial pressure associated with brain tumours, SVC obstruction, then a starting dose of 16mg/day is suggested, with gradual tapering to a maintenance dose in the single figures.

Smaller doses are recommended for the treatment of anorexia (eg dexamethasone 2–4mg daily). Corticosteroids should never be prescribed lightly, and their appropriateness and effectiveness should be monitored regularly. If after one week's treatment there is no improvement they should be discontinued. The lowest effective dose should be used, and this should be given as a single dose in the morning (unless hydrocortisone is being used), to prevent possible sleep disturbance. All patients should carry a steroid alert card and be aware of some of the basic facts about the use of steroid medication.

Route Corticosteroids are rapidly absorbed when given orally, so this remains the route of choice with most patients. Dexamethasone can be easily dissolved in water. Topical steroid preparations should be used if possible for inflammatory skin conditions, with the weakest effective preparation being used. The potential for systemic absorption of the more potent preparations with long-term usage should not be ignored. Corticosteroid preparations are available which are suitable for rectal administration, and these have a role in the management of haemorrhoids and the relief of tenesmus.

Subcutaneous use   Dexamethasone can be given by subcutaneous infusion if clinically indicated. The problem of precipitation with other drugs in a syringe can be avoided by mixing the dexamethasone with the other drugs at body temperature (warm syringe in the palm of the hand) rather than room temperature.

STEROIDS IN AIDS

Corticosteroids have a number of therapeutic applications in patients with AIDS but they also intensify the impairment of immune defences worsening the risk of opportunistic infections.

In Pneumocysits carinii pneumonia (PCP) treatment with corticosteroids (eg IV hydrocortisone 100mg QDS for 5 days) within 72 hours of beginning conventional therapy improves outcome and reduce mortality by 50% in moderate to severe episode (PaO2 <8kPA. on air). The current data do not indicate whether corticosteroids are beneficial for mild episodes.[31]

Every effort should be made to establish a definitive diagnosis of PCP in patients treated with corticosteroids. Pulmonary tuberculosis or fungal infection may mimic PCP and corticosteroids may cause initial improvement while the underlying infection would actually be worsening. Corticosteroids may accelerate the progression of cutaneous and pulmonary Kaposi's sarcoma by stimulating a Kaposi's growth factor. However where there is a very high suspicion of PCP in a very ill patient, corticosteroids are sometimes commenced without a definitive diagnosis because of the high mortality associated with the infection. Patients need to be monitored closely in this situation.

In patients cerebral lymphoma where there is significant cerebral oedema dexamathasone forms part of the chemotherapy regime.

CONCLUSION

Risks   The widespread applicability of corticosteroids in palliative care runs the risk that their use will become less carefully controlled. This would lead to serious consequences in terms of toxicity. A surprising number of patients taking corticosteroids are unaware of some of the basic precautions necessary while taking them.[30]

Benefits   It is essential, therefore, to have a sound understanding of the risks and benefits associated with the use of corticosteroids. Centres that have accumulated experience with corticosteroids for less common conditions should publish their series of cases or conduct proper controlled trials. In this way we will be able to take full advantage of this very useful class of drugs.

References:

1. Walsh D, Avashi J. Glucocorticoids in clinical oncology. Cleve Clin J Med 1992; 59: 505–15.
2. Coleman RE. Glucocorticoids in cancer therapy. Biotherapy 1992; 4(1): 37–44.
3. Bruera E, Roca E, Cedaro L, et al. Action of oral methylprednisolone in terminal cancer patients: a prospective randomized double-blind study. Cancer Treat Rep 1985; 69: 751–4.
4. Farr WC. The use of corticosteroids for symptom management in terminally ill patients. Am J Hosp Care 1990; 1: 41–6.
5. Swartz SL, Dluhy RG. Corticosteroids: clinical pharmacology and therapeutic use. Curr Ther 1978; 19: 145–70.
6. Twycross R. The risks and benefits of corticosteroids in advanced cancer. Drug Safety 1994; 11(3): 163–178.
7. Weissmann DE, Dufer D, Vogel V, et al. Corticosteroid toxicity in neuro-oncology patients. J Neurooncol 1987; 5: 125–8.
8. Spector TD, Sambrook PN. Steroid osteoporosis. BMJ 1993; 307: 519–20.
9. McCluskey J, Gutteridge DH. Avascular necrosis of bone after high doses of dexamethasone during neurosurgery. BMJ 1982; 284: 333–4.
10. Piper JM, Ray WA, Daugherty JR, et al. Corticosteroid use and peptic ulcer disease: role of nonsteroidal anti-inflammatory drugs. Ann Intern Med 1991; 114: 735–40.
11. Guslando M, Titobello A. Steroid ulcers: a myth revisited. BMJ 1992; 304: 655–6.
12. Ellershaw JE, Kelly MJ. Corticosteroids and peptic ulceration. Pall Med 1994;8: 222–8.
13. Strafl FC, Breitbart WS, Holland JC. Corticosteroids in cancer: neuropsychiatric complications. Cancer Invest 1989; 7(5): 479–91.
14. Hanks GW, Trueman T, Twycross RG. Corticosteroids in terminal cancer: a prospective analysis of current practice. Postgrad Med J 1983; 59: 702–6.
15. Watanabe S, Bruera E. Corticosteroids as adjuvant analgesics. J Pain Symp Management 1994; 9(7): 442–5.
16. Greenberg HS, Kim JH, Posner JB. Epidural spinal cord compression from metastatic tumour: results with a new treatment protocol. Ann Neurol 1979; 8: 361–6.

17. Sorensen S, Helweg-Larsen S, Mouridsen H, et al. Effect of high-dose dexamethasone in carcinomatous metastatic spinal cord compression treated with radiotherapy: a randomised trial. Eur J Cancer 1994; 30A(1): 22–7.

18. Heimdal K, Hirschberg H, Slettebo H, et al. High incidence of serious side-effects of high-dose dexamethasone treatment in patients with epidural spinal cord compression. J Neurooncol 1992; 12(2): 141–4.

19. Watts RW, Silagy CA. A meta-analysis on the efficacy of epidural corticosteroids in the treatment of sciatica. Anaesth Intens Care 1995; 23: 564–9.

20 Bruera E. Current pharmacological management of anorexia in cancer patients. Oncology 1992; 6(1): 125–30.

21. Loprinzi CL. Management of cancer anorexia/cachexia. Supp Care Cancer 1995; 3(2): 120–2.

22. Loprinzi CL, Johnson PA, Jensen M. Megestrol acetate for anorexia and cachexia. Oncology 1992; 49 Suppl 2: 46–9.

23. Vecht ChJ, Hovestadt A, Verbiest HBC, et al. Dose-effect relationship of dexamethasone on Karnofsky performance in metastatic brain tumours: a randomized study of doses 4, 8, and 16mg per day. Neurology 1994; 44: 675–80.

24. Weissmann DE, Janjan NA, Erickson B, et al. Twice-daily tapering dexamethasone treatment during cranial radiation for newly diagnosed brain metastases. J Neurooncol 1991; 11: 235–9.

25. Renaudin J, Fewer D, Wilson CB, et al. Dose dependency of Decadron in patients with partially excised brain tumours. J Neurosurg 1973; 39: 302–5.

26. Storlie JA, Buckner JC, Wiseman GA, et al. Prostate specific antigen levels and clinical response to low dose dexamethasone for hormone-refractory metastatic prostate carcinoma. Cancer 1995; 76(1): 96–100.

27. Kristensen B, Ejlertsen B, Holmegaard SN, et al. Prednisolone in the treatment of severe malignant hypercalcaemia in metastatic breast cancer: a randomized study. J Int Med 1992; 232(3): 237–45.

28. Gralla RJ. An outline of anti-emetic treatment. Eur J Cancer Clin Oncol 1989; 25: S7–11.

29. Parry H, Martin K. Single-dose IV dexamethasone: an effective anti-emetic in cancer chemotherapy. Cancer Chemother Pharmacol 1991; 28: 231–2.

30. Needham PR, Daley AG, Lennard RF. Steroids in advanced cancer: a survey of current practice. BMJ 1992; 305: 999.

31. Nelson TL, Eefinck-Scattenkerk JK, Jensen BN, et al. Adjunctive corticosteroid therapy for Pneumocystis carinii pneumonia in AIDS: a randomized European multicenter study. J. AIDS 1992; 5: 726–731.

32. Page RC, How to wean a patient off corticosteroids Prescribers Journal 1997; 37 No. 1: 11–16

Chapter 15

Confusion

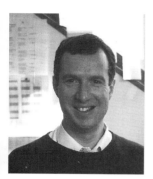

Dr Paul McNamara

Paul McNamara came the long way round, via palliative care jobs at Tunbridge Wells, Clapham, Oxford and Crawley, and is now Consultant at St Oswald's Hospice, Newcastle. Current interests include opioid rotation, and production of the Newcastle and North Tyneside Palliative Care Newsletter. Josephine (3 years) and William (18 months) ensure that home life is a complete break.

A DEFINITION

Confusion: A disorder affecting attention, level of consciousness and cognitive functions. It is acute or sub-acute in onset (usually acute) and is due to a medical cause. It causes global cerebral dysfunction and is characterized by fluctuation or waxing and waning of the symptoms. It is often reversible, except in the last 24–48 hours of life: ("terminal restlessness or terminal agitation").

Note: Other terms for confusion are:

● acute confusional state
● delirium.

The word confusion is used throughout this chapter.

INTRODUCTION

Confusion can be infectious. Confusion about diagnosis is common due to the too-easy 'labelling' of a patient who appears confused. And the huge range of possible aetiologies conjured up in the clinician's can cause confusion about the best therapeutic options.

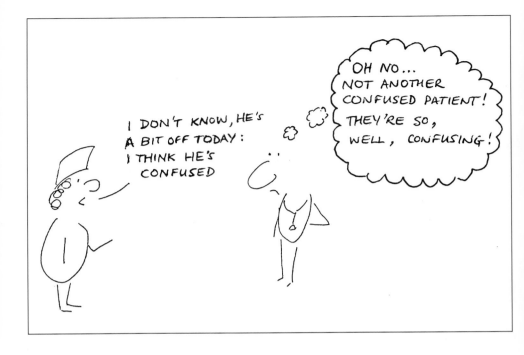

CHARACTERISTIC FEATURES OF CONFUSION (DSM IV)

Features of confusion

1. Disturbance of consciousness (i.e. reduced clarity of awareness of environment) with reduced ability to focus, sustain or shift attention.

2. A change in cognition (such as memory deficit, disorientation, language disturbance) or the development of a perceptual disturbance that is not accounted for by a pre-existing or evolving dementia.

3. The disturbance *develops over a short period of time* (usually hours to days) and tends to fluctuate during the course of the day.

EFFECTS OF CONFUSION

- Level of consciousness
- Attention
- Thinking
- Perception
- Memory
- Psychomotor behaviour
- Emotion
- Sleep-wake cycle

4. There is evidence from the history, physical examination or laboratory findings, that the disturbance is caused by the direct physiological consequences of a general medical condition.

Dementia In dementia, the mental effects are chronic, level of consciousness is unaffected (usually) and the memory loss is progressive and irreversible.

Depression can mimic dementia, but there is usually a rapid onset (comparatively) of the cognitive impairment, which tends not to be progressive. There is often a recent precipitant of the depressed mood (perhaps with a history of depression) and mental tests show better cognitive function than expected.

A MODEL OF CONFUSION

It can be helpful to have a simple mental model of what is happening to the patient, to better understand their point of view. This helps avoid the temptation to simply prescribe medication, without trying to understand the strangeness of the situation in which confused patients find themselves, which is often bewildering and frightening.

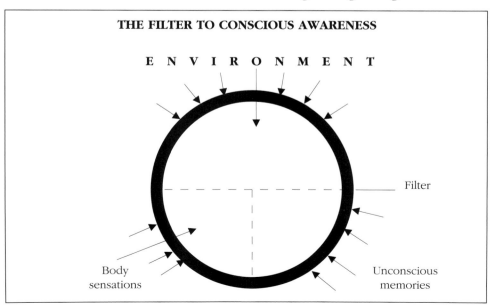

THE FILTER TO CONSCIOUS AWARENESS

E N V I R O N M E N T

Filter

Body sensations

Unconscious memories

The model[17] postulates filters which govern the entry of stimuli into consciousness, from the body, environment and unconscious.

When awake, stimuli are correctly attributed to their area of origin (environment or body) and the filter to the unconscious is strong.

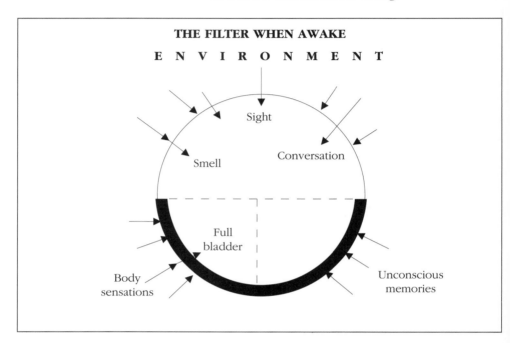

When asleep, the reverse situation holds, with the unconscious being the main source of stimuli. The filter to bodily or environmental stimuli is in place, and only a strong external stimulus would reach consciousness (eg heat may cause dreams about the desert).

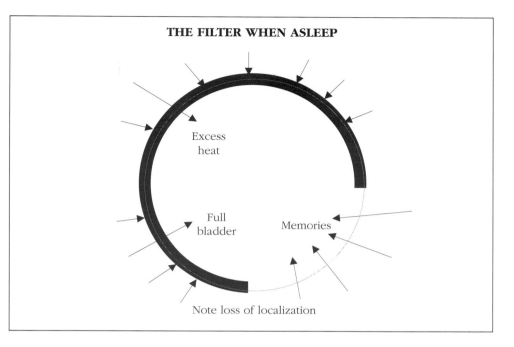

THE FILTER WHEN ASLEEP

Excess
heat

Full
bladder

Memories

Note loss of localization

In confusion, the filters are no longer effective in partitioning off recognisable areas. The patient finds it difficult to interpret whether stimuli are coming from the body, the environment or the unconscious. The unconscious stimuli can assume prominence (sometimes leading to hallucinations) and the world, understandably, then seems a very strange place.

The filter model explains why reducing unnecessary external stimuli, in calm, quiet surroundings, is part of good management.

Confusion can also be frightening and the "fight or flight" protective reflexes may come into play, making the patient seem hostile or aggressive.

Having some appreciation of this process can help us connect with patients who are confused. Our attempts to get through to[18] such patients and understand their reactions, will itself reassure and calm them. They will appear less strange to us, if we remember that they are responding appropriately to the world as it seems to them. The challenge for us is to try and understand something of their world and thereby to offer explanation and reassurance. Medication can help us in gaining this access, and helping restore some normality.

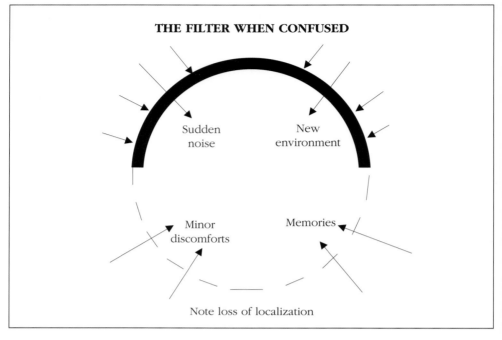

THE FILTER WHEN CONFUSED

Sudden
noise

New
environment

Minor
discomforts

Memories

Note loss of localization

Incidence of Confusion $10 - 27\%^2, 39\%^3, 57\%^4, 85\%^5$.

Take your pick! The above are quoted figures of the incidence of confusion in dying cancer patients. Except the 57% (dying AIDS patients). The 10 – 27% figure is the common range on an in-patient unit in my experience, although some days it feels like 85%!

PATHOPHYSIOLOGY

The pathophysiology of confusion is not clear cut. However here are a few of the theories.

1. Reduced cerebral oxidative metabolism. The level of consciousness in delirium correlates with the slowing of background activity on the EEG. This reflects change in the metabolism of cerebral neurones. Increased cerebral energy demands (pyrexia), increased cerebral neuroelectrical act- ivity (fear or pyrexia), or decreased cerebral energy supply (glucose or oxygen), may all precipitate delirium.

2. Neurotransmitter imbalance. Anticholinergics (known to cause delirium and hypoxia) reduce acetylcholine synthesis. Acetylcholine has a key role in attention, arousal and memory. It is thought that it is the balance of acetylcholine to dopamine that is important in the development of delirium.

3. Age-related cortical damage (or structural damage e.g. from brain metastases) may mean further small changes in the intracranial milieau can manifest as delirium.

CLINICAL CAUSES OF CONFUSION

Metabolic	Psychosocial	Physical	End Stage
Infection	Change of environment	Pain	Organ failure
Dehydration	Anxiety ± depression	Fatigue	Cancer
Drug withdrawal	Psychiatric illness	Trauma	
Biochemical disturbance		Cerebrovascular accident	
Hypoxia			
Hypercapnia			
Pain fatigue			
Hypoglycaemia			
Vitamin deficiency			

NB: Two or more causes may be present.

Discussion of causes

Infection – this is a prime cause of delirium. It should be suspected whether or not there is pyrexia, highlighting the importance of routinely examining the chest and a specimen of urine.

Pain and Fatigue – the distracting effect of pain is well known. This can lead people to misinterpret what is being said to them, or done for them, and therefore to behave defensively or inappropriately. Fatigue has a similar effect and together these effects are additive.

Drugs – see below

Dehydration – is less well tolerated in the elderly, where their delicate intracranial milieau can be easily disturbed.

Biochemical disturbance eg hypercalcaemia, uraemia, hyponatraemia.

DRUGS THAT CAN CAUSE CONFUSION

- **Anticholinergics**
  - Antihistamines
    eg diphenhydramine, cyclizine
  - Tricyclic anti-depressants
    eg. amitriptyline
  - Phenothiazines eg
    chlorpromazine, thioridazine
  - Antispasmodics
    eg hyoscine, oxybutynin
  - Anti-parkinsonian
    eg benzhexol
  - Anti-arrhythmics
    eg quinidine

- **Opioids**
  - morphine, fentanyl, buprenorphine
    (or withdrawal of these)

- **Hypnotics/Anxiolytics**
  - Benzodiazepines
    eg. diazepam, lorezepam
  - Barbiturates
    (or withdrawal of these)

- **Cardiac drugs**
  - Digoxin
  - Betablockers
  - Methyldopa
  - Diuretics

- **Cytotoxics**
  - Methotrexate
  - Ifosfamide

- **Antibiotics**
  - Aminoglycosides
  - Cephalosporins
  - Ciprofloxacin
  - Penicillins
  - Sulphonamides

- **Other drugs**
  - Corticosteroids
  - Cimetidine
  - NSAIDS
  - Acyclovir
  - Ranitidine
  - Anticonvulsants

Remember that cimetidine can practically double the half life of diazepam.

Change of environment - the disorientating effect of new surroundings can precipitate confusion. Admission to an inpatient unit, with the normal procedure of gaining consent either curtailed or bypassed and with little, if any, explanation or agreement from the patient (or entirely forgotten by the patient) may worsen confusion.

Alcohol/nicotine withdrawal – are easily overlooked, and benzodiazepine withdrawal can commonly contribute to the development of delirium.

Cancer – systemic effect or cerebral involvement.

Recent trauma – eg long bone fracture (with accompanying anaemia and hypotension) or subdural haematoma with raised intracranial pressure

Organ Failure – eg cardiac, liver, kidney etc.

Hypoxia – eg from respiratory or cardiac disease

Vitamin deficiency – including vitamin B1[6]

Differential Diagnosis ("Confusion about confusion")

Other possibilities to consider when a patient appears "confused" are:

- Not understanding in what is said – perhaps deaf, too anxious or ill to take it in
- Forgetful
- Disorientated in time and place – does not warrant the label "confused" if this is the only abnormality
- Misperceiving
- Hallucinations may be normal on going to sleep (hypnogogic hallucinations) or on waking (hypnopompic). These are more common with people taking sedatives. If these 'normal' hallucinations are not explained, they may cause anxiety, because people associate hallucinations with going mad.
- Vivid nightmares/sleep disturbance may reflect a person's unresolved fears eg about death, pain.

CLINICAL ASSESSMENT

History

History taking must include:

- duration of the change in mental state.
- associated changes eg medication, environment, infection, trauma, pain relief, vomiting, diarrhoea, dehydration.
- description of behaviour, eg paranoia, aggression.
- variability of the level of confusion – any diurnal pattern?

- nicotine and alcohol history.
- previous episodes and pre-existing mental state.
- what has been tried and its success, whether physical or medical interventions.

The history should be taken from the case notes *and* from the carers/family, medical and nursing colleagues involved (because the patient is unlikely to be able to give a reliable account).

Examination
- Content of speech
- Behaviour exhibited eg psychotic features, level of disruption
- Level of consciousness
- Signs of infection – chest, urine, skin (may not be pyrexial)
- Anoxia
- Dehydration
- Neurological examination
- Assess risk to self or staff

These points will help determine the need for urgent drug control of the situation.

Investigations
- Urine ward test, finger prick blood glucose
- FBC WCC differential
- Biochemistry including calcium and renal function
- C & S of infected sputum, wound swab etc.
- Drug levels of anticonvulsants, digoxin etc.
- Brain scan may occasionally be helpful, eg where treatable brain secondaries suspected.

Brain scan
The question of whether a brain scan is appropriate may be raised, and often a therapeutic trial of dexamethasone, (eg 16 mg for 5 days) can indicate whether or not brain metastases may be present. However, even when it is not appropriate to follow through with radiotherapy, it can be helpful to know definitely about cerebral metastases. CT scan or MRI are the investigations of choice. Both the patient and the relatives may be relieved to know that there is a brain tumour and an identifiable organic cause for the behavioural changes. Otherwise it may be felt that the patient has simply gone mad and this may carry a stigma with it. This knowledge often has placement implications also,

quite apart from its treatment possibilities. Response to dexamethasone, does not necessarily indicate the presence of cerebral metastases,[22] but may point to the therapeutic benefit of corticosteroids by some, as yet, unexplained mechanism.

MANAGEMENT

General management

1. Explanation is important:
   a) calmly to the patient of everything that is done and the proposed management. This may need to be explained repeatedly. Always assume that the patient does understand.
   b) to the family or carers
   c) to the clinical team caring for the patient and colleagues

   The time spent in explanation, especially to the carers and clinical team is time well spent, as confusion in any setting can be extremely disruptive. The team need to feel confident in the management plan, and well supported, especially when the behaviour exhibited by the patient is hostile or otherwise unpleasant.

Environment

2. Environment needs to be quiet, with
   - calm lighting
   - familiar faces
   - a small number of (familiar) staff involved in care
   - safety (avoid matches, sharp objects, high windows etc.)

3. Calming Influences - environment
   - touch (if this is soothing then massage may be calming also: this can be undertaken by members of the interdisciplinary team, or family)
   - soothing music
   - aromatherapy

   All of these calming influences are important, but the most important factor is the calmness of the clinical team caring for the patient. What is required seems to be a mixture of confidence with compassion.

Medical Management

1. Treat reversible causes if appropriate eg hypercalcaemia, infection, cardiac failure. Where there is dehydration simply encouraging the patient to drink may not be sufficient, and a period of parenteral rehydration may be necessary. In this context hypodermoclysis (SC infusion) may be safer than IV fluids.[7]

2. Stop 'suspected' drugs judiciously or reduce the dosage eg. corticosteroids. There has been some documented success with opioid rotation.[10]

Opioid rotation

Opioid rotation is a practice now increasingly adopted, following reports of its success in reducing the incidence of side effects, which include confusion.[8] Indications for change of opioid included cognitive failure (39%) and hallucinations (24%) as well as smaller groups with uncontrolled pain, myoclonus and nausea. Opioids used were morphine, as first choice, with mainly hydromorphone and methadone as alternatives, in these North American studies. In the above study, improvement in cognitive failure occurred in 29/42 (69%) and in 10/15 (66%) with hallucinations. In the UK, the availability of fentanyl in a transdermal patch delivery system has made this a popular alternative when morphine side effects are troublesome. Similar studies in the UK are being planned, to look more closely at the claims made for opiod rotation.

3. Drug treatment will probably be necessary where there is disruptive behaviour e.g. mania, restlessness, wandering, shouting or hitting out, or distressing anxiety, fear, paranoia or depression.

The presence of a calm supportive person together with the general approaches mentioned, is not always sufficient. Drug treatment may be necessary.

Core resources

The indications for drug treatment depend on both the severity of delirium and the care resources available. With few care resources (in a busy hospital ward, or accident and emergency department) early sedation may be a "damage limitation" exercise, in a hard pressed environment.

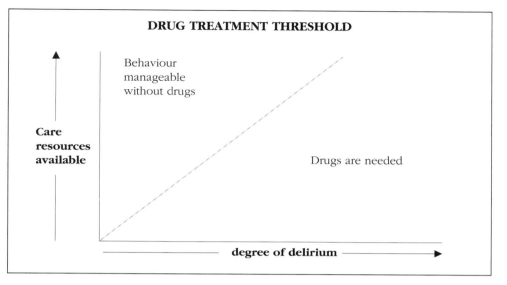

On the other hand, elderly care wards may have the expertise to cope with quite disruptive behaviour without recourse to drugs. In one such unit extensive use was made of aromatherapy oils and massage, to exert a strong calming effect, and transquillisers were rarely required. More needs to be known about such approaches.

Often however, confusion at home places great emotional strain upon the carers, even with a confident primary health care team and confident relatives/carers.

A specialist palliative care unit should have a high threshold for instigating drug treatment, as it has access to a multidisciplinary team and a spectrum of approaches. At the most basic (but often most effective) having the availability of a team member to be with the patient continuously can obviate the need for strong sedatives. This tends to be a nurse, but appropriately chosen volunteers have sometimes been used in this context, satisfactorily.

Reversible versus non-reversible confusion

Where the cause of the confusion is thought to be reversible, symptomatic treatment of the patient is still appropriate while the precipitating cause is addressed. Where the cause is irreversible, good symptomatic control is achievable, using the drugs which will be discussed below.

The non-drug measures mentioned additionally may be useful in both contexts.

DRUG MANAGEMENT

Drug management is often required early, whilst investigation and other management approaches are being initiated. Frequent review is mandatory to monitor the effects. As these drugs in themselves may cause confusion, they are not to be used lightly. Management is tailored to the individual as the effect of powerful drugs cannot be accurately predicted. The goals of treatment need to be defined at the outset and redefined as time goes by.

Keeping dying patients "settled and peaceful" may give rise to concern as to whether they are over-sedated, excluding further conscious inter-action, at a time when this may be important.

The question of sedation

This caveat is important to bear in mind in the drug management of delirium, where there may be influences to "settle" a patient quickly and keep them sedated. These may range from appropriate family or carer feelings to inappropriate staff reactions towards a "disruptive" or noisy patient who may be "upsetting" other patients. Family may say "You would not let a dog suffer like this", out of distress at the patient's perceived loss of dignity. Considerable time must be set aside by the main clinician to weigh up the factors and explain and educate the carers and staff where conflict of opinion arises. This is time well spent and is an integral and essential part of the overall manage-ment of the case.

THE IDEAL DRUG FOR TREATING CONFUSION

- Reduced agitation, paranoia and fear.
- Improved cognition
- Little sedation.
- Few anticholinergic side effects.
- Few respiratory or cardiovascular effects.
- Little effect on seizure threshold.
- Available orally, S/C, IM and IV.

Neuroleptics   The mainstays of drug management are the neuroleptics and the benzodiazepines. The neuroleptics are able to control psychotic behaviour.

Haloperidol   Haloperidol, a butyrophenone, has become the drug of choice for the reasons in the box below. Haloperidol has dopamine blocking qualities and this may help the postulated imbalance of central cholinergic and adrenergic neurotransmitters. The metabolism of haloperidol has wide inter-individual variation so frequent review is the key to achieving the optimum effect.

Akathisia   One relatively rare, but troublesome side effect of haloperidol is akathisia. This inability to sit still, or motor restlessness, should be considered where increasing the dose of haloperidol worsens the situation. The treatment is to withdraw the haloperidol and an anticholinergic drug may be required. If sedation as well as anti-psychotic effects are needed, thioridazine, chlorpromazine or methotrimeprazine may be more appropriate. The incidence of side effects increases with these drugs.

HALOPERIDOL

- Anxiolytic and anti-psychotic
- Starting dose 0.5 -5 mg oral, S/C, IM and IV
- Review effects (wide inter-individual metabolism variation)
- Usually 5 -15 mg is sufficient per 24 hours
- Limitations:
    - skin tolerability subcutaneously
    - relatively non-sedating
    - Parkinsonism
    - occasional akathisia

Thioridazine   Thioridazine (Melleril) is also anxiolytic and anti-psychotic but is slightly more sedating than haloperidol. The starting dose is 10–30mg orally, with a total of 30–100mg per 24 hours. Its use may be limited by the fact it is only available orally, and it has some hypotensive and anticholinergic side effects.

Methotrimeprazine   Methotrimeprazine is an alternative, if strong sedative activity is needed. It is possible to use a SC infusion (although skin irritation can occur). Methotrimeprazine shares many properties with chlorpromazine but is more sedating and its antiemetic properties are more "broad-spectrum".[19] It also has analgesic activity.[20]

METHOTRIMEPRAZINE

- Sedative anti-psychotic
- Starting dose 12.5–50 mg oral, S/C, IM, IV (usually 75–250 mg per 24 hours)
- Limitations:
    - skin reaction SC (reduced by mixing with normal saline (maximum dose 250–300 mg per 24 hours))[9]
    - excessive sedation
    - Hypotensive and extra-pyramidal side effects

Managing Confusion

A 69 year old man with carcinoma of the prostate and a degree of dementia was admitted in a confused state to a palliative care unit. He was found to have a urinary tract infection and antibiotic treatment improved his mental state. However, he remained suspicious of staff at times and occasionally agitated. His medication was adjusted (opioid reduced) and there seemed to be temporary improvement. However, he continued to exhibit some paranoia despite normal electrolytes and calcium. He was started on a low dose of haloperidol, 1.5 mg at night, and was able to be discharged home 10 days later with no recurrence of his confusion or paranoia. This case underlines the importance of treating simple causes (initially) for confusion and the beneficial effect of low dose haloperidol in abolishing mild psychotic features.

Benzodiazepines   Where "quiet sedation" is the goal, instead of changing to a more sedating major tranquiliser, eg haloperidol to methotrimeprazine (approximately twice as sedating as chlorpromazine), the addition of a short-acting benzodiazepine may be more logical, e.g. lorazepam or midazolam.

Benzodiazepines may be used to treat confusion on their own if there is no evidence of psychotic symptoms and it is mainly due to over-riding anxiety. However, a double blind randomised comparative trial, of haloperidol versus chlorpromazine, versus lorazepam demonstrated that lorazepam alone, in doses up to 8 mg /12 hours was ineffective in the treatment of confusion. There was a worsening of the confusion and the cognitive impairment, whereas both neuroleptic drugs in low dose (2 mg haloperidol per 24 hours) were highly effective in controlling the symptoms of confusion and improving cognitive function.[10]

Benzodiazepines may however be the drug of first choice in confusion due to alcohol withdrawal or hepatic encephalopathy. They have no anticholinergic or dopamine-blocking actions. They decrease anxiety associated with confusion and, unlike the neuroleptics, they raise seizure threshold.

LORAZEPAM

- Dose range: 0.5–2 mg sublingually, IV, IM or orally 1–4 hourly
- Swallowing lorazepam considerably slows its onset of action
- No active metabolites
    - conjugated in the liver (to inactive glucuronides)
    - excreted chiefly renally
- Limitations:
    - sedation
    - can worsen confusion

Diazepam   Diazepam, along with some of the other older benzodiazepines, eg chlordiazepoxide or flurazepam, has a long half-life and active metabolites. This can easily lead to accumulation and prolonged sedation

Terminal Agitation

A 53 year old lady with a grade IV glioma, after full discussion, decided to stop all medication as she "had had enough". The dexamethasone was reduced quickly from 16 mg daily to 8 mg to zero and she consistently refused any further steroid. 36 hours after reduction of the dexamethasone to zero, she became increasingly agitated and restless. She had no headache, and said she would have sedation only. Midazolam was started and escalated rapidly to over 200 mg/24 h. At this level she was well sedated, but mechanically it required frequent changes of the syringe in the syringe driver to keep up. Subsequently, in situations with comparable agitation we have added haloperidol which has precluded the dose of midazolam going above 120 mg. Methotrimeprazine is preferable if deeper sedation is indicated. The combination of midazolam with an anti-psychotic is valuable where there is any risk of fits.

leading one authority to liken its action to that of a tank: difficult to stop once it gets going![11] Used judiciously its long duration of action can be harnessed to give an anxiolytic effect the morning after a night time dose, but the risk is unwelcome sedation. IM diazepam is slowly absorbed, making this an inappropriate route of administration.

Midazolam

Midazolam is a newer, water soluble benzo-diazepine, that has the shortest half-life of the group, now in common use in palliative care. Its makes an excellent pre-med where sedation and amnesia is desirable for the duration of a short procedure eg in dentistry, casualty or endoscopy. It has been used for the control of delirium for some years in intensive care units where very large doses may be employed eg head injured patients (in one case up to 800 mg/24 hours IV). Since its first description[12] in palliative care, several reviews of midazolam have appeared[13-15] which are summarised below:

MIDAZOLAM USE IN PALLIATIVE CARE

- Sedation and amnesia for short procedures

  1 mg IV (0.5 mg if elderly or frail) and 0.5mg per 30 secs until desired effect

- Muscle stiffness and multifocal myoclonus

  2.5–5mg S/C 4 hourly before turning or 20–40mg S/C per 24 hours by continuous infusion

- Terminal agitation

  5–10mg S/C repeated at 30 minute intervals until noticeable effect. Then 30–60mg S/C per 24 hours by continuous infusion (the maximum dose may need to be as high as 200mg)

Midazolam has no clinically significant metabolites and can be readily titrated. Given SC, it is safe and effective, with no clinically significant hypotension or respiratory depression.

Tolerance to benzodiazepines

Tolerance to benzodiazepines is rare. In one study the median length of time on a midazolam syringe driver was 48 hours at the end of life.[15] However, in younger patients whose dying may occur over 1–2 weeks, increasingly high doses of midazolam may be needed, and may not control agitation. If methotrimeprazine has been tried or excluded, phenobarbitone provides a useful next step.

Phenobarbitone

Phenobarbitone has been used as a third line option, after lack of control with the above drugs (which is a rare event). The injection is oily and may cause skin irritation. A dose of 50–200mg SC followed by a continuous SC infusion of 200–800mg per 24 hours[16]). Phenobarbitone needs to be administered in a separate syringe driver as it does not mix with other drugs. Experience is limited with phenobarbitone in this context, but case reports suggest tachyphylaxis is less often a problem.

TERMINAL CONFUSION

The decision to treat underlying medical causes

There are a number of active measures that may be considered for a patient with confusion, eg IV antibiotics or parenteral rehydration. In deciding whether "resuscitation" of this type is warranted in a patient with an acute deterioration, the important factor to consider is how good the patients health and quality of life was before the deterioration. Is this a readily reversible situation, or is the deterioration signalling that the patient is now dying? The history is all important and the family and the GP may give the most reliable picture, perhaps together with serial indicators of the disease trend over the preceding days or weeks or months. For the independent 70 year old, riding their bicycle up until a week ago, the case for active measures is strong, compared with the bed bound, severely incapacitated 70 year old with a poor quality of life and prognosis. The urge to actively treat, automatically, may need to be weighed carefully, asking "What am I trying to achieve here, as my expected outcome?" Advance directives may give a lead on such questions, but usually, full discussion with the family/carers, plus the clinical team is indicated, to take account of their views and explain the treatment or non-treatment decision, and ensure that everyone understands the management plan.

Where the patient is "actively dying" (death expected in the next 24 – 48 hrs), the process causing the confusion, e.g. organ failure, may be ongoing and irreversible. In this situation, attempting to improve the cognitive function is no longer an appropriate goal and significant sedation may be required.

The question of terminal sedation

Is this really the best approach? Should not death be allowed to take its course "naturally"? It is helpful here to step back from the bedside and take account of the pros and cons of no treatment, close to death where confusion is common.

In some patients, rarely, all medication is refused, to retain control over the mind and body. If this is extended into the last days when consciousness may be diminishing naturally, uncontrolled confusion may occur.

NON – TREATMENT OF TERMINAL CONFUSION

Pros	Cons
• No medical "interference" during death • Death "as nature intended" • No mistaken belief by the relatives (or staff) that medication "hastened their end" or "changed" the patient in some way, so they were different	• Symptoms may be distressing to the patient and there may be loss of dignity • Symptoms may be distressing for the relatives (and for staff or other patients) • Bereavement implications (this is how the family will remember them)

Effect on the family

Terminal agitation can have a powerful effect on the family/carers into their bereavement. The wishes of the patient may need to be balanced with the needs of the family. Therapeutic manoevres in the terminal hours may be largely for the benefit of the family/carers, but are still valid eg drying noisy secretions with hyoscine to prevent "death rattle". Where there is distressing confusion, one of the duties of care should be to minimise its impact.

As mentioned, symptomatic treatment of the confusion is nearly always possible, using the drugs mentioned above.

Is there a role for Propofol?

Propofol has been put forward as an "ideal drug" for treating terminal agitated delirium.[21] It is an IV sedative hypnotic used for induction and maintenance of anaesthesia. Like midazolam it has a rapid onset of readily titratable sedative action which includes amnesia and anxiolysis, but its total body clearance is extremely rapid, and faster recovery than with midazolam is reported.

Also in its favour is its antiemetic action and it is antipuritic in cholestatic liver disease. Warnings are however given about its unpredictability of sedation, even with similar infusion rates. When opioids and propofol are used together, the plasma drug concentration may vary widely. (Concern has also been raised about propofol's impairment of the chemotactic motion of human leukocytes and therefore the risk of infections.) More needs to be known about this interesting drug before it can be recommended.

ETHICAL ISSUES

Sedation of the patient in palliative care can raise clinical and ethical concerns[23]. The divide between the utilitarian view (maximum well being or a minimum of suffering) and the moral view ("What is my obligation here?") need to be reconciled individually. These are rarely absolute standpoints, like black and white, and in reality the clinical situation usually contains many shades of grey.

A question of balance

Doctors who are unwilling to sedate in case they risk hastening death, or because of their moral standpoint, may need to develop more compassion for an agitated patient or anguished family.

Doctors who are "trigger happy" in their prescription of pharmacological sedation may need to develop an appreciation that a level of "upset", or even a perception of suffering, in its broader sense, is not necessarily something to eradicate. The medical-technological mastery of death and dying with sedation may prevent possible working through of painful emotions, or relationships, to resolution, or at least personal completeness. The prospect of death, with its finality, sometimes gives impetus to try to resolve conflicts or relationships, that may literally have been avoided all the patient's life. The kindly doctor who cannot allow any perception of suffering, may preclude, through sedation, this final opportunity for completion of relationships.

CONCLUSION

Making a diagnosis of the cause, or formulation of the most likely cause, is the key to management of confusion. Such a patient can present one of the more difficult clinical challenges and requires a careful approach, summarized below:

SUMMARY OF MANAGEMENT

- Accurate and focused history from the patient and carers
- Careful examination and some investigations
- Review current medication:
    - when each drug was started (and why)
    - whether the dosage has been altered (and why)
    - what medication has been stopped (and why)
- Consideration of alternative causes
- Assess whether emergency treatment is required, now
- Clear communication with
    - the patient
    - the family/carers
    - the multidisciplinary clinical team
- Frequent review of the response to any intervention

(With thanks to Dr Jenny Barraclough, and Dr Averil Stedeford, for their helpful comments and ideas).

References

1. American Pscyhiatric Association, Washington D.C., 1994. Diagnostic and Statistical Manual of Mental Disorders (4th ed.)
2. Stiefel F, Fainsinger R, Bruera E. Acuture Confusional States in Patients with Advanced Cancer. Journal of Pain Symptom Management 1992; 7: 94–98
3. Fainsinger R, MacEachern T, Hanson J, et al. Symptom Control during the last week of life as a Palliative Care Unit. Journal Pall. Care 1991; 7: 5–11
4. Fernandez F, Levy J K, Mansell P W. Management of delirium in terminally ill AIDS patients. Int. Journal Psychiatric Med. 1989; 19 (2): 162–172
5. Massie M J, Holland JC, Glass E. Delirium in terminally ill cancer patients. 1983. Am J Psychiatry 140: 1048–1050
6. Barbato M, Rodriguez P J. Thiamine deficiency in patients admitted to a palliative care unit. Pall. Med. 1994; 4: 320–324
7. Fainsinger R L, MacEachern T, Miller M J et al. The use of hypodermoclysis for rehydration in terminally ill cancer patients. Journal Pain Symptom Management 1994; 9: 298–302
8. De Stouz N B, Bruera E, Suarez-Almazor M. Opiod rotation for toxicity reduction in terminal cancer patients. Journal Pain Symptom Management 1995; 10: 378–384
9. Sykes N P, Oliver D J. Subcutaneous methotrimeprazine use in a hospice. Lancet 1987; 1: 393
10. Breitbart W, Passik S D. Psychiatric aspects of palliative care. In: Doyle D, Hanks G W, MacDonald N (eds). Oxford Textbook of Palliative Medicine, Oxford: Oxford University Press, 1993: 609 – 623

11. Regnard CFB. Personal communication
12. De Souza E, Jepson BA. Midazolam in terminal care (letter). Lancet 1988; 1: 67–68
13. Bottomley D M, Hanks G W. Subcutaneous midazolam infusion in palliative care. Journal Pain Symptom Management 1990; 50: 259–261
14. Amesbury BDW, Dunphy KP. The use of subcutaneous midazolam in the home care setting. Pal. Med. 1989; 3: 299–301
15. McNamara P, Minton M, Twycross RG. Use of midazolam in palliative care. Pall. Med. 1991; 5: 249–255
16. Proceedings of the Advanced Course in Pain and Symptom Management June 1993 Oxford
17 Stedeford A. Facing death. 2nd edition
18. Stedeford A, Regnard C. Confusional states, in Flow Diagrams in Advanced Cancer and other diseases. Ed. Regnard CFB. Churchill Livingston 1995
19. Proceedings of Advanced Course in pain and symptom management June 1995. Twycross R G Oxford and personal communication
20. Twycross R. Methotrimeprazine. Capter 21. Psychotropic drugs In Pain Relief in Advance Cancer 1994. Churchill Livingstone
21. Mercadente S, De Conno F, Ripamonti C. Propofol in Terminal Care.Journal of Pain Symp. Management 1995; 10: 639–642
22. Wilcock A, Twycross R G. Case report: confusion responding to dexamethasone in a patient with cancer of the prostate. Pall. Med. 1995; 9: 337–338
23. Fondras J C. Sedation and ethical contradiction. European Journal Pall. Care. 1996; 3: 17–20

Chapter 16

Nursing Care

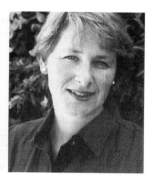

Raewyn Jenkins
Raewyn Jenkins is a Ward Manager at St Christopher's Hospice in London. She trained as a nurse in New Zealand and has worked for the past thirteen years in oncology, haematology and palliative care units in New Zealand and the United Kingdom. She took her Master's degree in Advanced Clinical Practice (Cancer Nursing) at the University of Surrey. She is particularly interested in the management of oral problems and the support needs of palliative care nurses.

This chapter is in two main parts. The first part describes organisational aspects of nursing for effective symptom control. The second discusses the management of a number of symptoms that are particularly challenging to the nurse. The main headings are:

1. Organizational aspects:
   - A Multi-disciplinary team approach
   - Team Nursing
   - Staff Support

2. Some challenging symptoms
   - Weakness and fatigue
   - Pressure areas and sores
   - Fungating wounds
   - Lymphoedema
   - Mouth problems.

Part 1: Organizational aspects

A MULTIDISCIPLINARY TEAM APPROACH

The concept of 'total pain' includes physical, emotional, social and spiritual components and this approach remains the corner-stone of symptom control in palliative care. Effective symptom control is unlikely unless the importance of each of the above dimensions is acknowledged. Clearly no one discipline possesses all the skills necessary to address the complexity of total pain; a multidisciplinary team approach is, therefore, essential. The purpose of the team is to function as a cohesive unit using the skills and resources of each discipline to develop and implement a joint plan of care.

An effective team is one that is skilled in communication. A weekly multidisciplinary case conference provides the most economical opportunity for the entire team to meet to review and plan care. However, situations change quickly and effective day-to-day handovers are also essential. Providing time for communicating from one shift to the next should be seen as a priority.

The use of a 'multidisciplinary liaison sheet' in the case notes can facilitate communication and collaboration between disciplines on a day to day basis. Each member of the team uses the liaison sheet to concisely document their involvement with the patient, family and other team members.

The Nurse as key-worker: Nurses are the best-placed members of the multidisciplinary team to establish supportive relationships with patients and families, collect baseline information, identify symptoms and initiate and monitor interventions.

The dying patient faced with loss of independence, increasing weakness, distressing physical symptoms and emotional pain is, clearly, in a fragile and vulnerable position. As such there may be times when he or his family are unable to represent their own needs and wishes, and require others to represent them.

The nurse who has developed a close relationship with a patient and family is often ideally placed to act as advocate for them, representing their concerns to the multidisciplinary team. While the key-worker may vary according to the needs of each situation it is often the nurse who coordinates the activities of the multidisciplinary team.

TEAM NURSING

In recent years there has been vigorous debate about the 'best' way to organise nursing care. The methods known as *primary nursing* and *team nursing* have received the most attention. However, there are many variations on these themes. Rather than promote 'the only' way of delivering nursing care it is for each nursing team to select the method that best meets the needs of the patients in their care. Good symptom control is enhanced by methods of nursing care that foster:

- Monitoring of symptoms;
- Effective channels of communication with the patient, family and multidisciplinary team
- Time to listen to the patients

Team nursing is one approach that meets the above criteria and complements the palliative care philosophy by its emphasis on team work and staff support while still allowing close nurse-patient relationships to develop.

There is more than one way of practising team nursing and what follows is just one example based on experience in a hospice setting.

TEAM NURSING

Small teams of nurses (6–7) are led by a team leader, who is experienced in palliative care. Teams are responsible for the nursing care of a small (4–6) group of patients and their families throughout their admission and, ideally, throughout any subsequent admission. The duty rota ensures even distribution of team nurses across shifts. In this way team nursing promotes continuity of care. The close nurse-patient relationships that develop allow for the provision of emotional care and support. Team nurses are responsible for presenting their patients at the weekly multidisciplinary case conference and reporting back changes in the patient's condition, meeting with families, planning discharges and liaising with other disciplines on a daily basis.

The team nurses also meet with families the day after the death of a patient to look back over the death and answer questions, to facilitate grieving, assess for risk in bereavement and to 'end' their relationship with the family. The results of a recent evaluation[1] within the hospice setting indicate that the continuity of care provided within team nursing facilitates good communication and promotes the development of close relationships with patients and families. Nurses also reported high levels of support from team colleagues, suggesting small teams foster a supportive work environment.

STAFF SUPPORT

Supporting patients and families through the 'total pain' of terminal illness presupposes a degree of emotional involvement which is inevitably demanding and draining for the professionals involved. The ability of caregivers to continue with this level of involvement depends on the development of solid support systems.

It is important to set aside time for team building. The working ward round should be supplemented by a weekly team meeting at which contentious issues can be debated, stresses shared and support given. It may be helpful at these meetings to remember those who have died in the past week, acknowledging that the death of certain patients will have particular significance for some team members who may have been more involved than others.

A recent study[2] with a small group of hospice nurses identified the use of a number of strategies that enabled them to cope with the constant death of their patients. These strategies included:

Terminating the relationship with the patient and family by, for example, being present at the time of death, spoken or silent 'goodbyes', laying out the body and spending time sharing the loss with the family following death. Strategies to end relationships enabled nurses to move on and reinvest in new relationships with other dying patients and their families.

Informal support from colleagues. The opportunity to talk, be listened to and be reassured informally by colleagues emerged as a major source of support. The hospice nurses in the study effectively supported each other from day to day and did not require formal, structured support systems. The importance of informal support needs to be acknowledged by managers who can do much to facilitate these supportive interactions by ensuring that sufficient time is made available. In addition to support from colleagues, the nurses used spouses, families and friends to talk through their feelings of loss.

Lifestyle management. Nurses in the study identified a number of activities outside their work environment that effectively helped them to cope with the constant losses they encountered at work. One of the most important aspects of lifestyle management seems to be the ability to separate home from work. A number of the nurses described 'unwinding rituals' they used to 'switch off' from work. Other methods of lifestyle management included: aerobics, gardening, music, dancing, swimming, reading, decorating, meditation, cooking and regular holidays. The nurses operated a 'pay back' system of stress management. They recognised that their work depleted their emotional energy so they developed ways of 'replenishing' themselves.

Part 2: Some Challenging Symptoms

WEAKNESS AND FATIGUE

The terms 'weakness' and 'fatigue' (along with others such as tiredness, lethargy and exhaustion) tend to be used synonymously by patients and carers to describe a general lack of energy. Like pain, weakness and fatigue are subjective phenomena and are difficult to define. Attempts to measure weakness and fatigue have tended to involve single items in symptom distress scales. Disease specific, multi-dimensional instruments with established reliability and validity are yet to be developed. Despite being recognised as the most frequently reported symptoms in patients with advanced cancer, mechanisms remain poorly understood. The potential causes, some of which may be reversible, are many and varied.

Causes of weakness and fatigue

- Drugs (opioids, benzodiazepines, tricyclic anti-depressants)
- Metabolic disturbances (hypercalcaemia)
- Electrolyte disturbances (hypokalaemia)
- Tumour load
- Anaemia
- Poor nutritional status
- Motor weakness
- Infection
- Lack of sleep
- Depression and anxiety

Management

Detailed patient assessment is necessary to establish the exact nature and impact of the weakness and/or fatigue for the individual patient. Encouraging patients, to use their own words to describe the problem is an important aspect of assessment because of the tendency to confuse the terms and use them interchangeably. Many of the commonly recommended interventions remain anecdotal and unevaluated by research. Studies have typically focused on patients receiving anti-cancer therapies and not on those with advanced cancer requiring palliative care. In the absence of research-based evidence, however, a combination of strategies tailored to the needs of the individual patient are most likely to be effective[4]. The strategies, which aim to help the patient cope both physically and emotionally, might include:

- Planned activity
- Energy conservation
- Emotional support
- Nutritional support

Planned activity

Exercise and activity should be encouraged within individual limitations. Even in far advanced cancer, patients benefit from physiotherapy and it is often possible to improve mobility and restore independence for a time. Goals, however, need to be realistic and patients and families may need guidance to adjust their expectations.

Energy conservation

Important activities should be scheduled during periods of least fatigue and non-essential activities eliminated. Periods of activity need to be interspersed with planned rest periods.

Emotional support

Adjusting psychologically to increasing physical weakness and dependence on others takes time. Constant anxiety about what lies ahead is immensely tiring and fatigue may be compounded by loss of sleep. Lack of, or misunderstood, information also generates stress and anxiety and careful regular explanations of what is happening can be enormously helpful in reducing anxiety and fatigue. Patients need opportunities and time to share their feelings of loss, anxiety and fear and feel that they are being listened to, understood and supported.

Nutritional support

Again there is little research-based information available on the nutritional needs of those with advanced cancer and it is clear that aggressive nutritional support is inappropriate, however, maintenance of adequate hydration and nutrition, including the use of oral supplements, for as long as possible may help alleviate weakness and fatigue. Appetite, energy levels and general well-being can be temporarily improved for some patients by using low-dose dexamethasone[3].

PRESSURE SORES

Pressure sores in the terminally ill patient may be an inevitable and distressing indication of advancing disease and physical deterioration. Causative factors include:

- Reduced mobility
- Weight loss
- Incontinence
- Sensory loss
- Poor nutritional status
- Anaemia
- Steroid therapy
- Cytotoxic therapy

Identification of Risk Factors

The Waterlow policy for assessing pressure sores[5] provides a numerical score of the risk of developing pressure sores. Of the currently available instruments it is thought to be the most sensitive for use in palliative care settings as it includes weighting for factors such as nutritional status, terminal cachexia, anaemia and steroid therapy.[6] The use of this assessment tool at regular intervals provides a systematic framework for preventative measures. The Waterlow policy is available in laminated pocket card form, easily incorporated into patient documentation (which are available from – see page 27) Newtons, Curland, Taunton, Somerset TA3 5SG.

Reduction of pressure

Once risk factors have been identified the most effective method of avoiding the development of sores is to relieve or reduce pressure. There is currently a plethora of pressure relieving equipment available, often with inadequate data to support its use. Potential buyers need to take the time to gather all the available information and use equipment on trial prior to purchase. Several palliative care units have established multidisciplinary working groups whose aim is to improve pressure area care by facilitating the sharing of information relating to current practice, recent research and product evaluation.

The most effective pressure-relieving systems utilise air to either redistribute pressure evenly or to vary the area under pressure. Pressure-relieving systems are available for each of the Waterlow risk categories. Lockyer-Stevens[7] and Willis[8] provide extensive and detailed reviews of currently available pressure relieving mattresses and seating products.

PRESSURE RELIEVING SYSTEMS

Waterlow Score	Mattress	Cushion
10–14 (At risk)	Foam mattress (eg Propad)	Foam cushion (eg Propad)
15–19 (High risk)	Alternating pressure overlay (eg AlphaXcell) Alternating pressure mattress	Foam and fluid cushion (eg Multitec)
20+ (Very High Risk)	Dynamic low air loss system (eg Pegasus) or Dynamic air flotation system (eg Nimbus II) (These are more sophisticated alternating pressure mattresses.)	Fluid filled cushion (eg Supatec) (eg Roho Quadro)

The most sophisticated pressure relieving system will only be effective if used in combination with good nursing care. The patient, family and nursing team, together, need to plan a realistic regime to meet the needs of the individual. Frequent changes of position, when lying and sitting (using lifting techniques that reduce shearing and friction) remain an essential component of effective nursing care. An alternative technique is the 30 tilt method, which involves less disturbance to the patient than traditional two hourly turning. The development of pressure sores may be related to poor nutritional status which, if appropriate, may be improved. Control of symptoms such as pain and dyspnoea helps maintain active mobility and may thereby prevent the development of pressure sores.

Preventing Pressure Sores

- Identify risk factors
- Reduce pressure on bony prominences
- Maintain skin integrity
- Maintain mobility whenever possible
- Relieve pain

Treatment of Pressure Sores

Despite the use of preventative measures some terminally ill patients do still develop pressure sores. The aims of care can be summarised as:

Aims of pressure sore care

● Maintain quality of life
● Promote potential healing
● Prevent further damage
● Relieve pain and discomfort
● Prevent infection
● Control odour and exudate
● Minimise bleeding

Management of pressure sores should be based on moist wound healing principles. Gilchrist and Corner[6] provide a detailed discussion of the management of pressure sores in terminally ill patients.

CHOICE OF DRESSING ACCORDING TO STAGE OF SORE

Stage	Dressing
1. Blanching hyperaemia (no broken skin)	* Vapour permeable adhesive film dressing * Replace every 5–7 days or as required
2. Non-blanching hyperaemia (superficial clean wound)	* *Hydrocolloid dressing* * Replace every 5–7 days or as required
3. Ulceration progress (subcutaneous tissue involved)	* Light to moderate exudate-as for stage 2 * Heavily exudating – *alginate-dressing* * Replace every 5–7 days or as required
4. Ulceration extends (subcutaneous fat involved)	* Pack with hydrocolloid paste and cover with hydrocolloid dressing or * Debride with hydrogel and cover with hydrocolloid dressing * Replace dressing as required
5. Infective necrosis (destruction of muscle occurs)	* Consider mechanical debridement or * Pack with alginate ribbon and cover with film dressing

Pressure sores can heal

Arthur was a 61 year old man with Motor Neurone Disease diagnosed five years earlier. He was admitted to the hospice for continuing care when his wife was no longer able to manage his care at home. On admission Arthur was virtually tetraplegic and chairbound. His major source of discomfort was sacral pain. On assessment he had a 5 x 5 cm reddened area with a black necrotic centre 1 cm in diameter. His initial Waterlow score was 19 (indicating a high risk). Arthur was nursed on an AlphaXcell mattress and a Roho cushion when in his chair. It was not possible to turn him so the 30 tilt was used during the night to relieve pressure. The pressure sore was dressed with Granuflex which was renewed weekly. By week 3 the necrotic area had been debrided leaving a yellow sloughy wound which was dressed with Kaltostat secured with film dressing. By week 4 the wound was clean but not healed so the dressing was changed to Thin Granuflex. By week 6 the sore was healed and Arthur's Waterlow score was 17. His sacrum subsequently remained intact until he died some five months later. The terminally ill are a special group of patients in that the deterioration of skin integrity and the subsequent development of pressure sores may be unavoidable. A systematic approach, such as that advocated by Waterlow, to the prevention and treatment of pressure sores is essential. Ensuring that the terminally ill patient remains comfortable is the primary aim of nursing care. A wide range of pressure relieving equipment is now available and its use in conjunction with moist wound treatment techniques mean that distressing symptoms can be controlled and quality of life maintained. This case study illustrates the potential for healing even when maintenance of mobility is impossible.

FUNGATING WOUNDS

A fungating lesion is a highly visible and emotionally distressing symbol of advancing disease and one that requires both skilled physical management and sensitive psychological care. To date little research has been undertaken on the management of fungating wounds and clinical practice largely relies on experience rather than on research based knowledge. The successful management of a patient with a fungating malignant wound provides a complex challenge for the multi-disciplinary team.

Assessment

Individualised patient assessment is essential before a wound management plan can be developed. Moody and Grocott[10] have developed a detailed framework for the assessment and management of fungating wounds which is also presented as an easy reference wall chart.

ASSESSMENT OF FUNGATING MALIGNANT WOUNDS

Patient Assessment	Wound Assessment
● Wound history	● Wound site and size
	● Pain
● Previous treatment	● Amount and nature of exudate
	● Presence of slough/necrotic tissue
● General health status	● Presence of infection
	● Odour
● Nutritional status	● Bleeding
	● Condition of surrounding skin
● Patient/carer's knowledge and acceptance of diagnosis and prognosis	
● Patient/carer's perception of impact of wound on daily life	
● Patient/carer's aims and expectations	
● Professional/lay support being provided	

Management

A fungating wound in a patient with advanced cancer is unlikely to heal. The prime aims of palliative management of a fungating lesion are symptom control at the site of the wound and improved of quality of life. It is essential that the patient and carer(s) be involved in developing the plan of care so that it clearly reflects their aims and priorities. The aims of care can be summarized as:

Aims when managing fungating malignant wounds

- Pain control
- Control of exudate
- Control of odour
- Control of bleeding
- Prevention of infection
- Fewest possible dressing changes
- Trauma-free dressing removal
- Cosmetic acceptability
- Improved quality of life

Modern dressings

Moist wound healing principles remain relevant to the palliative management of fungating lesions, even though healing is unlikely. Modern dressings have led to improved wound management as they do not adhere to the wound (thus allowing trauma-free removal). They also prevent infection, debride necrotic tissue and slough and are designed to be left in place for up to 7 days. However they are often only partially successful, particularly where there is profuse exudate and smell. Alternative dressings need to be developed in order to address these problems.[16]

SYMPTOM CONTROL AT THE WOUND SITE[9]

Symptom	Management
Pain	Regular analgesia may be inadequate during dressing changes Consider: • Short-acting analgesic (eg dextromoramide) • Topical anaesthetic agent (eg lignocaine) • Entonox
Exudate	High absorbency calcium alginate dressing covered with occlusive dressing
Slough	Debride with hydrocolloid paste and dressing or hydrogel
Bleeding	Calcium alginate dressing (haemostatic properties) Topical adrenaline 1 in 1000 solution
Odour/Infection	Topical metronidazole 1% gel or irrigate with IV metronidazole solution. Consider systemic antibiotics Mask odour with charcoal impregnated alginate or foam dressing

The skills of wound dressing

Susan was a 51 year old woman with a carcinoma of the left breast with extensive fungating local recurrence. She had been diagnosed six years previously and disease had progressed through chemotherapy, radiotherapy and hormone therapy. She was admitted to the hospice for pain control and assessment of the wound and associated lymphoedema. Susan was unmarried and had been living with her divorced sister and her three children since she became less well. An ulcerated chest wound of approximately 8 x 15 cm extended up towards the axilla. Susan was most distressed by pain during dressing changes, odour and excessive exudate soiling clothing. Her aims, in her own words, were: " not to be in pain, not to smell and to have the dressing done as early in the morning as possible". In addition to these aims the nurses hoped to reduce dressing changes to alternate days. Susan's regular analgesics and co-analgesics included: 1200 mg MST 12 hourly, Flurbiprofen SR 200 mg daily, Amitriptylline 100 mg at night. Dextromoramide 20 mg was given thirty minutes prior to dressing changes and a course of oral antibiotics given to combat infection and malodour. The new dressing regime consisted of: irrigation with 20 mls 1% lignocaine followed five minutes later by irrigation with intravenous metronidazole solution, Intrasite gel to sloughy areas, three to four sheets of Kaltostat forte secured with a large Granuflex dressing. Susan felt that pain control during dressing changes improved considerably. Odour was better controlled and not usually detectable except during dressing changes. It was usually possible to renew dressings on alternate days as the new regime was more effective in controlling exudate. This meant Susan was able to go home on weekend leave.

LYMPHOEDEMA

Lymphoedema involves swelling of a limb due to blocked or damaged lymphatics. In advancing cancer it is usually irreversible. Treatment is, therefore, ongoing and aims to:

- Reduce swelling and discomfort
- Improve movement in affected limb
- Prevent skin damage

Treatment has become specialised and complex and is usually undertaken by a skilled nurse or physiotherapist. It involves[11]:

- Compression
- Massage
- Skin care
- Exercise

Compression therapy

Compression therapy involves the application of pressure to the affected limb, thereby increasing the drainage of fluid and preventing new lymph formation. The effectiveness of compression therapy is monitored by regular limb measurements. Compression is provided by either:

- Containment hosiery for mild to moderate lymphoedema. Sleeves and stockings must be fitted correctly and smoothly applied. The garment size should be regularly reviewed. They should be worn all day but can be removed at night.
- Multilayer compression bandaging for severe lymphoedema or when the limb size and shape will not accommodate a compression garment. Bandaging involves 'wrapping' the limb in low stretch bandages (e.g Secure forte by Johnson and Johnson). Pressure should be graduated with more applied distally to encourage movement of fluid centrally. The skin of the swollen limb is usually protected with undercast padding beneath the compression bandages to even out the contours. Bandages are worn 24 hours a day and are renewed daily. Treatment usually lasts about two weeks. Kaye[12] provides a more detailed description of the bandaging technique.

- Intermittent External Pneumatic Compression Therapy (IEPCT) consists of a sleeve connected to a pump which inflates and deflates cyclically. The pumps are used in combination with compression hosiery for three to four hours a day for two weeks.

Massage
Relieves tightness by stimulating lymphatic drainage. The key principle behind massage is to 'clear the way ahead'[11] by beginning to massage in a non-oedematous quadrant of the trunk adjacent to the oedema. Fluid is then massaged away from the affected area using slow gentle strokes. Each massage session should last about fifteen minutes and should be done once or twice daily. A booklet that both patients and their carers may find helpful is 'Lymphoedema: advice on treatment'.[13] It gives step by step instruction in both arm and leg massage techniques.

Skin care
Oedematous skin is particularly vulnerable to dryness, splitting, blistering and subsequent infection. Careful skin hygiene and a daily application of unperfumed moisturising cream are essential preventative measures. Breaks in the skin should be dressed aseptically. The patient should be taught to recognise the early signs of infection and encouraged to seek treatment promptly.

Exercise
Exercise and movement prevent joint stiffness and help lymph drainage. Patients should, therefore, be encouraged to use their oedematous limb as normally as possible. The limb should be elevated and supported when the patient is resting. Again 'Lymphoedema: advice on treatment'[13] has a helpful diagrammatic section on arm and leg exercises.

MOUTH PROBLEMS

Mouth problems, despite being frequently identified as distressing symptoms by the terminally ill, have remained 'low profile' symptoms and much research is still required to identify appropriate and effective interventions for palliative care settings.

Assessment

Mouth care has long been considered the responsibility of nurses who usually select the tools and agents to use and the frequency with which mouth care is required. If mouth care is to be effective such decisions should be based on accurate oral assessment. A number of oral assessment guides have been developed. the most reliable and valid tool for use with cancer patients has been found to be that of Eilers, Bergen and Petersen.[14,15] This guide assesses oral status in 8 categories. Each category is allocated a score of 1–3 depending on the presence or absence of described symptoms. Total score is 8–24, 24 indicating severe oral problems.

ASSESSMENT OF MOUTH PROBLEMS	
	Score
● Voice	1–3
● Swallow	1–3
● Lips	1–3
● Tongue	1–3
● Saliva	1–3
● Mucous membranes	1–3
● Gums	1–3
● Teeth or dentures	1–3

Frequency of oral care

Frequency of oral care must be determined individually. 4 hourly mouth care has been shown to be effective in preventing infection but is not frequent enough to ensure the comfort of patients with reduced oral intake, or the unconscious, who may require 1–2 hourly mouth care.

The 5 main mouth problems experienced, often sequentially, by terminally ill patients are likely to be:

● Dry mouth
● Dirty Mouth
● Infection
● Pain
● Halitosis

Dry Mouth   A dry mouth is a common complaint in advanced cancer and may be related to dehydration, infection or drugs. Many of the drugs used in palliative care can cause a dry mouth, the drying effect is potentiated when two or more drugs with anticholinergic side-effects are taken concurrently. Reviewing medications can often alleviate some of the discomfort associated with a very dry mouth. It may be possible to reduce the dose of a drug or substitute a drug less likely to cause a dry mouth. For example, cyclizine to haloperidol.

DRUGS WITH ANTICHOLINERGIC SIDE EFFECTS

- Phenothiazines
- Tricyclic antidepressants
- Opioids
- Antiemetics
- Anticholinergics
- Diuretics

Interventions, which aim to either stimulate saliva production or replace saliva, include:

Stimulation of saliva
- Frequent sips of water, fruit juice or fizzy drink
- Mouth care before and after meals
- Sucking boiled sweets
- Sucking ice cubes (try fruit juices or gin & tonic)
- Sucking fresh pineapple chunks
- Artificial saliva
- Chewing gum
- Apply petroleum jelly to lips

Products containing glycerin, which has traditionally been used to lubricate the mouth, should be avoided as it may dehydrate oral tissue. Lemon, often used in combination with glycerin, may cause pain and exhaustion of the salivary glands.

Dirty Mouth   There is widespread agreement that oral debris is best removed using a small soft toothbrush and toothpaste. Rinsing the mouth with tap water following brushing aids the removal of debris and is refreshing without the drying effects associated with many commercial mouth washes, most of which are alcohol-based. A heavily coated tongue may, however, require one of the following interventions:

- Sodium bicarbonate solution (1 teaspoon to 1500mls warm water)
- Hydrogen peroxide solution (15mls to 200mls warm water – mix immediately prior to use)
- Effervescent vitamin C dissolved on the tongue (1/2 tablet)
- Sucking fresh pineapple chunks

Infection   Many terminally ill patients are immunosuppressed and are, therefore, susceptible to oral fungal infections. Oral thrush is usually treated with either a topical antifungal (nystatin) or a systemic anti-fungal (ketaconazole). If a topical agent is used the patient must be taught a 'rinse and swallow' technique and dentures must also be treated.

Pain   Oral pain is usually related to infection, stomatitis following radiotherapy or chemotherapy, or local tumour effects. Topical analgesics, available as both gels and mouthwashes, alongside regular systemic analgesia may provide additional pain relief.

Halitosis   Halitosis may be due to a dirty mouth, neglected oral hygiene following vomiting or upper respiratory or gastrointestinal tract infection. Whatever the cause, frequent careful mouth care is the key intervention.

Further Reading:

Regnard, C. Fitton, S. Mouth Care, In:Regnard, C. Hockley, J. eds. Flow Diagrams in Cancer and Other Diseases, London, Edward Arnold, 1995, 22–24.

The Macmillan Practice Development Unit, The Research Review Series, Managing oral care problems throughout the cancer illness trajectory. (Available from the Macmillan Practice Development Unit, Royal Marsden Hospital.)

References

1. Hatcliffe, S., Dawes, R. Implementing a vision for the future targets in a hospice. Nursing Standard, 1996, 10, 28, 44–46.

2. Jenkins, R. Grief in hospice nurses: an exploratory descriptive study (MSc thesis: University of Surrey). 1994.
3. Regnard, C. Mannix, K. Weakness and Fatigue. In Regnard, C. Hockley, J. eds. Flow Diagrams in Cancer and Other Diseases, London, Edward Arnold, 1995, 64–67.
4. Richardson, A. Fatigue in cancer patients: a review of the literature. European journal of Cancer Care, 1995, 4, 20–32.
5. Waterlow, J. Pressure Sore Prevention manual. Taunton, 1994. Copies of this manual and the Waterlow cards are obtainable from: Newtons, Curland, Taunton TA3 5SG, Somerset
6. Gilcrest, B. Corner, J. Pressure sores: prevention and management – a nursing perspective, Palliative Medicine, 1989, 3, 257–261.
7. Lockyer-Stevens, N. A developing information base for purchasing decisions: a review of pressure-relieving beds for at-risk patients, Professional Nurse, 1994, 9, 534–42.
8. Willis, J. Pressure-relief seating, Professional Nurse, 1995, 10, 713–721.
9. Saunders, J. Regnard, C. malignant Ulcers, In: Regnard, C. Hockley, J. eds. Flow Diagrams in Cancer and Other Diseases, London, Edward Arnold, 1995, 57–59.
10. Moody, M. Grocott, P. Let us extend our knowledge base: assessment and management of malignant fungating wounds, Professional Nurse, 1993, 8, 586–590.
11. Badger, C. Regnard, C. Oedema, In: Regnard, C. Hockley, J. eds. Flow Diagrams in Cancer and Other Diseases, London, Edward Arnold, 1995, 60–63.
12. Kaye, P. A to Z of Hospice and Palliative Medicine, Northampton, EPL Publications, 1994, 140.
13. Regnard, C. Badger, C. Mortimer, P. Lymphoedema: advice on treatment, Beaconsfield, Beaconsfield Publishers Ltd, 1991.
14. Eilers, J. Berger, A. Petersen, M. Development, Testing and Application of the Oral Assessment Guide, Oncology Nursing Forum, 1985, 15, 325–330.
15. Holmes, S., Mountain, E. Assessment of Oral Status: Evaluation of Three Oral Assessment Guides. Journal of Clinical Nursing, 1993, 2, 35–40.
16. Grocott, P. The Palliative Management of Fungating Malignant Wounds, Journal of Wound Care, 1995, 15, 240–242.

Chapter 17

The Terminal Phase

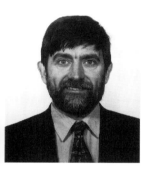

Dr Gerald Corcoran
Gerald Corcoran qualified from the London Medical College 1976. He is currently Macmillan Consultant in Palliative Medicine at Aintree Hospitals NHS Trust, Liverpool, and Medical Director, Woodlands Day Hospice. He has special interest in the organisation of palliative care services, nutrition and medical ethics.

WHAT IS THE TERMINAL PHASE?

The terminal phase of a person's illness refers to the stage where death is imminent, in a matter of hours or days. A person may have been considered to have a terminal illness for a year, but the advent of the terminal phase can still be an unpredicted event for both professionals and carers.

Care delivered during the terminal phase remains important for the dying person, but also the carers and relatives.[1] It is their view of the manner of dying which can have major effects on their subsequent bereavement. For the health professional, involvement in the terminal phase of a person's life can sometimes be intimidating and challenging. However, given the correct training and support within a team framework, care for the dying person and carers can be a very rewarding experience.

"Medicalisation of dying"   The term "medicalisation of dying" is often used in a derogatory sense to imply that even within palliative care the prime focus of care has become pharmacological symptom control e.g. using a cocktail of drugs delivered by a syringe driver. In contrast, many ill people and their carers have

personal memories of others who have died badly in terms of poor symptom control and in pain. Thus no apology should be made for being familiar with a small group of drugs, that can be used alone or in combination to gain symptom control for those that require such drugs. Health professionals should be confident to use such medication appropriately, to respond to the dynamic situation as a person dies.

It is clear, however, that symptom control alone is only part of the care necessary for dying people and their carers. Anticipation, co-ordination of services, explanation, comfort and support for patient and family are all important aspects of care in the terminal phase.[2]

THE TERMINAL PHASE IN DIFFERENT SETTINGS

Most people spend most of the last year of life at home, but many die in a hospital, hospice or nursing home. In many studies, bereaved carers have expressed disappointment that their relative did not stay at home to die. The reasons for this perceived failure of care are many, some being outside the remit of Health Care Services. Demographic changes mean people are now living alone or in pensioner-only households, and families are scattered. Employment difficulties restrict the availability of family members to supervise care over 24 hours. Also there is now a greater emphasis on professional support to care for a dying person at home. The greater emphasis on professional care, has developed at a time when continuity of care in the community is proving difficult to maintain.

Hospital Care

Hospital wards have changed in character over recent years. Lengths of stay on the wards are much reduced with a high turnover of patients. Organisation pressures from increasing numbers of emergency admissions are placing great demands on professional staff. Nevertheless, the acute hospital ward setting remains an important setting for dying people in the foreseeable future.

Facilities for families to stay with dying relatives remain inadequate in most general hospitals.

Distressed carers can be frequently seen fluxing between the day room and the patient's bed across busy corridors.

Most families require support and some degree of supervision during this difficult time. Even if carers are keen to do a lot of the caring or even nursing duties, it is very important that nursing staff frequently enquire about their concerns. Families need to have the reassurance that advice is on hand promptly if there is any change in the condition of the dying person.

For many carers, being present at the time of death is very important to them. Thus they become frightened to leave the ward and will often seek reassurance from staff to see that it is "safe" for them to have a rest period. With good communication between staff members and with regular assessment of the dying person it is usually possible to give proper guidance to carers.

Availability of analgesics is not usually a problem in the hospital setting, but other drugs commonly used for the dying person, such as hyoscine, methotrimeprazine and midazolam should also be available as stock on most wards. For the restless or agitated patient it is unacceptable to incur delays in treatment while ordering drugs from Pharmacy.

Information-giving to relatives following assessment by medical staff remains an important aspect of care.

Nursing home care

Many people are now dying in *nursing homes*. There is increasing pressure for medium term care (2 weeks to 4 months) for many frail people. Complex funding arrangements and assessment are making transfer from hospital to nursing home and indeed home to nursing home very difficult to arrange at times. Attention should be made to the skill-mix of staff within nursing homes and educational programmes should be in place, so that staff are familiar with the principles of symptom control. Specialist palliative care staff should also be available to give appropriate advice to nursing home staff.

The phase of illness should be regularly assessed so that adequate care plans can be made. Families,

General Practitioners and nursing staff, should all have sufficient information to judge the most appropriate course of action in the event of any deterioration. Unnecessary transfer to hospital can be avoided by adequate consideration of the likely outcomes of treatment.

Hospice Care

The hospice setting accounts for approximately 18% of all cancer deaths.[4] Hospices have the advantage of skilled professional staff and usually very good facilities for both patients and their families. However, hospices and specialist palliative care inpatient units are likely to experience greater pressures, as they become more integrated into the health service within any district. It is difficult to accept patients into a hospice on an urgent basis, who are not known to the hospice staff if there is a lack of information about the patient's condition. For those patients well-known to the palliative care services, (eg attending day hospice or previously an inpatient) it is very reasonable to expect, the hospice or specialist inpatient to have a flexible admission policy to accept such patients back for terminal care if the need arises.

Home Care

Home care can frequently continue until a late stage if there is an assurance that it would be possible to admit the dying person promptly if the need arises. However, such arrangements depend on the availability of a bed, and also on the staffing arrangements and availability of medical advice out of hours and at short-notice.

Requirements for Home Care

Thorpe has outlined the necessary requirements to enable more people to die at home[3]:

- a 24 hour District Nursing Service
- adequate sitting service
- confident GP's
- availability of drugs
- availability of aids and adaptations
- access to specialist advice
- ongoing education for professional staff

RECOGNISING THE TERMINAL PHASE

Many people with a terminal illness have a substantial time within the palliative phase of illness where palliative interventions can improve their symptoms and quality of life. Surgery, chemotherapy and radiotherapy can have significant roles for palliation.[5]

Acute deterioration

An acute condition in someone with far advanced disease requires assessment and diagnosis to determine the appropriate course of action. It is important for all involved professionals to have been up-dated with the patient's progress as promptly as possible. Conditions such as septicaemia or metabolic disturbance (including uraemia or dehydration) are potentially reversible situations which may be a complication of a recent treatment. Prompt treatment in such circumstances may enable the person to recover for another beneficial period of life. It may be important to transfer such a person to hospital for intervention. However, if the person has been steadily deteriorating over a clear period of time, it may be inappropriate to attempt to reverse these new conditions. The emphasis of treatment becomes symptom control and terminal care. The need for transfer of such a person for further intervention becomes less and arrangements become more focused on the preferred setting for delivering terminal care.

Recognizing deterioration

Many people enter the terminal phase gradually over a period of days. They become weaker, less interested in their surroundings, eat and drink less and sleep for extended periods.

ENTERING THE TERMINAL PHASE
● Weaker
● Loss of interest
● East and drink less
● Sleep more

Although, carers and families may notice this deterioration they may not appreciate its significance. There may have been other cycles of deterioration and recovery and carers may not appreciate that death is imminent.

Whether the deterioration is acute or gradual, it is important for the health professional to establish the significance of this phase of illness with the carers, so they understand the process of care, as well as the likely outcome. Carers may ask many varied questions about feeding, hydration, antibiotic therapy and further oncology treatment. Urgent transfers back to an acute hospital setting or dissatisfaction with the medical management can occur purely through lack of understanding that the terminal phase has developed.

BEFORE THE TIME COMES

Fears

Many patients know that they have a serious advancing illness and some are able to voice their concerns about their future deterioration. A common theme for such people is that they are worried about their mode of death. There may be a particular symptom which worries them more than any other e.g. dying "fighting for breath" or "the terrible pain at the end". It is important for the health professional to try and elicit these concerns and deal with them frankly.

Explanation

Explanation of the medication or techniques used to ease symptoms can often reassure the person. Frequently the doctor and nurse also find it helpful to know about these concerns, so they can deal with the symptoms promptly if they arise. During such discussions the patient may indicate that they do not wish their dying to be unduly prolonged by medical intervention. Again, doctors and nurses should respond openly and frankly and discuss the likely interventions which are available.

The question of resuscitation

It is possible to raise the question of resuscitation in the event of sudden cardio-respiratory arrest during these conversations and patients can clearly give their view. On other occasions, the patient's views about resuscitation can be easily inferred from the conversation without asking directly about resuscitation. Families and carers can be involved in these discussions and although it is often painful and emotionally draining for them they gain an important insight into the wishes of their dying relative.[7,8]

Unfinished business

Some people are less open with their concerns, but clearly understand that they are dying. Carers and staff often perceive that the person is troubled and anxious. Their anxiety can often be related to some "unfinished business" in their lives e.g. decisions about a will, an unresolved conflict or difficult family relationship or a business worry. They, too, may be anxious about their mode of death, but are not volunteering these concerns. It is important for staff to be alert to these problems. If ignored, patients may become more withdrawn and anxious. They develop insomnia with bad dreams and nightmares and even have paranoid ideas if problems are unresolved. Dreams and nightmares can often relate to bad experiences and anxieties and are important signs of unresolved conflicts.

Many personal situations are impossible to resolve within the time remaining for a particular person. The appreciation of such unresolved matters is helpful for the clinician in planning treatment. It seems that such unresolved problems can often result in restlessness and terminal anguish.

Not every dying person is fully aware of their serious condition and still others actively discourage professionals from giving them information. The terminal phase of illness is certainly not the time to deliver complicated information. It is important to have built up a degree of trust so that the dying person's questions or concerns can be answered appropriately. The opportunity to deal with major outstanding issues in a person's life usually lies within the palliative phase of illness. Procrastination about these issues can often lead to them being left unresolved.

WHEN THE TIME COMES

Recognizing the terminal phase

The terminal phase can occur with an acute event or gradually over days or even hours. The deterioration is often not detected by the patient themselves. However, it is important for families and carers to be aware of the seriousness of the situation.

In a hospital setting it is becoming accepted practise for nursing staff to enquire about the resuscitation status of all patients on a ward. The decision not to resuscitate should be made by a senior member of the medical staff after consulting the multidisciplinary team.[9] The question of resuscitation should also be discussed with the patient's families and carers. It is often not possible to have such a detailed conversation with the patient at this time, although as mentioned earlier, previous discussions with the patient may have indicated his wishes.

Resuscitation policy

Families find discussion about resuscitation very painful and burdensome. Families should not be given the impression that it is their decision alone and it is often much more preferable for them to feel that they agree with a decision which has been made by health care professionals. Guidelines for decisions concerning resuscitation are based on consideration of the likelihood of success of an attempt at resuscitation and also whether it is in the best interests of the person with a far advanced progressive disease.

Although, the question of a resuscitation policy may not be as relevant in other settings such as nursing home, hospice or home, discussion about resuscitation can often stimulate an understanding about the phase of illness of a particular person. Dying patients are still unnecessarily transferred to A&E Departments if they suddenly collapse in a nursing home or in their own home. Such inappropriate admissions can be avoided by prior discussion of relevant future care (If the time comes for you to need more nursing help, where would you like to be?).

SYMPTOM CONTROL IN THE TERMINAL PHASE

There are 3 important steps for controlling symptoms control in the dying patient:

● Rationalising regular medication.
● Anticipating the route of drug administration.
● Ensuring availability of parental medication.

1. Rationalising Regular Medication

Many dying patients continue to tolerate oral medication. However, the burden of taking many tablets should be reduced and regular medication can be discontinued e.g. Thyroxine, anti-hypertensives, Iron, oral hyperglycaemics and hormones, are unlikely to benefit the person at this stage.

2. Route of Administration

As the person deteriorates oral medication may become more difficult to administer. It is therefore important to prescribe alternative routes of administration, i.e. rectal or parentral (subcutaneous, intramuscular) but also to prescribe medication for new symptoms which may arise.

Inability to take oral medication in the dying patient is a common indication for delivering drugs via a syringe driver. It is very important to mention this possibility to families, who may come to blame the syringe driver medication for rapid deterioration into unconsciousness if they have not been forewarned. Other families can suspect that much greater doses of drugs are being delivered by the syringe driver, rather than a mere conversion of necessary medication by a different route of administration.

Starting a syringe driver should not be an automatic response to managing a dying patient. If a person is deteriorating rapidly, medication by intermittent injection may be sufficient rather than starting a syringe driver within one or two hours of death.

3. Availability of Parenteral Medication

It is necessary to anticipate the possible use of a small number of drugs which are commonly used in the terminal phase. At home it would be necessary for these drugs to be prescribed in good time, so that difficulties obtaining medication out of hours or at weekends can be avoided. The medication must also be prescribed on the appropriate form so that District Nurses can administer these drugs appropriately. With adequate training and discussion amongst team members, it is usually possible for the doctors to write appropriate dose ranges for particular drugs to allow for changing circumstances.

In other settings, easy availability of the required medications leads to greater confidence by staff, so that they are used appropriately and effectively.

COMMON SYMPTOMS IN THE TERMINAL PHASE

A survey of 200 consecutive hospice patients revealed the following frequency of symptoms recorded in the last 48 hours of life.[15]

Symptom	Frequency %
Noisy and moist breathing	56%
Pain	51%
Restlessness and agitation	42%
Incontinence of urine	32%
Dyspnoea	22%
Retention of urine	21%
Sweating	14%
Nausea and Vomiting	14%
Jerking, twitching, plucking	12%
Confusion	9%

Pain   Regular analgesia is still needed in the terminal phase. However, unless an acute event occurs analgesic requirements do not usually increase rapidly or significantly.[10] The route of administration may alter, but the dose range of analgesics usually remains within a factor of one. If bone pain or neuropathic pain has previously been a significant problem some adjustments may be necessary, particularly if oral medication such as amitriptyline or NSAIDs cannot be taken. Use of NSAIDs suppositories can be beneficial at this time.

Nursing measures are very important for pain control at this stage. Pressure relieving mattresses and more specialised beds can greatly help the problems of nursing a patient who has pain on movement. The timely use of a urinary catheter can also ease pain and discomfort by reducing the need to move a patient from the bed.

Nausea and Vomiting

Nausea and vomiting can be a potent cause of restlessness for a dying patient and should be avoided by the use of regular antiemetic therapy. Vomiting can be very distressing for the carers as well, who may be with the patient for extensive periods.

Gastric dilatation can occur spontaneously or as a result of upper GI obstruction. If this problem develops gradually, octreotide and hyoscine can be useful medication to reduce upper GI secretions.[11,12] However, the distressing syndrome of restlessness, abdominal distension, projectile vomiting or more commonly reflux of stagnant fluid into the mouth should be recognised. In these circumstances passage of a fine bore nasogastric tube can frequently drain 1–2 litres of fluid at once. Leaving the tube in situ and on free drainage often settles the patient without the need for extra sedation.

Anxiety, Restlessness and Agitation

This triad of symptoms can be the most challenging for clinicians to control.[13] Poor control can be stressful for patient, families and health professionals. The major importance of these symptoms is their effect on the perception of suffering of the dying person. Restlessness and agitation can often be taken as signs that the person is in pain. Carers and professionals alike often respond by escalating the dose of strong opioids. Unfortunately, this can lead to further agitation and confusion in the dying person. Myoclonic jerks can be interpreted as the person jumping with pain.

It is important to consider the potentially reversible causes of distress. Namely: constipation, retention of urine, infection, metabolic disorders (hypercalcaemia, uraemia) gastric dilatation and fear.

Anxiety and restlessness can be eased by introducing benzodiazepines (diazepam or midazolam) in addition to appropriate analgesia. Benzodiazepines are also useful for easing breathlessness and as an anti-convulsant.

Agitated and confused patients may require sedation with an anti-psychotic such as haloperidol or methotrimepazine.

Hyoscine hydrobromide is a useful agent for control of excess chest secretions.

Acute deterioration can occur through major haemorrhage or difficulties with airway. The possibility of this situation arising is often heralded by a warning (eg a bleed or difficulty with a tracheostomy tube) and it is important for the team to consider their care plan in advance.

The principle objective of care is to relieve distress and fear for the patient and is best achieved by creating amnesia with sedation. SC or IV midazolam (and occasionally hyoscine) provide prompt relief of distress. Strong analgesics are often not necessary in these emergencies and can lead to delays in administering medication.

DRUGS COMMONLY USED IN THE TERMINAL PHASE*

	Subcutaneous dose\24 hours
Diamorphine	50% of 24 hour oral morphine
Cyclizine	150mg
Haloperidol	1.5mg-10mg
Methotrimeprazine	25mgs-150mgs
Midazolam	10mg-60mgs
Hyoscine Hydrobromide	400–2400 mcg
Hyoscine Butylbromide (Buscopan)	20mgs – 60mgs

Note: Diazepam, Prochlorperazine, Chlorpromazine are not suitable for use in syringe-drivers. Oral Morphine 2–4 hourly can still be given for breakthrough pain
* Unlicensed use of drugs is common in Palliative Care. There is a wide experience of usage in hospices and specialist palliative care services.

THE QUESTION OF HYDRATION

Patients dying of cancer can become gradually dehydrated during the last 48 hours. The most common symptom is a dry mouth which can be treated by regular mouth care. Such patients rarely

369 THE TERMINAL PHASE

complain of thirst. If dying patients do complain of thirst then an increase in fluid intake is usually indicated (whether oral, nasogastric, SC or IV).

Diagnostic errors can occur. Careful clinical assessment is essential to exclude other causes of dehydration (eg severe vomiting, overtreatment with diuretics, hypercalcaemia or excessive sedation), because treatment with IV fluids may significantly improve the patient's prognosis.[16]

A common question from relatives (particularly from some cultural and religious groups) is whether the patient should be given fluids. Obviously the answer is yes, if there is any question that the patient is dying from dehydration due to reversible cause rather than advanced and progressing cancer. For most patients however giving IV fluids does not improve their physical comfort, mental state or prognosis. There are no definitive studies on the effect of IV fluids on prognosis in patients dying of cancer, but even if the prognosis is extended by a few days, the question arises is the intervention prolonging life or prolonging the dying process?[17]

Subcutaneous fluids

If the relatives are very distressed by the lack of fluid intake in an unconscious (or sedated) patient a sensible clinical compromise can be to give SC fluids, usually 1L per 24 hours. If the tube is primed with hyaluronidase the fluid disperses more easily under the skin. It can be helpful to give the infusion intermittently (eg during the night) which can make it easier for the family to face the decision of discontinuing fluid therapy.

Discuss with relatives

It is extremely important to re-assess the situation daily, to discuss the situation with relatives, to listen to their concerns and to explain the option of fluids in terms of the potential benefits versus disadvantages. One of many factors to consider is that IV cannulas (or any medical equipment) can cause a feeling of distance for relatives at a time when emotional closeness is often particularly important.

CONSIDERING THE FAMILY

It is important to be aware of the needs of the extended family as well as the main carer, or partner. Grand-parents, brothers, sisters and friends, all need support at this time. Documenting a family tree is an invaluable way of understanding the potential myriad of relationships within a family, so that the needs of all those affected can be addressed.

Confidentiality within families should be respected if requested by the dying person or main carer since tensions within carers can easily arise particularly if difficult relationships have not been resolved. *Lines of communication* should be established within the families, so that health professionals are not overwhelmed by multiple enquiries.

Main carers are often distracted by anxiety about other family members (eg elderly parents or young children) and may need help in giving them information. Carers are protective towards more vulnerable members of family and want to shield them from distress. Unfortunately, this can sometimes give rise to feelings of exclusion and professionals may need to give reassurance and encouragement, so that all family members who need to be with the dying person can be.

The death of a loved one is of a profoundly distressing event in any person's life and the role of the professional can only be one of support. Families should be encouraged to grieve with each other. Such distress can be alleviated, to a certain degree, if everyone is fully aware of the events as they unfold. Repeated explanation and information about rationale of therapy is frequently helpful for families in their recognition of the inevitability of the relative's death.

CONSIDERING THE STAFF

Caring for the dying can be very stressful for health professionals as well as for carers. Specialist palliative care staff may have gained the experience of caring for many dying people and may be more confident in dealing with distressed families and carers. Nevertheless even experienced staff can still be left with feelings of inadequacy after caring for someone with multiple problems. Such stresses can be even greater on staff with only occasional experience of such difficult situations.

Availability of appropriate medication is important, but staff need the understanding and confidence to use the medication in the appropriate way. Equally they need to be aware of the needs and concerns of families at this difficult time.

Much of these difficulties can be alleviated through staff team meetings where topics, such as relief of restlessness, agitation and acute collapse are discussed. Staff should not feel isolated in their actions. For instance, doctors prescribe medication but nurses may administer the drugs. It is important for all team members to be comfortable with the management in relation to approaches to treatment, information for families and use of appropriate medication.

AT THE TIME OF DEATH

In today's society, witnessing a death is an unfamiliar experience to many. It is important for families to have guidance at the time of death, tailored to the different settings.

As our society becomes more multi-cultural, it is also important for staff to take account of the needs of different cultural and religious traditions sur-rounding a person's death. Staff should enquire about any particular rituals or customs, such as special clothing or prayers at time of death.

In whatever setting, carers may be unfamiliar with the process of certification, registration and arrangements for funerals. In the case of industrial related disease, it is important that families are forewarned of the necessity for referral to the Coroner and probable post mortem examination.

For expected deaths at home or in nursing homes sufficient information should be available to deputising services to avoid unwarranted referral to the Coroner's Officer. Doctors confirming death need to know that a death certificate can be issued by a doctor familiar with the person's circumstance. When the proper arrangements have not been made, the involvement of police and the unnecessary removal of the body to a mortuary pending enquiries, can be an added avoidable distress for families.

Families often derive comfort from health professionals attending funerals. Equally staff may also find it beneficial to attend the funeral of someone with whom they have been closely involved professionally.

THE QUESTION OF EUTHANASIA

Requests for medically assisted death are only rarely persistent and repeated. Many such requests occur in the palliative phase of a person's illness and are prompted by the need for reassurance about adequate symptom control in the future or "when the time comes". Frank discussions about the likely course of the disease and measures to gain symptom control usually help to allay fears.

During the terminal phase, euthanasia can become more of an issue for carers and the families rather than for the dying person themselves. Many carers and relatives are keen for the dying process not to be unduly prolonged. Their concern is often voiced in terms of there being "only a shell remaining" or "it is not the person I knew". It is important for staff to support carers in their distress and to acknowledge that this is a very difficult time for those close to the dying person. It is often helpful to point out to them the improvements in symptom control, which are being achieved in this changing situation. It reassures families that significant symptoms are being dealt with.

Many staff are keen to control difficult symptoms, but do not want to be associated with "mercy killing". Fear of this association can lead to reluctance to use medication in the appropriate way. Medication used to control symptoms cannot be equated with euthanasia (where the medication is given with the intention of causing death.)

Colin's Story

Colin was a 40 year old man with recurrent colonic carcinoma referred to the Palliative Care Team for symptom control. In the past he had undergone right hemicolectomy and subsequent ileotransverse by-pass for adenocarcinoma of the colon. He had a large abdominal mass with a discharging entro-cutaneous fistula on to his abdominal wall.

He complained of pain in his right loin, radiating across his lower abdomen. His abdominal pain was controlled with MST 120mgs bd and Amitriptyline 25mgs at night. He took occasional Morphine Sulphate for breakthrough pain.

Having gained symptom control Colin was discharged home from the surgical ward. Socially, he was unmarried and lived with his elderly father, but had a large extended family. Colin understood that he had a far advanced progressing cancer. He was encouraged by the pain control having been gained relatively easily and was looking forward to a little more time.

Colin subsequently required two further admissions for symptom control. He developed acute breathlessness, secondary to recurrent anaemia and he found this symptom very frightening. He had confidence in the ward staff and prompt re-admission was arranged on each occasion. His symptoms settled after blood transfusion and a short-time in the ward.

Two months later he became anaemic again, was breathless on exertion and had developed gross oedema of abdomen and both legs over a few days. Colin readily accepted the offer of a further admission for assessment and symptom control.

Upon admission he was clearly anaemic and had increasing abdominal distension and peripheral oedema, and it became clear that Colin was convinced that he was going to die within the next 24 hours. He preferred to sleep in the chair rather than go to bed, fearing imminent death. His other main fear was that the peripheral oedema would extend proximally so that he would die fighting for his breath.

It was necessary to talk very frankly with him about these symptoms and fears and the therapeutic options were explained to him. Colin did not die within the first 24 hours. After talking to the Chaplain he decided to be Confirmed. He also expressed a wish to go home again, but recognised that his gross oedema would cause difficult nursing problems at home. In many ways he felt safe on the ward and had the confidence of the nursing staff. He accepted urinary catheterisation before it became too difficult due to genital oedema. Three days after admission arrangements were made for Colin to be confirmed by his Anglican Bishop in the day room of the surgical ward. He was well enough to have a small celebration afterwards with his family.

Although becoming weaker, Colin was still keen to return home for a short time. With the help of the ambulance service he went home at 10.00 am and returned to the ward at 3.00 pm on the same day.

On return to the ward Colin was clearly delighted to have been home for what he recognised to be the last time. However, the whole process had exhausted him and he started to sleep for prolonged periods.

24 hours later, he was becoming breathless at rest with retained chest secretions. He required to be nursed in bed and was having difficulty with oral medications. His analgesic requirements had not altered over 3 months and he was taking 240mgs of Morphine in 24 hours. This was duly converted to Diamorphine 80mgs via a syringe driver and Hyoscine 1200mcgs per 24 hours was also added to the driver. Midazolam 5mgs subcutaneously was given on the four occasions over the next 24 hours for intermittent restlessness.

7 days after admission, 3 days after being confirmed and 2 days after returning home for the last time, Colin died without distress with his relatives present.

References

1. Fakhoury W, McCarthy M, Addington-Hall J. The effects of the clinical characteristics of dying cancer patients on informal caregivers satisfaction with palliative care. Palliat Med 1997; 11: 107–115.
2. Groves K. How I'd like to be treated if I was terminally ill. Br Med J 1995; 311: 1691–1693.
3. Thorpe G. Enabling more dying people to remain at home. Br Med J 1993; 307: 915–918.
4. Eve A, Smith A, Tebbit P. Hospice and palliative care in the UK 1994–5, including a summary of trends 1990–5. Palliat Med 1997: 11: 31–43.
5. Ashby M, Stoffell B. Therapeutic ratio and defined phases: proposal of ethical framework for palliative care. Br Med J 1991; 303: 1322–1324.
6. Twycross RG, Lichter I. The terminal phase. In: Doyle D, Hanks GWC, MacDonald N. eds Oxford Textbook of Palliative Medicine. Oxford University Press, 1993: 651–661.
7. Schade S, Muslin H. Do not resuscitate decisions: discussions with patients. J Med Ethics 1989; 15: 186–190.
8. Mead G, Turnbull C. Cardiopulmonary resuscitation in the elderly: patients' and relatives' views. J Med Ethics 1995; 21: 39–44.
9. Doyal L, Wilsher D. Withholding cardiopulmonary resuscitation: proposals for formal guidelines. Br Med J 1993: 306: 1593–1596.
10. Scott JF, Viola RA, Buckley G. Pain control during the last week of life in a palliative care unit. J Palliat Care 1992; 8: 73.
11. Ripamonti C. Malignant bowel obstruction in advanced and terminal cancer patients. Eur J Palliat Care 1994; 1: 16–19.
12. Riley J, Fallon M. Octreotide in terminal malignant obstruction of the gastrointestinal tract. Eur J Palliat Care 1994; 1: 23–25.
13. Store P, Phillips C, Spruyt O, Waight C. A comparison of the use of sedatives in a hospital support team and in a hospice. Palliat Med 1997; 11: 140–144.
14. de Raeve L. Dignity and integrity at the end of life. Int J Palliat Nursing 1996; 2: 71–76.
15. Lichter I, Hunt E The last 48 hours of life Journal of Palliative Care 6:4/1990;7-15
16. Craig GM. On withholding nutrition and hydration in the terminally ill: has palliative medicine gone too far? Journal of medical ethics 1994; 20: 139-143.
17. Dunlop RJ, Ellershaw JE, Baines MJ, Sykes N, Saunders CM.On withholding nutrition and hydration in the terminally ill: has palliative medicine gone too far? Journal Medical Ethics 1995; 21: 141-143

Chapter 18

Palliative Care –
The Next 10 years

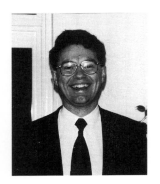

Dr Robert Dunlop
Robert Dunlop trained at Otago Medical School New Zealand, graduating in 1979. He is now Medical Director of St Christopher's Hospice in London. His special interests include neuropathic pain, the role of cytokines in the symptoms of advanced cancer and the future development of the Specialty of Palliative Medicine.

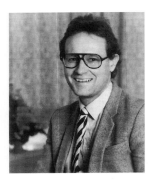

Dr Peter Kaye
Peter Kaye is Consultant in Palliative Medicine at Cynthia Spencer Hospice, Northampton, a Fellow of the Royal College of Physicians and a Member of the Royal College of General Practitioners. He has a special interest in the psychological aspects of illness.

INTRODUCTION

Despite the advent of gene therapy, it seems unlikely that accurate prophecy will become a human attribute for the foreseeable future. Medicine is changing rapidly, and any prediction about what the future may hold obviously runs the risk of being very wrong. Who could have predicted the AIDS epidemic? Nevertheless it is possible to make educated guesses about the direction we seem to be taking, both in medicine and within the relatively new speciality of Palliative Medicine. But first some history might help, because (to paraphrase Winston Churchill when he once addressed the Royal College of Physicians) if you want to look forwards, it helps to look back.

THE HISTORICAL PERSPECTIVE

Palliative care is not a new idea. In a sense all medical care was palliative before about 150 years ago, because very little could be done to cure anything (and most attempts, such as blood letting and surgery for bladder stone, were pretty barbaric). And then, after 2000 years of stasis, medicine started to become increasingly scientific and cure-orientated. Scientific understanding about the body began with Harvey's description of the circulation in 1628. The speed of new developments increased steadily from around the beginning of the 19th Century following Laennec's invention of the stethoscope in 1816. But it took another 100 years for patients to begin to feel the benefits, starting with the discovery of the sulphonamides in 1932. The following 30 years saw an explosion of new drugs and clinical skills, with medicine increasingly focused on its new-found ability to cure.

Neglect of the dying

It is often said that the neglect of the dying resulted from the scientific advances in medicine. As doctors developed more cures, the dying became failures and were ignored. This is one factor, but the focus on cure is not just driven by doctors blinded by technological achievement. It is fuelled at least as much by patients (even in the 12th Century, people flocked to St Bartholomew's Hospital after stories of remarkable cures). History teaches that the terminally ill have always been ignored. As far back as 1544, surgeons at St Bartholomew's Hospital had to establish which patients were curable and which were incurable, so that incurable patients would not be admitted. During the Great Plague, doctors abandoned the care of the dying to the nurses and apothecaries. The reasons for doctors deserting the terminally ill are undoubtedly complex, reflecting personal and professional issues. While it is possible to address some of the professional issues, the deep-seated personal fear of dying will always leave the dying vulnerable.

In 1967 when Christian Barnaard successfully transplanted the first heart his surgical teamed cheered. A new era of hope had dawned on the expectations of doctors and the public. But alongside the increasingly technological interest of the medical profession, hospice care (and eventually the new speciality of Palliative Medicine) emerged to focus on the special needs of the dying – "an idea whose time had come". St Christopher's Hospice in Sydenham was founded by Cicely Saunders and opened in 1967, and was the first purpose-built research and teaching hospice. It became the model for many other hospices; the focal point for a movement which has spread around the world. Saunder's concept of "Total Pain" embracing the physical emotional, social and spiritual aspects of distress led to the development of multi-disciplinary professional teams to meet the complex and changing needs of patients and their relatives.

Also in the 1960's, Elizabeth Kubler-Ross in the US showed that talking about dying to dying patients did not make them feel worse.[1] In fact, it made them feel much better, and her work provided professionals with a new way to help incurable patients. – you just talk with them. She raised the expectation that patients could be 'helped' to accept that they were going to die, and this became a key aim for many working in palliative care. Kubler Ross's model of the psychological reaction to dying (denial and isolation, anger, bargaining, depression and acceptance) mirrored similar models being developed by Colin Murray-Parkes and others studying grief and loss, and led to increased interest in ways of providing psychological support.

THE FUTURE OF MEDICINE

The future of Palliative Medicine will obviously be related to the wider context of the future of Medical care as a whole. Before considering the future of the speciality, we will briefly consider some of the wider developments in Medicine, because no doubt many of them will influence Palliative Care.

The world population

The world population is set to increase from 6,000 million to around 8,000 million by the year 2025. What will medical science have to offer to control the birth rate, or will it be left to governments to stem the tide. Millions of children in the poorer countries continue to die from preventable diseases: measles, diphtheria, cholera, tetanus, influenza and polio – preventable by simple vaccination programmes. How will society prioritise the health needs of populations? Will palliative care continue to receive support and funding?

Global warming

Global warming may change the distribution of the mosquito, spreading it again to more temperate latitudes, and may bring drug-resistant malaria to the West (which might indirectly benefit the poorer countries where it predominates, because no doubt the search for a solution to the worldwide scourge of malaria would then be accelerated). Global warming would probably also allow the spread of the tetse fly and sleeping sickness, and also bilharzia, leishmaniasis, yellow fever, dengue fever and many other conditions. Might Palliative care become involved with diseases once considered tropical?

Viral epidemics

Viral epidemics are likely to occur in the future. An example is the post-World War One influenza epidemic that killed more people than the war. The recent AIDS epidemic has confirmed their potential for a dramatic global impact. The Marburg and Ebola viruses have already caused scares. Health-care professionals working in Africa have observed other lethal viral-like illnesses. It and other new viral disease appears will the Hospice movement respond in the same way as it did when AIDS was first recognised?

Drug resistance

Drug resistant bacterial infections are becoming more troublesome. Multiple resistant Staphylococcus Aureus (MRSA) is the most widely recognised although its clinical effects are usually irksome rather than life-threatening. However, other bacteria are acquiring multiple drug resistance, such as enterococci. More potent antibiotics are being developed but the widespread use of these in clinical and veterinary practice will limit new advances. Will the widespread presence of multiple drug resistant organisms undermine some of the gains made in transplantation, especially bone marrow, and the use of prostheses?

Another significant development is multiple drug resistant tuberculosis (MDRTB). Health professionals have died as a result of MDRTB. Many of the hospices set up in the late 19th Century were built for the victims of consumption. Will hospices of the future again be caring for victims of TB?

Economic factors

Economic factors are increasingly defining patterns of healthcare. The growing cost of investi- gations and treatments is outstripping the capacity of countries which fund healthcare from taxation. In the USA, private healthcare insurers are also trying to constrain expenditure. The income- generating workforce (which pays taxes or health care insurance) is decreasing compared with the elderly who need most care. This will increase the pressure for euthanasia on the already vulnerable elderly. The quality of longer-term care will remain a problem, not just for the elderly but also for the severely disabled.

In the UK, private insurance is still only taken by a minority. Will the perceived decline in NHS standards of care, especially waiting times, lead to a majority of people having private insurance? Will health care insurers seriously consider including palliative care as suitable for reimbursement? How would palliative care services cope with this possibility, for example charging for individual patients?

Community care

Reduction in acute hospital beds is likely. The NHS has recently targeted patients in long-stay beds for discharge. Community-care 'packages' have enabled more people to be cared for at home but the social services/healthcare interface remains contentious. Will the current levels of community care be sustainable? One result of decreasing acute hospital beds is the need for more nursing home beds. In the USA, acute hospitals are only used for urgent diagnostic work and treatments. This has lead some nursing homes to specialise, for example coronary in care, rehabilitation, and hospice inpatient care.

Expectations of care

Patient and family expectations continue to rise. This trend has been accelerated by the Patient Charter. People are wanting to participate more fully in decision-making. The decision by one doctor to withhold or withdraw treatment will not preclude patients from seeking further opinions. The recent events following the withdrawal of funding to treat child "B" are a cogent reminder of the changing relationship between doctors, patients, and healthcare funders. Palliative care services are being exposed to these trends as well, not just specialist hospital teams who are more likely to be involved with patients seeking active treatment.

Computers

Computers will continue to change the way medical information is stored and moved around. The Internet will grow, Electronic biosensors will enable more body fluids to be chemically analysed ("intelligent toilets" may even be able to relay news of any blood or protein in your excretions straight to your doctor's surgery!)

The computer-design of drugs, modelled in 3–D, to interact with specific receptor sites or hormones, will increasingly replace the present system of routine screening of massive numbers of natural or synthetic chemicals for biological activity. Hopefully we will develop newer drugs with fewer side-effects, acting on specific receptors wherever possible.

New treatments

New drug developments will effect more cures or significantly improve the quality of life for incurable diseases. However, there is the prospect of treatments which will prolong life without reducing the need for care. For example, new therapies for motor neurone disease can extend survival but they only slow the inevitable progression.

Treatment-induced diseases

Treatment-induced diseases have become more complex, throwing up new and interesting challenges to palliative care such as graft versus host disease (GVHD). Many patients have benefited from bone marrow transplantation in the face of otherwise incurable disease. However, a few patients have suffered terribly from GVHD, for example coughing up the entire lining of the oesophagus. What new diseases might gene therapy give rise to? Will transplantation of immune-neutral organs from animals introduce new diseases from the host?

Monoclonal antibodies

Monoclonal antibodies may be increasingly used to deliver drugs to specific sites in the body, or to neutralize the body's own chemicals (such as Tumour Necrosis Factor).

Transplanted fetal tissue

Transplanted fetal tissue may be increasingly used to replace damaged or diseased adult tissue in conditions such as Parkinson's disease, diabetes, Alzheimer's and even myocardial infacts.

Keyhole surgery

Keyhole surgery, using endoscopes passed through one hole and surgical instruments through another, will develop further. It can currently be used to repair hernias, close fallopian tubes and to remove of gall bladder, appendix, kidneys, sections of bowel or uterus. Robots will be increasingly used to improve precision of surgical techniques. Some of these techniques may become appropriate in controlling symptoms.

Gene therapy

Gene therapy, for the delivery of normal genes (via altered viruses and other methods) which can now be given to replace abnormal genes will develop, and will enable the treatment and possibly cure of a growing number of illnesses caused by single gene defects, and possibly other conditions as well. Introduced genes often function poorly, do not reach sufficient of the appropriate cells, or shut off after time. More work is needed to improve effectiveness.

Medical education

Medical education will increasingly incorporate computer-assisted teaching for anatomy and the use of virtual reality techniques to teach the handling of sophisticated medical equipment, but will also hopefully develop video-feedback of consultations and the use of group discussions and other techniques to help teach counselling skills to all doctors.

Evidence-based medical care and purchasing of medical care will increase the need for relevant record keeping and statistical analysis of medical care.

THE FUTURE OF PALLIATIVE MEDICINE

Palliative Care Services have expanded rapidly in recent years.

GROWTH OF PALLIATIVE CARE SERVICES IN THE UK

Inpatient hospices:	3 – 200 over the past 30 years
Macmillan nurses:	0 – 400 over the past 15 years
Hospital Support teams:	0 – 250 over the past 15 years

There are now over 4,500 palliative services in more than 76 countries.

In 1989 Palliative Medicine became a recognised medical speciality in the UK.Currently, hospice inpatient units care for about 15% of all cancer patients who die in the UK. Estimates suggest that around 40–50% of terminally ill cancer patients receive specialist home care services.

Future growth of services

The trend in the growth of hospice inpatient units appears to have slowed, reflecting in part the expense of establishing and running them. Many people still fear admission to a hospice, and 50% of all patients and families who are offered admission will refuse. Specialist home care services are likely to grow more quickly. More hospital support teams will fuel this growth, by encouraging more and earlier discharges from hospital. The importance of Palliative Care has recently been emphasised by the Calman-Hine report (1995) which emphasisis the need to incorporate good quality palliative care within improved services for all patients with cancer.

The scope of Palliative Care

With its roots in the Hospice Movement, the focus of palliative care historically has been on patients with far-advanced cancer. This is changing. Palliative care teams are rightly being involved earlier and earlier in the care of patients with cancer. We are also beginning to see that the principles extend to patients with non-malignant conditions that are also progressive and life-threatening (and there are 2 such patients for every 1 with advanced cancer). Palliative Care Teams will have to become more and more aware of developments in oncology and general medicine. This book contains a tutorial on AIDS, but any future editions will need to cover other progressive medical conditions: neurological, cardio-vascular, gastro-intestinal, renal and pulmonary.

Non cancer patients

The prospect of serving non-cancer patients as well as cancer patients is daunting. The sheer number of patients 3 times the number of cancer deaths) seems overwhelming. However, closer analysis suggests that the role of specialist Palliative Care services will not be required for the entire population. Many people with non-malignant conditions die 'suddenly', with no or little warning. Sudden death from cardiac arrest is one example, as is fatal CVA, broncho-pneumonia, etc. Another large subset of non-cancer patients are disabled for many years, for example with multiple sclerosis, chronic bronchitis/ emphysema, etc. The proportion of patients who follow a similar course to cancer patients is much smaller than expected.

Palliative Care services may have to develop a consultancy approach, providing symptom control and other advice and then stepping back when the problem is resolved. Hospital support teams could provide more symptom control for patients admitted acutely to hospital. Home care teams could visit patients who deteriorate in nursing homes. For chronic illnesses.

Ethnic groups

Minority ethnic groups are making more use of Palliative Care services. The relative proportion of people from minority ethnic groups who get cancer is lower but will increase in the future. Services must adapt to the different needs and expectations.

How will Palliative Care practitioners cope with examples like the Nepalese family whose 11 year old boy was dying of a brain tumour where the family believed that if they even thought that he would die then this would kill him?

Symptom control

Symptom Control may become more challenging in the light of new diseases and the effects of other treatments. New advances will be made in the understanding of patho-physiological processes underlying symptoms. This will enable more specific treatments to be developed. Palliative care specialists must remain alert to new options developed in other fields of medicine. Many of our current symptom control measures exploit "side-effects" of drugs designed to treat other conditions.

Complementary therapies

Complementary therapies are becoming more sophisticated. The mind-body connection is now recognised. Even non-specific "holistic" treatments may have specific effects on symptoms. Just as links are needed with other fields of medical research, Palliative Care must continue to encourage appropriate links with specialists in Complementary therapies. Massage, aromatherapy, art therapy and reminiscence work (biography therapy) have all proved useful. More research is needed.

Palliative Surgery, radiotherapy, and chemotherapy

Palliative surgery, radiotherapy, and chemotherapy are evolving constantly. If the current pattern of advances in these anti-cancer modalities continues, treatments will become more highly selective, more expensive, and more likely to be used in combination. Careful assessment of new palliative chemotherapy regimes will continue, using multi-centre trials and meta-analysis, focusing on quality of life issues rather than simply on response rates. The costs of treatments will rise, both from the increased use of adjuvant treatments for example and from the costs of new therapies, with little survival advantage.

Some advances have important applications for palliative care. The variety of stents has improved, along with ease of insertion. Brachytherapy can be used to palliate difficult problems such as recurrent oesophageal cancer. Advances in endorscopic key-hole surgery may make surgical intervention feasible for control of some symptoms even in advanced disease.

New treatments

New anti-cancer drugs will be designed (probably using molecular design by computer graphics) to interfere with specific targets of DNA replication and transcription in tumour cells, and to interfere with the process of micro-metastases. Bone marrow support by growth factors or grafting techniques may improve response rates. *Growth factors* may prove useful in managing some palliative care patients. For example, thrombopoeitin might be used to minimise symptoms from severe thrombocytopenia associated with marrow failure in advanced breast or prostate cancer.

High dose chemotherapy

The use of very intensive *high-dose chemotherapy* with stem cell transplants, for patients with early chemo-sensitive disease (eg, breast cancer) may improve survival in well-motivated patients. If a major breakthrough occurs in cancer treatments, patients with cancer may live longer. The development of triple therapy for HIV offers a model of what might happen. The need for Palliative Care services could be reduced (some specialist AIDS hospices have reported a 50% decrease in bed usage since triple therapy became available). However, the patients will still die (death and taxes being the only certainties in life), albeit later. Thus, an initial down-turn in activity would be followed by a return to normal levels of activity, with the risk that Government funding would be removed while the service activity was temporarily reduced.

Gene therapy may eventually become available for common cancers. Our understanding of oncogenes and tumour suppressor genes will expand, and gene transfer (using viruses to insert new DNA into cells) may develop from a laboratory technique to a clinical treatment.

Nursing specialisation

Nursing specialisation is a logical extension of multi-skilling in Palliative Care. Nursing has always been the corner-stone of Palliative Care. The work of Professor Jessica Corner illustrates how nurses can play a more active role in managing symptoms by non-pharmacological means. At St Christopher's Hospice, nurses have been more involved in the admission process, carrying out nurse-led admissions.

Audit

Audit is essential for improving patient care. New audit tools are being developed that can be used in any setting. Postal questionnaires may help to evaluate services by obtaining relatives views after patients have died. This can highlight deficiencies in non-specialist services. Organisational audit may come to be required of all services which receive Government funding.

Research

Research is difficult in palliative care. Academic units will improve the quality of research but multi-centre studies will be needed to overcome low accrual rates. Quality of life measurements are being evolved to capture some of the existential issues that are affected by Palliative Care. Service provision issues will need careful study if Government intervention is to be effective.

Counselling psychotherapy

Counselling\psychotherapy skills need to be developed more systematically. Issues of sexuality in Palliative Care and bereavement support for children are two key areas of concern. Palliative Care practitioners need to become more expert in managing group interviews. The knowledge and skills developed in the fields of Family Therapy and Group Psycho-analytic Therapy have much to teach Palliative Care professionals.

Group psychotherapy can prolong survival in breast cancer. Speigal's work showed that 40 women with breast cancer who had weekly psycho-therapy (for 90 minutes) for a year survived twice as long as 40 matched women (after 10 years follow-up).[3] The effects of psychotherapy on quality of life (as well as tumour response) should be further explored.

Teaching and education

Teaching and education has always been important, spreading the expertise of Palliative Care. Undergraduate teaching has been limited by over-crowded curricula and many junior doctors still arrive on the wards with little of no training even in basic symptom control. However, medical school Deans are realising that doctor/patient com-

388 PALLIATIVE MEDICINE – THE NEXT 10 YEARS

munication must be improved. Postgraduate oppor-tunities have increased with the new Specialist Register schemes and with the new academic departments. New teaching methods such as CD ROM and interactive video-conferencing will enable more people to learn about Palliative Care or be supported in their practice. The importance of Palliative Medicine will be validated in the eyes of doctors when questions on it regularly appear in medical and postgraduate examination papers.

The Internet enables patients and families to gain more information. Even now they ask about new treatments that are available overseas. Patient groups will provide encouragement and support for some. Palliative Care practitioners can also use the Internet to communicate about difficult cases, new advances and meetings.

Ethical issues

Ethical issues will continue to be at the forefront of Palliative Care. The euthanasia debate grows more worrying, as the highly organised pro- euthanasia lobby seek to exploit every opportunity to legalise 'mercy-killing'. The Northern Territories experience in Australia exposed how easily euthanasia can be legalised if specialist Palliative Care services are not available or are slow to speak out.

Informed consent is having an effect on Palliative care as medical services become more patient\consumer led. Younger patients particularly want to be involved in decision-making, not always accepting what we think is 'best' for them. We need to understand more about what 'informed consent' means and the extent and limits of its usefulness. Advanced Directives (legal instructions written by a patient in case they become unable to com-municate) are a useful communication tool but the medico-legal implications still need to be further explored.

Organ donation

Organ donation is still needed for transplantation, and recipients benefit enormously. Yet many patients who want to donate organs do not end up doing so. The planning and communication of organ donation needs improving. Corneas, Heart valves (and kidneys from patients with primary brain tumours) can all be donated.[2]

Spiritual aspects

Spiritual aspects are fundamental to Palliative Care. Patients' belief systems (religious, spiritual, philosophical, humanist or none) surely affect their priorities and their ability to deal with the losses and crises of a progressive illness. There is a lot we still need to understand and explore. Which methods of spiritual support are effective? Kearney has raised the fear that Palliative Medicine physicians were ignoring spiritual care in favour of becoming 'symptomatologists'.[4] More work is needed to develop the concept of soul pain, and the indepth work that is needed to address it.

The place of hospices

The place of hospices within Society is already changing. More patients are requesting admission on the basis that a relative or friend received care in the past. Many hospices now support patients having active treatments, for rehabilitation, and for respite. This will slowly overcome the idea that hospices are places where people only go to die. If current trends continue, specialist palliative care services will become the major providers of cancer care within the Health Service. The combined effect of hospices, hospital support teams and home care teams will be to free up acute hospital beds. Specialist services need to dovetail together to achieve this and work more closely with Primary Health Care Teams and Cancer Units/Centres.

Calman-Hine

The Calman-Hine report has encouraged centralisation of many anti-cancer services, particularly radiotherapy. This can cause problems for patients with advanced cancer, particularly if they live some distance and only require single fraction for bone metastases. Will low cost 'low-tech' radiotherapy machines be made more locally available in the future for this group of patients?

Funding

Funding is likely to remain the major constraint to the growth of Palliative Care. No-one knows what the limit of community support is for hospices, provided that the services expand gradually as community awareness grows. Government support is always going to be constrained. Will the effects of hospital support teams in reducing hospital admissions and length of stay be recognised, particularly as no pot of money ever appears at the end of any financial year as a result? What will be the effect of expensive new anti-cancer treatments, or even the wider application of existing treatments such as adjuvant 5FU for colorectal cancer? As the impact of Palliative Care grows, some form of explicit rationing may be necessary. It is interesting to note that the Oregon Health Plan, based on evaluations by professional and lay groups strongly favour the funding of 'comfort care'. The plan prioritised health problems in order to rationalise funding and conditions below number 578 on the list can have treatment denied. Comfort care is placed at number 260.[5]

CONCLUSION

Thirty years after the founding of St Christopher's Palliative Care has become a speciality with a major impact on Health Care. The next 10 years holds many opportunities and threats. Medical expertise is developing faster than at any time in history, and there are likely to be improvements in procedures, equipment and drugs. However, the plight of the dying and their families will always remain. The challenge is to ensure that the fundamental tenets of the speciality are maintained and strength- ened irrespective of the evolving circumstances.

REFERENCES

1. Kubler-Ross E. On Death and Dying. Tavistock Publications. London. 1970.
2. Peters D, Sutcliffe J. Organ donation: the hospice perspective. Palliative Medicine 1992; 6: 212–216
3. Spiegal D et al. "Effect of psycho-social treatment on survival of patients with metastatic breast cancer". Lancet (1989) 2, p888–91
4. Kearney M. Palliative medicine – just another speciality? Palliative Medicine 1992; 6: 39–46.
5. Bodenheimer MD. The Oregon health Plan – Lessons for the Nation. N Engl J Med 1997; 337: 651–5.

FURTHER READING

The Future for Palliative Care. Ed David Clark. 1993. Open University Press. Buckingham Philadelphia.

Index

OTHER BOOKS AVAILABLE FROM EPL PUBLICATIONS:

A-Z OF HOSPICE AND PALLIATIVE MEDICINE (272 pages)
by Peter Kaye, Price £21.50

A-Z POCKETBOOK OF SYMPTOM CONTROL (128 pages)
by Peter Kaye, Price £12

BREAKING BAD NEWS - A 10 STEP APPROACH (28 pages)
by Peter Kaye, Price £4.50

Send a cheque, payable to EPL Publications, to:

EPL Publications
41 Park Avenue North,
Northampton NN3 2HT

Book sent by return of post (Post and Package FREE in UK).